Contents

IV. Physical Activity in the Prevention of Cardiovascular Disease and Other CVD Risk Factors

V. Secondary Prevention of Cardiovascular Disease and Cardiac Rehabilitation

VI. Successful Approaches to Adopting and Maintaining a Physically Active Lifestyle

Books are to be returned on or before
the last date below.

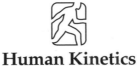

Human Kinetics

LIVERPOOL
JOHN MOORES UNIVERSITY
AVRIL ROBARTS LRC
TEL. 0151 231 4022

Library of Congress Cataloging-in-Publication Data

Physical activity and cardiovascular health : a national consensus /
  [edited by]
      p. cm.
    Includes bibliographical references and index.
    ISBN 0-88011-610-2
    1. Cardiovascular system--Diseases--Prevention--Congresses.
    2. Cardiovascular system--Diseases--Exercise therapy--Congresses.
    I. Leon, Arthur S.
    [DNLM: 1. Cardiovascular Diseases--prevention & control--United
States--congresses.   2. Exercise--congresses.   3. Health Status
Indicators--United States--congresses.   4. Physical Fitness-
-congresses.   WG 120 P578 1997]
    RA645.C34P49   1997
    616.1'05--dc21
    DNLM/DLC
    for Library of Congress   96-50955
                                                              CIP

ISBN: 0-88011-610-2
Copyright © 1997 by Human Kinetics, Inc.

Developmental Editors: Nanette Smith, Kirby Mittelmeier; **Assistant Editors:** Henry Woolsey, Jennifer Stallard; **Editorial Assistant:** Coree Schutter; **Copyeditor:** Dena Popara; **Proofreader:** Erin Cler; **Indexer:** Theresa Schaefer; **Graphic Designer:** Keith Blomberg; **Graphic Artist:** Tara Welsch; **Illustrator:** Sara Wolfsmith; **Photo Editor:** Boyd La Foon; **Cover Designer:** Keith Blomberg; **Printer:** United Graphics

Printed in the United States of America   10   9   8   7   6   5   4   3   2   1

Human Kinetics
Web site: http://www.humankinetics.com/

United States: Human Kinetics, P.O. Box 5076, Champaign, IL 61825-5076
1-800-747-4457
e-mail: humank@hkusa.com

Canada: Human Kinetics, Box 24040, Windsor, ON N8Y 4Y9
1-800-465-7301 (in Canada only)
e-mail: humank@hkcanada.com

Europe: Human Kinetics, P.O. Box IW14, Leeds LS16 6TR, United Kingdom
(44) 1132 781708
e-mail: humank@hkeurope.com

Australia: Human Kinetics, 57A Price Avenue, Lower Mitcham, South Australia 5062
(08) 277 1555
e-mail: humank@hkaustralia.com

New Zealand: Human Kinetics, P.O. Box 105-231, Auckland 1
(09) 523 3462
e-mail: humank@hknewz.com

Foreword

The past three decades have witnessed dramatic reductions in age-adjusted cardiovascular disease mortality in the United States. People are living longer with less disease. Improvement in population levels of cardiovascular risk factors, specifically cigarette smoking, blood lipids, hypertension, and better medical care underlie these changes.

Nevertheless, coronary heart disease is still the leading cause of mortality, with stroke ranking third. Much remains to be done. Improved control of the classical risk factors is one important approach; however, other factors are emerging. Specifically, physical inactivity and obesity have gained increasing interest because they have been identified both in aggravating the classical risk factors and as being independent predictors of cardiovascular disease. Unfortunately, while some risk factors have improved, population levels, physical inactivity, and obesity have increased in recent decades.

Better evidence for a relationship of physical inactivity with disease is the result of several decades of work. The evidence has gradually accumulated as more systematic research has accumulated on physical inactivity. The quality of work has improved and small, highly selected studies have been replaced by larger population investigations. Knowledge has increased on the importance of physical activity in both healthy and diseased individuals. These many observations were reviewed at the 1995 NIH Consensus Development Conference on Physical Activity and Cardiovascular Health. At that conference, the answers to the following questions were sought:

1. What is the health burden of a sedentary lifestyle on the population?
2. What type, intensity, and quantity of physical activity are important to prevent cardiovascular disease?
3. What are the benefits and risks of different types of physical activity for people who already have cardiovascular disease?
4. What are the successful approaches to adopting and maintaining a physically active lifestyle?
5. What are the important questions for future research?

The proceedings in this book include 30 papers reviewing the research contributions in this field. The initial chapters describe the burden of physical inactivity on population health. Here the authors reviewed epidemiologic studies documenting associations of physical inactivity with subsequent disease patterns. The burden of disease attributable to physical inactivity provides estimates of likely outcomes if the population were to return to more active lifestyles.

The results of the clinical trials of the effects physical activity has on cardiovascular disease were reviewed. Mechanisms by which physical activity affects health were considered. These remain issues of debate. Even more important, the issue of the relative benefits of moderate versus vigorous physical activity are presented. This question was an important one for the Panel's deliberations.

Because physical activity does not act in an independent fashion on cardiovascular disease, its association to other risk factors is discussed, including body size, lipids, blood pressure, clotting factors, and diabetes. There appears to be a beneficial effect of regular physical activity on each of these well-known risk characteristics. The real and potential negative effects of various physical activity, including injury and sudden death, are considered.

While much of the work described focuses on physical activity as a primary prevention measure, its use in cardiac rehabilitation is also presented. New research demonstrates the benefits of a variety of strategies for encouraging physical activity among patients with known cardiovascular disease. It is also apparent that these programs are prescribed infrequently by physicians.

Finally, the challenges to changing physical activity in US society are considered. While specific subgroups and their unique needs are reviewed, the necessity for broad national programs to facilitate and encourage regular physical activity in citizens are presented. This is perhaps the greatest challenge in an increasingly mechanized and labor-saving society.

The Panel reviewed these many state-of-the-art scientific presentations. The report is included with these proceedings. It stresses the need for increasing regular physical activity among US citizens. The benefits for cardiovascular disease prevention are also clear. The Panel concluded that regular daily physical activity at a moderate level was most likely to be a successful and effective public-health intervention. They also concluded that specific programs needed to be developed for different portions of society based on age, gender, ethnic group, and ability. If such changes occur, the benefits to the public health will be substantial. This book, which reviews the scientific evidence, provides the basis for recommending those changes.

Russell V. Luepker, MD, MS
Chairperson of the Consensus Development Panel
Minneapolis, Minnesota

Foreword

Despite impressive progress in research and prevention, cardiovascular disease is still the leading cause of morbidity and mortality in the United States where it is responsible for more than 40% of all deaths. Scientific research supported by the National Heart, Lung, and Blood Institute (NHLBI) and others has shown that physical activity influences cardiovascular health both directly and indirectly. For instance, physical activity improves blood lipids and blood pressure, helps control weight, and makes clot formation less likely.

Those who are sedentary run the highest risk for coronary heart disease. It is estimated that about 20,000 fewer deaths a year would occur in the United States if half of those who are sedentary would engage in a low-intensity activity a few times weekly.

Furthermore, research shows that physical activity even helps those who already have heart disease. For example, regular physical activity improves chances of survival and well-being after a heart attack.

Yet, as the evidence has mounted of physical activity's benefits, confusion and questions have also arisen. How much physical activity is needed for cardiovascular health? Must the activity be done in one continuous period or can it be done in separate periods throughout the day? Should the activity be vigorous or moderate? What's the difference between an activity done for fitness and one done for cardiovascular health? Do environmental problems, such as smog or heat, cancel any good effects from a physical activity? What is the risk of injury?

The answers to these questions are vital to Americans' health. For Americans to adopt a healthier lifestyle to reduce their risk of heart disease, they need guidelines about what to do. For health-care professionals to give advise about physical activity, they also must know what activities are best for the public and for special groups such as cardiac patients, children, and the elderly.

To provide such guidelines the NHLBI, the NIH Office of Medical Applications of Research, and others convened a non-Federal expert panel to review the latest scientific evidence and offer recommendations.

The urgency to have such recommendations was demonstrated in part by the rapid and overwhelming response that met the announcement of the conference: About 1,500 people registered to attend. Since the conference, many more people have requested the recommendations and other information about the benefits of physical activity.

The Panel's statement was published in the July 17, 1996, issue of the *Journal of the American Medical Association* and in the Department of Health and Human Services' (DHHS) Surgeon General's Report on Physical Activity and Health, also issued in the summer of 1996. This present volume makes available the full conference proceedings.

The NHLBI wishes to thank those who helped support the conference, including other institutes, centers, and divisions of the National Institutes of Health, as well as the Centers for Disease Control and Prevention, and the President's Council on Physical Fitness and Sports. I want to express a special thanks to the NIH Office of Medical Applications of Research for its assistance in managing the conference.

As noted in the DHHS *Healthy People 2000*, blueprint for the nation's health, one of today's most important public health challenges is moving our society from being sedentary to being more physically active. The recommendations from this conference offer Americans the chance to take a big step toward that healthier future.

Claude Lenfant, MD
Director
National Heart, Lung, and Blood Institute

List of Contributors

Steven N. Blair, PED
Director of Research, Director,
Epidemiology and Clinical
Applications
Cooper Institute for Aerobics
Research
Dallas, Texas

James A. Blumenthal, PhD
Professor, Division of Medical
Psychology
Department of Psychiatry
Duke University Medical Center
Durham, North Carolina

Claude Bouchard, PhD
Professor
Physical Activity Sciences Laboratory
Laval University
Sainte Foy, Quebec, Canada

David Braddock, PhD
Institute on Disability and Human
Development
University of Illinois, Chicago
Chicago, IL

David M. Buchner, MD, MPH
Professor of Health Services and
Medicine
Department of Health and Community
Medicine
University of Washington
Seattle, Washington

Karen J. Calfas, PhD
San Diego University
San Diego, California University of
California-San Diego
La Jolla, California

Carl J. Caspersen, PhD, MPH
Physical Activity Epidemiologist
Cardiovascular Health Studies Branch

Division of Chronic Disease Control
and Community Intervention
National Center for Chronic Disease
Prevention and Health Promotion
Centers for Disease Control and
Prevention
Atlanta, Georgia

Patricia M. Dubbert, PhD
Chief, Psychology Service
Jackson Veterans Affairs Medical
Center
Professor, Psychiatry and Human
Behavior
University of Mississippi School of
Medicine
Jackson, Mississippi

E. Randy Eichner, MD
Professor of Medicine
Hematology—Oncology Section
Department of Medicine
University of Oklahoma Health
Sciences Center
Oklahoma City, Oklahoma

Barry A. Franklin, PhD
Director, Cardiac Rehabilitation and
Exercise Laboratories
William Beaumont Hospital
Beaumont Rehabilitation and Health
Center
Royal Oak, Michigan
Professor of Physiology
Wayne State University School of
Medicine
Detroit, Michigan

Elizabeth D. Gullette, MA
Duke University Medical Center
Durham, North Carolina

James M. Hagberg, PhD
Professor of Medicine

Division of Preventive Cardiology
Department of Medicine
University of Pittsburgh Medical
Center
Pittsburgh, Pennsylvania

William L. Haskell, PhD
Professor, Division of Cardiology
Department of Medicine
Stanford University School of
Medicine
Palo Alto, California

James O. Hill, PhD
Associate Professor of Pediatrics
Associate Director, Center for Human
Nutrition
School of Medicine
University of Colorado Health
Sciences Center
Denver, Colorado

Harold W. Kohl III, PhD
Director of Research, Sports Medicine
Baylor Sports Medicine Institute
Baylor College of Medicine
Houston, Texas

Andrea M. Kriska, PhD
Assistant Professor
Department of Epidemiology
Graduate School of Public Health
University of Pittsburgh
Pittsburgh, Pennsylvania

I-Min Lee, MD, ScD, MBBS
Assistant Professor of Medicine
Harvard Medical School
Assistant Professor of Epidemiology
Harvard School of Public Health
Boston, Massachusetts

Arthur S. Leon, MD, MS, FACSM,
FACC
Henry L. Taylor Professorship in
Exercise Science and Health
Enhancement

Division of Kinesiology
School of Kinesiology and Leisure
Studies
College of Education
University of Minnesota
Minneapolis, Minnesota

Barbara J. Long, MD, MPH
University of Pittsburgh
Pittsburgh, Pennsylvania

Bess H. Marcus, PhD
Associate Professor of Psychiatry and
Human Behavior
Division of Behavioral and Preventive
Medicine
Department of Psychiatry
The Miriam Hospital and Brown
University School of Medicine
Providence, Rhode Island

Nancy Houston Miller, RN, BSN
Associate Director
Stanford Cardiac Rehabilitation
Program
Stanford University School of
Medicine
Stanford, California

Geoffrey E. Moore, MD
Assistant Professor of Medicine
Director, Cardiopulmonary
Rehabilitation
University of Pittsburgh Medical
Center
Pittsburgh, Pennsylvania

Melissa Napolitano, MA
Duke University Medical Center
Durham, North Carolina

Neil B. Oldridge, PhD
Professor
Department of Health Sciences
School of Allied Health Professions
University of Wisconsin
Milwaukee, Wisconsin

Ralph S. Paffenbarger, Jr.,m MD. PhD
Stanford University School of
Medicine
Stanford, California
Harvard School of Public Health
Cambridge, Massachusetts

Russell R. Pate, PhD
Chairman, Department of Exercise
Science
School of Public Health
University of South Carolina
Columbia, South Carolina

Kevin Patrick, MD, MS
Director, Project PACE
Associate Clinical Professor of Family
and Preventive Medicine
University of California-San Diego
Adjunct Professor of Public Health
San Diego State University
San Diego, California

Kenneth E. Powell, MD, MPH
Associate Director for Science
Division of Violence Prevention
National Center for Injury Prevention
and Control
Centers for Disease Control and
Prevention
Atlanta, Georgia

James H. Rimmer, PhD
Visiting Professor
Institute on Disability and Human
Development
University of Illinois, Chicago
Chicago, Illinois
Northern Illinois University
Debalk, Illinois

James F. Sallis, PhD
San diego State University
San Diego, California

Robert S. Schwartz, MD
Professor of Medicine

Division of Gerontology and Geriatric
Medicine
Department of Internal Medicine
Harborview Medical Center
University of Washington
Seattle, Washington

Roy J. Shephard, MD, PhD, DPE
Professor Emeritus of Applied
Physiology
Department of Preventive Medicine
and Biostatistics
School of Physical and Health
Education
University of Toronto
Health Studies Programme
Brock University
Toronto, Ontario, Canada

L. Kent Smith, MD, MPH
Medical Director
Preventive Medicine Program/
Ambulatory Drug Research
Department of Cardiology
Arizona Heart Institute
Phoenix, Arizona

Marcia L. Stefanick, PhD
Senior Research Scientist
Stanford Center for Research in
Disease Prevention
Department of Medicine
Stanford University School of
Medicine
Stanford, California

Renata Szczepanski, PhD
Duke University Medical Center
Durham, North Carolina

Paul D. Thompson, MD
Professor of Medicine
Division of Cardiology
Department of Medicine
University of Pittsburgh Heart
Institute
Pittsburgh, Pennsylvania

Wilma J. Wooten, MD, MPH
University of California-San Diego
La Jolla, California

Deborah Rohm Young, PhD
Assistant Professor
The Johns Hopkins Center for Health
Promotion
The Johns Hopkins School of Medi-
cine
Baltimore, Maryland

Matthew M. Zack, MD, MPH
Health Care and Aging Studies Branch
National Center for Chronic Disease
Prevention and Health Promotion
Centers for Disease Control and
Prevention
Atlanta, GA

Preface

This book provides the reader with an explanation of the format and deliberations involved in a National Institutes of Health (NIH) consensus development process; detailed summaries of the presentations of each of the principal speakers; and the final consensus statement on the contribution of physical activity to cardiovascular health, along with limitations of the current data and areas of required additional research. The major topic areas covered in the conference and these proceedings are the following:

- An overview of the contributions of physical activity and other lifestyle habits to health in America
- The burden of physical inactivity to health in the United States
- Current issues related to the type and intensity of physical activity required for prevention of cardiovascular disease
- The effects of physical activity on other risk factors for cardiovascular disease
- The contributions of physical activity to rehabilitation and secondary prevention of cardiovascular disease
- Behavioral and sociocultural determinants of adaptation and maintenance of a physically active lifestyle in the general population and in various population subgroups, including women, minority groups, youth, seniors, and disabled persons
- The potential impact of health-care providers in promoting physical activity
- Recommendations for how communities can promote physical activity for their citizens of all ages
- The final consensus statement document

The conclusions and recommendations from this conference should be of great value not only to health-care providers, but also to those groups responsible for formulating health practice and research policy guidelines, as well as to the general public. The conclusion by the Consensus Development Panel that physical inactivity is a major risk factor is very rewarding for conference participants like myself who have dedicated our academic careers to this area of research.

Arthur S. Leon, MD

May 1, 1996

Acknowledgments

This Consensus Development Conference on Physical Activity and Cardiovascular Health was held on the NIH Campus in Bethesda, Maryland, December 18 to 20, 1995. The primary sponsors for the Conference were the National Heart, and Blood Institute (NHLBI) and the NIH Office of Medical Applications of Research. The Conference was cosponsored by the National Institute of Child Health and Human Development, National Institute on Aging, National Institute of Arthritis and Musculoskeletal and Skin Diseases, National Institute of Diabetes and Digestive and Kidney Diseases, National Institute of Nursing Research, Office of Research on Women's Health and the Office of Disease Prevention of the NIH, the Centers for Disease Control and Prevention and the President's Council on Physical Fitness and Sports. This was the 101st Consensus Development Conference held by the NIH since the establishment of the Consensus Development Program in 1977.

Deepest appreciation is expressed to Karen A. Donato, MS, RD Coordinator, Nutrition Education and Special Initiatives Office of Prevention, Education and Control, NHLBI, and John H. Ferguson, MD, Director, Office of Medical Applications of Research, NIH, for organizing the program for the conference and to Technical Resources International (TRI), Rockville, MD, for assisting with conference logistics.

Introduction: Charge to the Panel

John H. Ferguson MD
Director, Office of Medical Applications of Research

The process followed at the Consensus Development Conference was started 18 years ago and has been used by many countries around the world. The process was designed to assess medical technologies where data exist but controversy remains or where gaps exist between current knowledge and practice. As a part of the process, exercises were structured to assess medical procedures by resolving controversies and to disseminate new information to the health-care community, sometimes called technology assessment and technology transfer.

The conclusions and recommendations from these conferences are used not only by health practitioners, but also by groups charged with formulating practice guidelines and health policy decisions and the general public. The essence of this process is the convening of a knowledgeable panel, whose members have not themselves been intimately involved in the research of the particular topic and who are not federal government employees. A major attribute of this process is that the evaluation of the data, the conclusions and recommendations appearing in the final statement are produced by this expert panel, which has been chosen to have no intellectual or financial stake in the issues. The panel then hears expert testimony from those who researched the subject. These conferences are always conducted in public. Thus, they combine elements of a jury proceeding with those of a scientific and a town meeting. During the lengthy discussion periods, and on the last day of the conference when the entire statement was read, participants had a chance to comment, raise questions, and critique the document. This public "peer review" was an important part of the process and we encouraged all to take part.

Over the past 25 years, the United States has experienced steady declines in the death toll from cardiovascular disease (CVD), primarily in coronary heart disease and stroke. Lifestyle improvements by the American public and better control of the risk factors for heart disease and stroke have been a major factor in this decline. Despite these declines, heart disease remains the number one and stroke the number three leading causes of death. Cardiovascular disease has many causes with several modifiable risk factors including high blood pressure, high blood cholesterol, obesity, smoking, diabetes, and physical inactivity. In contrast to the positive trends observed with the reduction of high blood pressure and high blood cholesterol, overweight and physical inactivity have been on the increase.

In light of these trends, the accumulating evidence of the risk of cardiovascular disease associated with a sedentary lifestyle and the role of physical activity in the prevention and treatment of CVD and other CVD risk factors need to be examined. A majority of adults report that they exercise sporadically or not at all. Similarly, data suggest that adolescents are less active than they were a decade ago.

Physical activity not only independently protects against the development of CVD but also can appropriately modify the CVD risk factors of blood pressure, cholesterol, diabetes, and overweight. The type, frequency, and intensity of the physical activity, however, remains controversial. Some experts suggest that moderate forms of physical activity can help prevent cardiovascular disease, while others suggest it must be vigorous and sustained.

Physical activity is also important in the treatment and management of patients with CVD or its risk factors, including patients who have stable angina, have suffered a myocardial infarction or have heart failure. Additionally, physical activity is an important component of cardiac rehabilitation; however, questions remain regarding the type, frequency, and intensity needed for patients.

We need to understand what variables influence the adoption of a physically active lifestyle by various population groups including children, adolescents, adults, the elderly, and minority populations. Various intervention strategies may need specific targeting to those groups. Different environments, such as schools, work sites, health-care settings, and family structures, need to be examined for their roles in promoting physical activity. In addition, costs and availability of adequate resources can influence the adoption of a physically active lifestyle.

This book provides the scientific data that will inform attempts to assist health-care providers and patients who need answers to the important questions that have been posed.

The consensus process that was followed served as a public forum to weigh issues in medical care for which there is a scientific data base. The presentation by experts of the best available data weighed by a non-biased panel composed of scientists and lay representatives and discussed in public session has been a very forceful tool for assessing controversial medical technologies.

By supporting this conference and others like it, the NIH aims to assist health professionals and the public in obtaining and evaluating the most up-to-date and accurate information available on controversial topics in medicine. What was learned in those three conference days is being disseminated broadly as this book attests. The Panel's statement has also been published by a major medical journal, and it will be printed by the Federal Government and distributed as part of an intensive effort to reach the widest possible audience.

NIH Consensus Statement

NIH Consensus Statements are prepared by a nonadvocate, non-Federal panel of experts, based on (1) presentations by investigators working in areas relevant to the consensus questions during a two-day public session; (2) questions and statements from conference attendees during open discussion periods that are part of the public session; and (3) closed deliberations by the panel during the remainder of the second day and the morning of the third. This statement is an independent report of the panel and is not a policy statement of the NIH or the Federal Government.

Over the past 25 years, the United States has experienced steady declines in the age-adjusted death toll from cardiovascular disease (CVD), primarily in mortality caused by coronary heart disease and stroke. Lifestyle improvements by the American public and better control of the risk factors for heart disease and stroke have been major factors in these declines. Nonetheless, heart disease remains the leading cause of death, and stroke the third leading cause of death.

Coronary heart disease and stroke have multiple causes. Modifiable risk factors include smoking, high blood pressure, blood lipids, obesity, diabetes, and physical inactivity. In contrast to the positive US national trends observed in decreased cigarette smoking, high blood pressure, and high blood cholesterol, improvement has not been seen in the areas of obesity and physical inactivity. Indeed, automation and other technologies have contributed greatly to lessening physical activity at work and home.

The purpose of this conference was to examine the accumulating evidence on the role of physical activity in the prevention and treatment of CVD and its risk factors.

Physical activity in this statement is defined as "bodily movement produced by skeletal muscles that requires energy expenditure and produces progressive healthy benefits." Exercise, a type of physical activity, is defined as "a planned, structured, and repetitive bodily movement done to improve or maintain one or more components of physical fitness." Physical inactivity denotes a level of activity less than that needed to maintain good health.

Physical inactivity afflicts most Americans. Exertion has been systematically engineered out of most occupations. In 1991, 54% of adults reported little or no regular leisure physical activity. Data from the 1990 Youth Risk Behavior Survey show that most teenagers in grades 9 through 12 are not performing at least 20 minutes of vigorous activity at least three or more times per week. About 50% of students reported that they are not enrolled in physical education classes.

Physical activity protects against the development of CVD and also favorably modifies CVD risk factors, including high blood pressure, blood lipids, insulin resistance, and obesity. The unique contributions of type, frequency, and intensity of physical activity that are needed, however, remain controversial.

Physical activity is also important in the treatment and management of patients with CVD or increased risk, including those who have hypertension, stable angina, a prior myocardial infarction, peripheral vascular disease, or heart failure. Physical activity is an important component of cardiac rehabilitation, and people with CVD may benefit from participation. In addition to potential advantages, questions remain regarding benefits, risks, and costs associated with becoming physically active.

Adopting and maintaining a physically active lifestyle is influenced by many variables, such as socioeconomic status, cultural influences, age, and health status. There is a need to understand how such variables influence the adoption of this behavior at the individual level. Various intervention strategies might be more or less useful for encouraging individuals from different backgrounds to adopt and adhere to a physically active lifestyle. Different environments, such as schools, work sites, health-care settings, the home, and other settings, can play a role in promoting physical activity. There is also need to advance understanding of these community-level factors.

To address these and related issues, the National Heart, Lung, and Blood Institute and the NIH Office of Medical Applications of Research convened a Consensus Development Conference on Physical Activity and Cardiovascular Health. The conference was cosponsored by the National Institute of Child Health and Human Development, the National Institute on Aging, the National Institute of Arthritis and Musculoskeletal and Skin Diseases, the National Institute of Diabetes and Digestive and Kidney Diseases, the National Institute of Nursing Research, the Office of Research on Women's Health, the Office of Disease Prevention of the NIH, the Centers for Disease Control and Prevention, and the President's Council on Physical Fitness and Sports.

The conference brought together specialists in medicine, exercise physiology, health behavior, epidemiology, nutrition, physical therapy, and nursing, as well as representatives from the public. After one and one-half days of presentations and audience discussion, an independent, non-Federal consensus panel weighed the scientific evidence and developed a draft statement that addressed the following questions:

- What is the health burden of a sedentary lifestyle on the population?
- What type, intensity, and quantity of physical activity are important to prevent cardiovascular disease?
- What are the benefits and risks of different types of physical activity for people with cardiovascular disease?
- What are the successful approaches to adopting and maintaining a physically active lifestyle?
- What are the important questions for future research?

What Is the Health Burden of a Sedentary Lifestyle on the Population?

Physical inactivity among the US population is now widespread. Four national surveillance programs have documented that about one in four adults (more women than men) currently have sedentary lifestyles with no leisure-time physical activity. An additional one-third of adults are insufficiently active to achieve a healthful level of physical fitness. The prevalence of inactivity varies by age, ethnicity, and geographic region and is common in all demographic groups. Change in physical exertion associated with occupation has not been systematically measured in this country; however, because of automation, it has declined markedly during this century.

As young children grow older, girls become less active than do boys, and children become far less active as they move through adolescence. Obesity is increasing among children and is presumably related to physical inactivity. There are also data indicating that obese children and adolescents have a high risk of becoming obese adults, where obesity is related to coronary artery disease, hypertension, and diabetes. Thus, the prevention of childhood obesity has the potential of helping prevent hypertension and atherosclerosis, which are the major causes of CVD in adults. Seventy percent of 12-year-old children report participation in vigorous physical activity; by age 21, participation at this level of intensity is seen in only 42% of men and 30% of women. As adults continue to age, their physical activity levels continue to decline.

Although knowledge about physical inactivity as a risk factor for cardiovascular disease has come mainly from investigations of middle-aged, white men, more limited evidence from studies in women and other populations suggests that the findings are similar in these groups. In the meantime, and based on current knowledge, we must note that physically inactive Americans occur disproportionately among those who are not well-educated and who live under unfavorable social circumstances.

Physical activity has been demonstrated to be directly related to physical fitness. Although the means of measuring physical activity have varied between studies (i.e., there is no standardization of measures), evidence indicates that physical inactivity and lack of physical fitness are directly associated with increased mortality from CVD. The increase in mortality is not entirely explained by physical inactivity's association with elevated blood pressure, smoking, and lipids.

There is an inverse relationship between measures of physical activity and indices of obesity in most US population studies. Only a few studies have examined the relationship between physical activity and body-fat distribution, and these suggest an inverse relationship between levels of physical activity and visceral fat. There is evidence that weight loss can be produced through increased physical activity and that the addition of physical activity to dietary energy restriction can increase, and help to maintain, the loss of body weight and body fat mass.

Middle-aged and older men and women who engage in regular physical activity have significantly higher high-density lipoprotein (HDL) cholesterol levels than do those who are sedentary. When the exercise training has extended to at least 12 weeks, beneficial HDL cholesterol level changes were reported.

In most studies of endurance exercise training of individuals with hypertension, a decrease in systolic and diastolic blood pressure has been observed. Insulin resistance is also improved with endurance exercise.

A number of factors that affect thrombotic function—including hematocrit, fibrinogen, platelet function, and fibrinolysis—are related to the risk of CVD. Regular endurance exercise lowers the risk related to these factors.

The lack of physical fitness and the burden of CVD rests most heavily on the least active. In addition to its powerful impact on the cardiovascular system, physical inactivity is also associated with other adverse health effects, including osteoporosis, diabetes, and some cancers.

What Type, Intensity, and Quantity of Physical Activity Are Important to Prevent Cardiovascular Disease?

Activity that reduces CVD risk factors and confers the many other health benefits does not require a structured or vigorous exercise program. Because the majority of benefits of physical activity can be gained by performing moderate-intensity activities outside of formal exercise, such activity is the emphasis for these recommendations. The amount and type of physical activity needed for health benefits or optimal health are a concern due to limited time and to the lifestyle demands competing for the attention of most Americans. The amounts and types of physical activity that are needed to prevent disease and promote health must, therefore, be clearly communicated, and effective strategies must be developed to promote physical activity to the public.

The quantitative relationship between the level of activity or fitness and the magnitude of cardiovascular benefit may extend across the full range of activity. A moderate level of physical activity confers health benefits. However, physical activity must be performed regularly to maintain these effects. Moderate-intensity activity performed by previously sedentary individuals results in significant improvement in many health-related outcomes. Activities of low to moderate intensity are more likely to be continued than are high-intensity activities.

Some evidence suggests lowered mortality with more vigorous activity, but further research is needed to more specifically define safe and effective levels. The most active individuals have lower cardiovascular morbidity and mortality rates than do those who are least active; however, most of the benefit appears to be accounted for by comparing the least-active individuals to the moderately active. Further increases in the intensity or amount of activity produce further benefits in some, but not all, parameters of risk. High-intensity activity is also associated with an increased risk of injury, discontinuation of activity, or acute cardiac events during the activity. Current low rates of regular activity in Americans may be partially due to the misperception of many that vigorous, continuous exercise is necessary to reap health benefits. Many people, for example, fail to appreciate walking as "exercise" or to recognize the substantial benefits of short bouts (at least 10 minutes) of moderate-level activity. Examples of moderate activity include brisk walking, cycling, swimming, home repair, and yard work.   \

We recommend that all people in the United States increase their regular physical activity to a level appropriate to their capacities, needs, and interests. We recommend that all children and adults should set a long-term goal to accumulate at least 30 minutes or more of moderate-intensity physical activity on most, preferably all, days of the week. Intermittent or shorter bouts of activity (at least 10 minutes), including occupational and nonoccupational tasks and those of daily living, also have similar cardiovascular and health benefits if they are performed at a level of moderate intensity (such as brisk walking) and accumulate to 30 minutes per day. People who currently meet the recommended minimal standards may derive additional health and fitness benefits from becoming more physically active or including more vigorous activity.

The frequency, intensity, and duration of activity are interrelated. The number of episodes of activity recommended depends on the intensity and/or duration of the activity: higher-intensity or longer-duration activity could be performed approximately three times weekly and achieve cardiovascular benefits, but low-intensity or shorter-duration activities should be performed more often to achieve cardiovascular benefits.

The type of activity is best determined by the individual's preferences and what will be sustained. Exercise, or a structured program of activity, is a subset of activity that may encourage interest and allow for more intensive participation. People who perform more formal exercise (i.e., structured or planned exercise programs) can accumulate this daily total through a variety of recreational or sports activities. People who are currently sedentary or minimally active should gradually build up to the recommended goal of 30 minutes of moderate activity daily by adding a few minutes each day until reaching their personal goal to reduce the risk associated with suddenly increasing the amount or intensity of exercise. (The defined levels of effort depend on individual characteristics, such as baseline fitness and health status.)

Developing muscular strength and joint flexibility are also important components for an overall activity program to improve one's ability to perform tasks and to reduce the potential for injury. Upper extremity and resistance (strength) training can improve muscular function, and evidence suggests that there may be cardiovascular benefits, especially in older patients or those with underlying CVD, but further research and guidelines are needed. Older people or those who have been deconditioned from recent inactivity or illness may particularly benefit from resistance training due to the benefits in accomplishing tasks of daily living. Resistance training may contribute to better balance, coordination, and agility that may help prevent falls in the elderly.

Physical activity has risks as well as benefits. The most common adverse effects of activity are related to musculoskeletal injury and are usually mild and self-limited. The risk of injury increases with increased intensity, frequency, and duration of activity and is also dependent on the type of activity. Exercise-related injuries can be reduced by moderating these parameters. A more serious but rare complication of activity is myocardial infarction or sudden cardiac death. Although persons who engage in vigorous physical activity have a slight increase in risk of sudden cardiac death during activity, the health benefits outweigh this risk and lead to an overall risk reduction.

In children and young adults, exertion-related deaths are uncommon and are generally related to congenital heart defects (e.g., hypertrophic cardiomyopathy, Marfan's syndrome, severe aortic valve stenosis, prolonged QT syndromes, cardiac conduction abnormalities) or to acquired myocarditis. It is recommended that patients with those conditions remain active but not participate in vigorous or competitive athletics.

Because the risks of activity are very low compared with the health benefits, most adults do not need medical consultation or pretesting before starting a moderate-intensity physical activity program. However, those with CVD and men over 40 and women over 50 years of age with multiple cardiovascular risk factors who contemplate a program of vigorous activity should have a medical evaluation prior to initiating their program.

What Are the Benefits and Risks of Different Types of Physical Activity for People With Cardiovascular Disease?

More than 10 million Americans are afflicted with clinically significant CVD, including myocardial infarction, angina pectoris, peripheral vascular disease, and congestive heart failure. In addition, more than 300 000 patients per year are currently subjected to coronary artery bypass surgery and a similar number to percutaneous transluminal coronary angioplasty. Increase in physical activity appears to benefit each of these groups. Such benefits include reduction in cardiovascular mortality, reduction of symptoms, improvement in exercise tolerance and functional capacity, and improvement in psychological well-being and quality of life.

Several studies have shown that exercise training programs significantly reduce overall mortality, as well as death due to myocardial infarction. The reported reductions in mortality have been particularly great—approximating 25%—in those who participated in cardiac rehabilitation programs that included control of other cardiovascular risk factors. Rehabilitation programs using both moderate and vigorous physical activity have been associated with reductions in fatal cardiac events, although uncertainty exists regarding the minimal or optimal level and duration of exercise required to achieve beneficial effects. Data are also inadequate to determine whether stroke incidence is affected by physical activity or exercise training.

The risk of death during medically supervised cardiac exercise training programs is very low. However, those who exercise infrequently and have poor functional capacity may be at somewhat higher risk. All patients with coronary heart disease (CHD) should have a medical evaluation prior to participation in a vigorous exercise program.

Appropriately prescribed and conducted exercise training programs improve exercise tolerance and physical fitness in patients with coronary heart disease. Moderate as well as vigorous exercise training regimens are of value. Patients with low basal levels of exercise capacity experience the greatest functional benefits, even at relatively modest levels of physical activity. Patients with angina pectoris typically experience improvement in angina in association with a reduction in effort-induced myocardial ischemia, presumably as a result of decreased myocardial oxygen demand and increased work capacity.

Patients with congestive heart failure also appear to have improvement in symptoms, exercise capacity, and functional well-being in response to exercise training, even though left ventricular systolic function appears to be unaffected. The exercise program needs to be tailored to the needs of these patients and monitored adequately in view of the marked predisposition of these patients to ischemic events and arrhythmias.

Cardiac rehabilitation exercise training often improves skeletal muscle strength and work capacity and, when combined with appropriate nutritional changes, may result in greater fat oxidation and acceleration of fat and weight loss. In addition, such training generally results in improvement in measures of psychological status, social adjustment, and functional capacity. However, cardiac rehabilitation exercise training exerts less influence on rates of return to work than do many nonexercise variables, including employer attitudes, prior employment status, and economic incentives. Because of the need for various interventions to improve health status and reduce cardiovascular risk factors, multifactorial intervention programs—including nutritional changes and medications—should be provided.

Cardiac rehabilitation programs have traditionally been institutional and group-based (e.g., hospitals, clinics, community centers). Referral and enrollment rates have been relatively low, generally ranging from 10% to 25% of patients with CVD. Referral rates are lower for women than for men and lower for nonwhites than for whites. Restructured, home-based programs have the potential to provide rehabilitative services to a wider population. Home-based programs incorporating limited hospital visits with regular mail or telephone follow-up by a nurse case manager have demonstrated significant increases in functional capacity, smoking cessation, and improvement in blood lipids. A range of options exists in cardiac rehabilitation, including site, number of visits, monitoring, and other services.

There are clear medical and economic reasons for carrying out cardiac rehabilitation efforts. Optimal outcomes are achieved when exercise training is combined with educational messages and feedback about changing lifestyle. Patients who participate in cardiac rehabilitation programs show a lower incidence of rehospitalization and lower charges per hospitalization. Cardiac rehabilitation, therefore, is a cost-efficient therapeutic modality that should be used more frequently.

What Are the Successful Approaches to Adopting and Maintaining a Physically Active Lifestyle?

The cardiovascular benefits and physiological reactions to physical activity appear to be similar among diverse population subgroups defined by age, gender, income, region of residence, ethnic background, and health status. However, the behavioral and attitudinal factors that influence the motivation for, and ability to sustain, physical activity are strongly determined by social experiences, cultural background, and physical and health status. For example, perceptions of appropriate physical activity differ by gender, age, weight, marital status, family roles and responsibilities, disability, and social class. Thus, the following general guidelines will need to be further specified and elaborated when planning with or prescribing for specific individuals and population groups.

Available data suggest that physical activity need not be strenuous and is more likely to be initiated and maintained if the individual

- perceives a net benefit,
- chooses an enjoyable activity,
- feels competent doing the activity,
- feels safe doing the activity,
- can easily access the activity on a regular basis,
- can fit the activity into the daily schedule,
- feels that the activity does not generate financial or social costs that he or she is unwilling to bear,
- experiences a minimum of negative consequences (e.g., loss of time, negative peer pressure, and problems with self-identity),
- is able to successfully address issues of competing time demands, and
- recognizes the need to balance the use of labor-saving devices (e.g., power lawn mowers, golf carts, automobiles) and sedentary activities (e.g., watching television, use of computers) with activities that involve a higher level of physical exertion.

Other people in the individual's social environment can influence the adoption and maintenance of physical activity. Health-care providers play a key role in promoting smoking cessation and other risk-reduction behaviors. Preliminary evidence suggests that this also applies to physical activity. It is highly probable that people will be more likely to increase their physical activity if their health-care provider counsels them to do so. Providers can do this effectively by learning to recognize stages of behavior change, to communicate the need for increased activity, to assist the patient in initiating activity, and to follow up appropriately.

Family and friends also can be important sources of support for behavior change. For example, spouses or friends can serve as "buddies," joining in the physical activity; or a spouse could offer to take on a household task, giving his or her mate time to engage in physical activity. Parents can support their children's activity by providing transportation, praise, encouragement, and by participating in activities with their children.

Work sites have the potential to encourage increased physical activity by offering opportunities, reminders, and rewards for doing so. For example, an appropriate indoor area could be set aside to enable walking during lunch hours. Signs placed near elevators can encourage the use of the stairs instead. Discounts on parking fees could be offered to employees who elect to park in remote lots and walk.

Schools are another community resource for increasing physical activity, particularly given the urgent need to develop strategies that affect children and adolescents. As noted previously, there is now clear evidence that US children and adolescents have become more obese. There is also evidence that obese children and adolescents exercise less than do their leaner peers. All schools should provide opportunities for physical activities that

- are appropriate and enjoyable for children of all skill levels and are not limited to competitive sports or physical education classes;
- appeal to girls and boys, as well as to youngsters from diverse backgrounds;
- can serve as a foundation for activities throughout life; and
- are offered on a daily basis.

Successful approaches may involve mass education strategies or changes in institutional policies or community variables. In some cases (e.g., schools, work sites), policy-level interventions may be necessary to enable people to achieve and maintain an adequate level of activity. Policy changes that increase opportunities for physical activity can facilitate activity maintenance for motivated individuals and increase readiness to change among the less motivated. As in other areas of health promotion, mass communication strategies should be used to promote physical activity. These strategies should include a variety of mainstream channels and techniques to reach diverse audiences that get their information in different ways (e.g., TV, newspaper, radio, Internet).

What Are the Important Considerations for Future Research?

The following are important considerations for future research:

- Carry out controlled, randomized clinical trials to test the effect of adding increased physical activity to multifactorial behavioral intervention among adults for the primary prevention of CVD morbidity (including multiple CVD endpoints of myocardial infarction, angina pectoris, stroke, and peripheral vascular disease and mortality). Studies should include adequate numbers of women, lower socioeconomic populations, and minority groups.

- Carry out controlled, randomized clinical trials among inactive children and adolescents to test the effects of increased physical activity on CVD risk factor levels, including obesity. The effects of intensity, frequency, and duration of increased physical activity should be examined in such studies.
- Maintain surveillance of physical activity levels in the US population by age, gender, geographic, and socioeconomic measures.
- Develop better methods for analysis and quantification of activity. These methods should be applicable to both work and leisure-time measurements and provide direct quantitative estimates of activity.
- Develop more accurate means for cost-benefit analysis as a means of comparing activity to other forms of treatment and prevention of CVD.
- Conduct experiments designed to explore intensity-time relations for design of activity programs.
- Conduct basic research necessary to define the mechanisms by which activity affects CVD, including changes in metabolism as well as cardiac and vascular effects. This will provide new insights into cardiovascular biology that may have broader implications than for other clinical outcomes.
- Link activity effects to alterations in the quality of life as well as to mortality and morbidity.
- Examine the effects of physical activity and cardiac rehabilitation programs on morbidity and mortality in elderly individuals.
- Conduct research on the social and psychological factors that influence adoption of a more active lifestyle and the maintenance of that behavior change throughout life.
- Conduct research on the development of activity preferences and behaviors across the life span, addressing decline in activity with increasing age and ways to alter or reverse this decline.
- Determine optimal level of physical activity with regard to intensity, frequency, and duration.
- Perform more research on the relationships between cardiovascular risk factors, physical activity, and family history.

Conclusions

Accumulating scientific evidence indicates that physical inactivity is a major risk factor for cardiovascular disease. Moderate levels of regular physical activity confer significant health benefits. Unfortunately, most Americans have little or no physical activity in their daily lives.

All Americans should engage in regular physical activity at a level appropriate to their capacity, needs, and interest. All children and adults should set a goal of accumulating at least 30 minutes of moderate-intensity physical activity on most, and preferably all, days of the week. Those who currently meet these standards may derive additional health and fitness benefits by becoming more physically active or including more vigorous activity.

Cardiac rehabilitation programs that combine physical activity with reduction in other risk factors should be widely applied to those with known CVD. There are medical and cost benefits to well-designed rehabilitation programs that are lost because of these programs' limited use.

Individuals with CVD and men over 40 or women over 50 with multiple cardiovascular risk factors should have a medical evaluation prior to embarking on a vigorous exercise program.

The Panel recognizes the importance of individual and societal factors in initiating and sustaining regular physical activity. The Panel makes several recommendations, including the following:

- Develop programs to teach health-care providers how to communicate to patients the importance of regular physical activity.
- Establish community support for regular physical activity, with environmental and policy changes at schools, work sites, community centers, and other locations.
- Initiate a coordinated national campaign to encourage regular activity involving a consortium of collaborating health organizations.

The implementation of the recommendations in this statement has considerable potential to improve the health and well-being of American citizens.

Part I

AN OVERVIEW OF THE FIELD

Physical Activity, Lifestyle, and Cardiovascular Health

William L. Haskell
Stanford University School of Medicine, Stanford, California, USA

The concept that a sedentary lifestyle leads to an increase in the clinical manifestations of coronary heart disease (CHD), especially myocardial infarction and sudden death, has become generally accepted by the general public and health-care professionals. Most often, the idea has been expressed that regular physical activity, in conjunction with other risk-reducing behaviors, will help protect against an initial clinical cardiac event *(primary prevention)*; will aid in the recovery of patients following myocardial infarction, coronary artery bypass surgery, or angioplasty *(cardiac rehabilitation)*; and will reduce the risk of recurrent cardiac events *(secondary prevention)*.

Evidence relating the level of habitual physical activity to the risk of CHD has been derived from a variety of sources, including animal studies, clinical impressions, observational surveys of the general population or special groups, and experimental studies in which the exercise of subjects assigned to "treatment" was increased in relation to sedentary control subjects. Not one of these studies provides irrefutable evidence of a causal relationship between exercise status and CHD pathology, even though many sources of information do generally support such a contention. Until the basic biologic process of atherosclerosis at the molecular level has been established, it is highly unlikely that any study of exercise will definitively demonstrate a cause-and-effect relationship.

This situation is not unique to our understanding of the preventive role of physical activity as it relates to CHD since it applies to all other lifestyle risk factors. Additional observational studies will only provide more data on associations or demonstrate the predictive value of an active lifestyle. No plans presently exist to initiate a randomized, controlled trial of adequate design to determine the impact of habitual exercise on the rate of initial CHD clinical events. Thus, it appears that over the next decade, decisions regarding the use of exercise as a preventive modality for CHD will have to be based primarily on information currently available.

Physical Activity and the Primary Prevention of Coronary Heart Disease

During the past half-century, as many as 70 studies have been published reporting on the association between habitual level of physical activity or level of endurance fitness and the prevalence or incidence of initial clinical manifestations of CHD, especially myocardial infarction and sudden cardiac death.[1] These studies have included the determination of on-the-job or leisure-time activity in free-living populations of many men and a few women, with activity classifications based on job category, self-report questionnaires, or interviewer determinations. Manifestations of CHD were established by examination of death certificates, hospital or physician records, questionnaires completed by the subjects or physicians, and medical evaluations conducted by the investigators. Reported activity levels ranged from daily caloric expenditures exceeding 6,000 kilocalories (kcal) per day in Finnish lumberjacks at one extreme, to very sedentary civil servant managers and postal clerks at the other.

Studies have been conducted in major industrial environments as well as in rural or primitive living areas. As a result of the diverse protocols used in the various studies—including sample-selection procedures, physical activity classification methods, clinical event determination criteria, and statistical treatment of the data— it is not possible to collate the results into a single summary statement or interpretation. However, certain findings, although not universally obtained, occur frequently enough to warrant the formulation of preliminary conclusions to use as a basis for recommendations to health professionals and to the general public and for planning future research.

More Active Persons Appear to Be at Lower Risk

The general impression obtained as the result of a comprehensive review of the scientific reports containing data on the primary preventive effect of physical activity is that more active people develop less CHD than their inactive counterparts, and when they do develop CHD, it occurs at a later age and tends to be less severe.[1] The results of the numerous reports are quite variable, with some studies demonstrating a highly significant beneficial effect of exercise,[2-4] others showing a favorable but nonsignificant trend in favor of the more active,[5,6] and some showing no difference in CHD rates.[7,8] Recent reports also have demonstrated that an increase in activity or fitness by middle-aged or older men is associated with lower mortality rates than for men who remain unfit or inactive.[9,10] Of major importance is the consistent finding that being physically active *does not increase* an individual's risk of CHD.

No specific study characteristics can be identified that explain the differences in results among the various studies, but in some cases the physical activity measure is not very accurate or reliable and the activity gradient among the population is quite small.[2] Also, with populations in which CHD mortality is exceptionally high and in which major risk factors such as hypercholesterolemia, hypertension, and cigarette smoking are prevalent, even very high levels of physical activity do not appear to exert a major protective effect. Finnish lumberjacks are an example of physically active individuals in whom CHD risk remains high.[11] These results argue strongly for a multifactor approach to CHD prevention.

Moderate Amounts of Exercise May Be Protective

The characteristics of physical activity required to provide benefit have not been well defined, but a wide variety of activities performed at moderate intensity or higher on most days appear to be of value. The recommendations for use of physical activity to improve cardiovascular health should be based on a systematic and thoughtful consideration of the best scientific information available that address what types and amounts of physical activity provide specific health benefits.

A striking feature of many studies that demonstrate a reduced CHD risk for more active individuals is that the greatest difference in risk is achieved between those people who do almost nothing and those who perform a moderate amount of exercise on a regular basis. Much smaller differentials in risk are observed when moderately active individuals are compared with the most active participants.[1,2,12]

The amount of activity, in both intensity and duration, that is associated with a decrease in CHD clinical manifestations varies substantially among the different reports. Several studies have observed significant differences in CHD indicators with quite small differences in habitual activity level at a relativity low intensity,[2,13] whereas other authors interpret their data to indicate that a threshold of higher intensity or amount of activity is needed in order to obtain a benefit.[3,14,15]

The types of activity performed by the more active groups included brisk walking on level ground or up stairs, lifting and carrying light objects, lifting heavy objects, operating machinery or appliances, light and heavy gardening, performing home maintenance or repairs, and participating in active games and sports. The results of several studies, however, indicate that an intensity threshold of approximately 7 kcal/min may exist, with exercise more vigorous than this providing greater protection than a similar amount of less vigorous activity.[14-16] Of greatest benefit seems to be large muscle dynamic, or *aerobic,* activity that substantially increases cardiac output (volume load on the heart) with rather small increases in mean arterial blood pressure (pressure load on the heart). Such activity is in contrast to heavy resistance, or *isometric,* exercise, which substantially increases arterial blood pressure with a relatively small increase in cardiac output.

Physical Fitness and Primary Prevention

Studies published over the past decade have observed that men and women with higher levels of cardiovascular or endurance fitness as measured by submaximal or maximal exercise tests experience less CHD and all-cause mortality over the next 3 to 16 years than their less-fit counterparts.[17-20] If a higher level of habitual activity causes a reduction in cardiovascular morbidity and mortality, then a similar association should be observed with an accurate and reliable measure of fitness. The results of these studies are very similar to the results of many of the studies of physical activity, in that the greatest differences in CHD mortality occur between the least-fit and the moderately fit persons as compared to the differences observed between moderately fit and high-fit persons.

Secondary Prevention of Coronary Heart Disease

As with primary prevention, there is no definitive study that demonstrates a significant reduction in new cardiac events as a result of exercise training in patients with established CHD. But in addition to studies that have simply compared morbidity or mortality rates in active with inactive cardiac patients, controlled experimental trials have been conducted in which myocardial infarction patients have been randomly assigned to exercise and control groups. Here again, the trend in mortality favors the more physically active patients, with benefits apparently derived from an increase in caloric expenditure of no more than 300 to 400 kcal per session three to four times per week at a moderate intensity (60%-75% of $\dot{V}O_2max$). All of the studies published, which show either no differences or lower mortality rates in the active population, have either design or implementation flaws that prohibit a definitive conclusion that an increase in exercise reduces the future likelihood of recurrent myocardial infarction, cardiac arrest, or sudden cardiac death.

Randomized clinical trials of cardiac rehabilitation following hospitalization for myocardial infarction usually have demonstrated a tendency for lower mortality in treated patients, but a statistically significant reduction occurred in only one trial. To overcome the problem of inadequate power of any one study to detect small but clinically important benefits on cardiovascular morbidity and mortality in randomized trials of rehabilitation, a meta-analysis was performed on the combined results of ten clinical trials.[21] All of the trials were required to have good documentation of myocardial infarction, randomization of patients, a rehabilitation program lasting at least six weeks, follow-up for 24 months or longer, and comprehensive documentation of outcome. Data collected on a total of 4 347 patients were analyzed. The pooled odds ratio of 0.76 (95% confidence interval, 0.63-0.92) for all-cause deaths and of 0.75 (95% confidence interval, 0.62-0.93) for cardiovascular death were significantly lower for the rehabilitation group than for the control group, with no significant difference for recurrent myocardial infarction. A similar review, but evaluating a total of 22 randomized trials of rehabilitation after myocardial infarction, reached a very similar conclusion.[22]

Mechanisms of Action by Physical Activity to Reduce CHD Clinical Events

There are substantial data supporting biological plausibility for an increase in physical activity causing a reduction in CHD.[23] An increase in endurance-type physical activity produces a wide variety of biological responses that could reduce clinical

CHD events or the underlying disease process, but which of these changes actually contribute to reduced mortality has not been established. Many of the changes produced by endurance-type physical activity that may help protect against CHD are summarized in Table 1.

Other Health Benefits of Physical Activity

In addition to a physically active lifestyle being related to reduced CHD and all-cause mortality, physical activity status is inversely associated with reduced mortality due to stroke, adult-onset diabetes mellitus, and selected site-specific cancers.[24] A lower incidence of hypertension has been reported in more active older persons, and elevated endurance exercise training tends to lower systemic arterial blood pressure. Most of these data have been collected on white men.[25] Adherence to appropriate exercise training regimens can improve skeletal muscle strength and endurance, cardiorespiratory endurance, joint range of motion, and balance in older persons, leading to enhanced functional capacity and possibly greater independence. More active people, especially patients with chronic disorders, report less anxiety and depression and a better general sense of well-being than do sedentary persons.

Overall, the human body tends to function closer to an optimal level of physical and psychological health and performance when it participates on most days in moderate or vigorous physical activity that requires the use of major muscle groups. Despite these benefits being achievable by most people at relatively little financial cost or health risk, and requiring only about 2% of their time, it appears that no more than 25% of adult Americans meet the current physical activity-CVD health recommendations. However, the results of surveys have demonstrated that most Americans consider physical activity important for maintaining optimal health.[26]

Summary of Research to Date

Results of animal, experimental, clinical, and epidemiological research support the hypothesis that more physically active individuals have greater resistance to the development of coronary atherosclerosis and its clinical manifestations. At average rates of energy expenditure of less than 7 kcal/min, a daily expenditure of 300 to 500 kcal above that expended by inactive peers is associated with a lower risk of CHD. Above 7 kcal/min, it appears that less activity needs to be performed, probably no more than 200 to 300 kcal at least every other day. Large-muscle dynamic exercise that requires a substantial increase in calorie expenditure and places a greater volume than pressure load on the myocardium appears to be most useful in providing protection. Many of the benefits are achieved at exercise intensities that are well within the capacity of most people, and the cardiovascular risks of health-oriented exercise are minimal. Both job-related and leisure-time activity seem to provide benefit, with only recent activity making a contribution: No credits or advantages appear to be gained from being more active earlier in life. The

Table 1.   Biologic Mechanisms by Which Exercise May Contribute to the Primary or Secondary Prevention of Coronary Heart Disease*

Maintain or increase myocardial oxygen supply
   Delay progression of coronary atherosclerosis (possible)
      Improve lipoprotein profile (increase HDL-C/LDL-C ratio, decrease triglycerides) (probable)
      Improve carbohydrate metabolism (increase insulin sensitivity) (probable)
      Decrease platelet aggregation and increase fibrinolysis (probable)
      Decrease adiposity (usually)
   Increase coronary collateral vascularization (unlikely)
   Increase epicardial artery diameter (possible)
   Increase coronary blood flow (myocardial perfusion) or distribution (possible)

Decrease myocardial work and oxygen demand
   Decrease heart rate at rest and submaximal exercise (usually)
   Decrease systolic and mean systemic arterial pressure during submaximal exercise (usually) and at rest (usually)
   Decrease cardiac output during submaximal exercise (probable)
   Decrease circulating plasma catecholamine levels (decrease sympathetic tone) at rest (probable) and at submaximal exercise (usually)

Increase myocardial function
   Increase stroke volume at rest and in submaximal and maximal exercise (likely)
   Increase ejection fraction at rest and during exercise (likely)
   Increase intrinsic myocardial contractility (possible)
   Increase myocardial function resulting from decreased "afterload" (probable)
   Increase myocardial hypertrophy (probable); but this may not reduce CHD risk

Increase electrical stability of myocardium
   Decrease regional ischemia or at submaximal exercise (possible)
   Decrease catecholamines in myocardium at rest (possible) and at submaximal exercise (probable)
   Increase ventricular fibrillation threshold due to reduction of cyclic AMP (possible)

---

*Expression of likelihood that effect will occur for an individual participating in endurance-type training program for 16 weeks or longer at 65% to 80% of functional capacity for 25 minutes or longer per session (300 kilocalories) for three or more sessions per week ranges from unlikely, possible, likely, probable, to usually.

Abbreviations: HDL-C = high-density lipoprotein cholesterol; LDL-C = low-density lipoprotein cholesterol; CHD = coronary heart disease; AMP = adenosine monophosphate.

Adapted from Haskell (reference 23).

benefits of exercise in terms of reducing CHD risk occur at all ages for men over 40, but the advantages have not been adequately studied for women or younger men.

Needed Research

To confirm the substantial observational data supporting an inverse association between physical activity status and CHD mortality, a randomized trial of CHD primary prevention would be of significant value for evaluating the causality of this relation. Costs, design limitations, and logistics make the successful conduct of such a study unlikely. Additional longitudinal observational studies of adequate size and duration with clinical outcomes are needed in women and ethnic minorities. Studies of how and what genes are activated by physical activity to produce various biological changes would help in understanding issues of dose-response. Improvements in physical activity measurement methodology are needed, as well as in intervention methodologies.

References

1. Berlin JA, Colditz GA. A meta-analysis of physical activity in the prevention of coronary heart disease. *Am J Epidemiol.* 1990;132:612-626.

2. Shapiro S, Weinblatt E, Frank CW, Sager, RV. Incidence of coronary heart disease in a population insured for medical care (HIP). *Am J Public Health* (Suppl). 1969;59:1-101.

3. Paffenbarger RS, Wing AL, Hyde RT. Physical activity as an index of heart attack in college alumni. *Am J Epidemiol.* 1978;108:161-175.

4. Morris JN, Pollard R, Everitt MG, Chave SPW. Vigorous exercise in leisure time: Protection against coronary heart disease. *Lancet.* 1980;8206:1207-1210.

5. Costas R, Garcia-Palmieri MR, Nazario E, Sorlie P. Relation of lipids, weight and physical activity to incidence of coronary heart disease: The Puerto Rico Heart Study. *Am J Cardiol.* 1978;42:653-658.

6. Salonen JT, Puska P, Tuomilehto J. Physical activity and risk of myocardial infarction, cerebral stroke and death: A longitudinal study in Eastern Finland. *Am J Epidemiol.* 1982;115:526-537.

7. Chapman JM, Massey FJ. The interrelationship of serum cholesterol, hypertension, body weight and risk of coronary disease. *J Chronic Dis.* 1964;17:33-42.

8. Paul O, Lepper MH, Phelan W, Dupertuis GW et al. A longitudinal study of coronary heart disease. *Circulation.* 1963;28:20-31.

9. Paffenbarger RS, Hyde RT, Wing AL, Lee I-M, Jung DL, Kamperet JR. The association of changes in physical activity level and other life-style characteristics with mortality among men. *N Engl J Med.* 1993;328:538-545.

10. Blair SN, Kohl HW, Barlow CE, Paffenbarger RS, Gibbions LW, Macera CA. Changes in physical fitness and all-cause mortality. *J Am Med Assoc.* 1995;273:1093-1098.

11. Karvonen MJ, Rautaharju PM, Orma E et al. Heart disease and employment: Cardiovascular studies on lumberjacks. *J Occup Med.* 1961;3:49-55.

12. Leon AS, Cornett J, Jacobs DR, Rauramaa R. Leisure-time physical activity levels and risk of coronary heart disease and death: The multiple risk factor intervention trial. *J Am Med Assoc.* 1987;258:2388-2395.

13. Kahn HA. The relationship of reported coronary heart disease mortality to physical activity of work. *Am J Public Health.* 1963;53:1058-1067.

14. Cassel J, Heyden S, Bartel AG et al. Occupation and physical activity and coronary heart disease. *Arch Int Med.* 1971;128:920-928.

15. Morris JN, Clayton DG, Everitt MG, Semmence AM, Burgess EH. Exercise in leisure time: Coronary attack and death rates. *Br Heart J.* 1990;63:325-334.

16. Lee I-M, Hsieh C-C, Paffenbarger RS Jr. Exercise intensity and longevity in men: The Harvard alumni health study. *J Am Med Assoc.* 1995;273:1179-1184.

17. Ekelund LG, Haskell WL, Johnson JL, Wholey FS, Criqui MH, Sheps DS. Physical fitness as a prevention of cardiovascular mortality in asymptomatic North American men. *N Eng J Med.* 1988;319:1279-1284.

18. Blair SN, Kohl HW, Paffenbarger RS, Clark DG, Cooper KH, Gibbons LW. Physical fitness and all-cause mortality: A prospective study in healthy men and women. *J Am Med Assoc.* 1989;262:2395-2401.

19. Sandvik L, Erikssen J, Thaulow E, Erickssen G, Mundal R, Rodahl K. Physical fitness as a predictor of mortality among healthy middle-aged Norwegian men. *N Engl J Med.* 1993;228:533-537.

20. Lakka TA, Venäläinen JM, Rauramaa R, Salonen R, Tuomilehto J, Salonen JT. Relation of leisure-time physical activity and cardiorespiratory fitness to the risk of acute myocardial infarction. *N Engl J Med.* 1994;330:1549-1554.

21. Oldridge NB, Guyatt GH, Fisher ME, Rimm AA. Cardiac rehabilitation after myocardial infarction: Combined exercise of randomized clinical trials. *J Am Med Assoc.* 1988;260:945-950.

22. O'Conner GT, Boving JE, Yusuf S et al. An overview of randomized trials of rehabilitation with exercise after myocardial infarction. *Circulation.* 1989;80:234-244.

23. Haskell WL. Mechanisms by which physical activity may enhance the clinical status of cardiac patients. In M.L. Pollock & D.H. Schmidt (Eds): *Heart Disease and Rehabilitation* (2d edition). New York: John Wiley & Sons, 1985, pp 276-296.

24. Bouchard C, Shephard RJ, Stephens, T (Eds): *Physical activity, physical fitness and health: International proceedings and consensus statement.* Champaign, IL: Human Kinetics, 1994.

25. Fagard RH, Tipton CM. Physical activity, fitness and hypertension. In Bouchard C, Shephard RJ, Stephens, T (Eds): *Physical activity, physical fitness and health: International proceedings and consensus statement.* Champaign, IL: Human Kinetics, 1994, pp 633-655.

26. Thornbery OT, Wilson RW, Golden P. *Health promotion and disease prevention provisional data from the National Health Interview Survey, United States, January-June, 1985. Advanced data from vital statistics* (126). Hyattsville, MD: Public Health Service. September 19,1986.

Part II

BURDEN OF PHYSICAL INACTIVITY TO THE POPULATION'S HEALTH

What Is the Magnitude of Risk for Cardiovascular Disease Associated With Sedentary Living Habits?

Harold W. Kohl III
Baylor College of Medicine, Houston, Texas, USA

Since the seminal work by Morris and colleagues,[1] more than 40 years of research in the area of physical activity and health has led to recent conclusions that physical inactivity is causally related to the risk of cardiovascular disease (CVD).[2,3] This conclusion is based on research findings from a variety of sources and depends largely on the integration of information regarding the strength, consistency, temporality, and reported biologic gradients between measures of physical activity or inactivity and CVD outcomes. The purpose of this paper is to briefly summarize the magnitude of risk of CVD associated with sedentary living habits to which four decades of research has led us and to highlight gaps in current knowledge. CVD outcomes considered here are limited to observational studies of morbidity and mortality and include stroke and coronary heart disease (CHD). Studies in which clinical measures of the physiologic status of important circulatory system vessels have been evaluated are not included.

Association of Inactivity With Risk

Existing comprehensive reviews of the association of physical inactivity with CVD risk have focused on the various frequent manifestations of CVD.[4,5] Specifically, reported results have related physical activity, assessed at one point in time, to morbidity or mortality outcomes some years later. Typically, physical activity has been measured in doses obtained from either occupational exposure or leisure-time pursuits. Early studies (predominantly through 1970) relied on occupational assessment, while in later years studies have predominantly assessed leisure-time physical activity.

In a quantitative meta-analysis, Berlin et al.[4] estimated that there is an approximate doubling of CHD risk among inactive persons when they are compared with their active peers. Among the studies evaluating occupational physical activity, inactivity is associated with a 90% increased risk of CHD death (RR = 1.90, 95% confidence interval = 1.6-2.8) relative to those classified as active. Among the studies of nonoccupational physical activity, inactivity is associated with a 60% increased risk of CHD mortality (RR = 1.6, 95% confidence interval = 1.2-2.2). Figure 1 summarizes the findings of Berlin et al.

The role that physical activity and fitness may play in the risk of stroke is not as clear, however. When CHD and stroke are studied independently, the inverse asso-

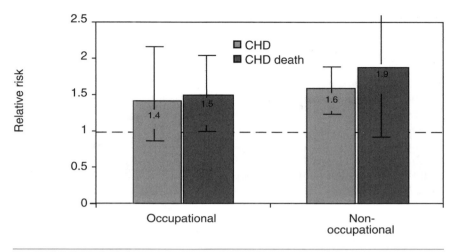

Figure 1.   Pooled relative-risk estimates of CHD from studies with two group physical-activity exposure categories.

Adapted from Berlin et al. 1990 (references 4).

ciation is readily apparent for CHD but not for stroke. Many studies designed to detect a dose-response gradient for stroke have been unable to do so, and in fact there is some suggestion of a nonlinear, U-shaped relation.[5] Although stroke is a cardiovascular disease, a much larger proportion of the burden of CVD is attributable to CHD. Therefore, the discrepant results seen between studies of all CVD and studies of stroke alone may be attributed to the large proportion of CVD that is actually CHD in origin. More work is needed to determine if physical activity and fitness are related to risk of stroke as they are to risk of CHD.

Ethnicity, Sex, and Age

No studies of physical activity or fitness and CVD have focused specifically on minority populations. Moreover, few have included any ethnic group other than whites, and those that have rarely have reported the results stratified by ethnic status. The physiologic rationale as to why the relationships should or could differ among ethnic groups are lacking, but differential distributions of potential confounding factors or effect modifiers among the various ethnic groups could possibly affect the magnitude of associations among these groups.

Studies of physical activity and CHD in women are not as prevalent as those done with men, and the results of those studies that have been performed are not nearly as consistent as those done for men. This has been attributed to a differential validity of physical activity assessment instruments between men and women.[6] Existing data on women regarding physical fitness and CVD mortality do show a consistency with the results found in men. Although it is difficult to imagine a physiologically valid rationale as to why any relationships should be different between men and women for CVD outcomes, the inconsistencies should be rectified.

When results are stratified by age, there is remarkable consistency in the inverse association between physical inactivity and CVD risk across this strata. In most studies, the inverse relation is consistent across all age groups. In fact, several studies report stronger associations between physical activity or physical fitness and CVD mortality among older participants than in younger ones. Most studies have not, however, adequately assessed lifetime (cumulative) exposure of physical activity and how that relates to risk of CVD. Rather, they have focused on a contemporary (single point estimate) assessment of physical activity. Figure 2 highlights age-specific mortality rates by physical activity index as observed in the College Alumni Study.[7]

Effects of Increase in Physical Activity

Although cardiorespiratory fitness is a physiologic attribute, it can be modified by physical activity and inactivity. Studies of fitness and CVD have shown consistent results with a clear inverse dose-response gradient across the spectrum of fitness levels and risk of CVD death.[8,9] Although there is a genetic contribution to fitness as well as to one's capacity to change fitness, studies of changes in physical fitness nonetheless show that improvements in fitness result in a lower risk of CVD death. No published studies on physical fitness and stroke exist.

One possible, although indirect, mechanism through which physical inactivity or physical unfitness has been hypothesized to lower the risk of CVD is by acting

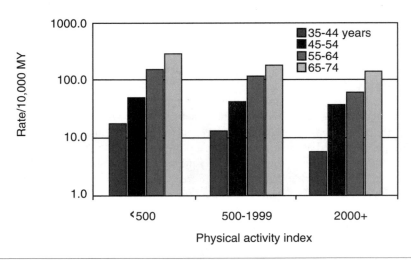

Figure 2.   Age-specific incidence of CHD by physical-activity index in 6-10 year follow-up, male Harvard alumni.

Adapted from Paffenbarger et al. 1978 (reference 7).

through other CVD risk factors (e.g., high blood pressure, high cholesterol, over-weight, diabetes mellitus, smoking habit). Existing clinical data suggest an inverse relation between physical activity and physical fitness and the risks of hypertension, overweight, and diabetes mellitus. In general, null associations have been reported between physical activity and physical fitness and serum total cholesterol and cigarette smoking habit. Although such indirect relations are possible (and perhaps even likely in some individuals), multivariable results in studies examining all characteristics simultaneously report that the associations of physical activity and physical fitness with risk of CVD are statistically independent of other factors. This leads to the conclusion that the mechanisms through which physical activity and physical fitness may be operating are at least partially independent of other CVD risk factors.

Conclusions

Although physical inactivity is causally related to the risk of mortality due to CHD, several unresolved issues are apparent when considering the relationships among physical activity, physical fitness, and CVD. First, are physical activity, physical fitness, or some combination of both related to risk of CVD and CHD? Although physical activity is a behavior, it has many physiological effects on the circulatory, metabolic, and musculoskeletal systems. Most studies have used measures of physical activity rather than fitness, and only two studies have jointly assessed both, with mixed results. The crudeness of existing physical activity measures as well as the genetic contributions to physical fitness and ability to change physical fitness continue to plague existing research. More work, with better measures of physical activity and concurrent measurement of physical fitness, is necessary to help quantify the environmental versus genetic contributions to reduced risk of CVD and CHD.

Second, there are few data on changes in physical activity or physical fitness as they relate to CVD risk. All studies but one have relied on a single, baseline measure of physical activity or fitness and related that measure to risk of CVD or CHD sometime in the future.[10] Follow-up periods in existing studies extend to 25 years. It is therefore more difficult to interpret these long-term follow-up studies without some measure of change during the course of the study. Behavioral changes and alterations in health status and the like are more likely to occur with longer periods of follow-up observation; without an assessment other than that which was taken at baseline, there is a substantial probability that misclassification will occur.

There are no population-based observational studies that address the appropriate physical activity profile necessary to reduce the risk of CVD. There is convincing evidence in existing data of a dose-response relation between physical activity and physical fitness and the risk of CVD and CHD. This has been translated in current recommendations so that physical activity of moderate intensity is sufficient to provide reduced risk of CVD and CHD. What is unavailable, however, is an assessment of the optimal manner in which that dose should be accumulated (i.e., type, intensity, frequency of bouts, duration of bouts, and various interactions). There is no direct evidence that accumulation of a total dose of physical activity over an extended period of time at a relatively low intensity provides any protection against an increased risk of CVD or CHD. More work is needed to determine the type of exercise dose that is necessary for various population subgroups.

Studies in women and minority groups are glaringly lacking. Initial cohort studies of CVD and CHD were begun in white men for convenience and because of the disproportionate disease burden in men compared with women. The inertia of tradition apparently has made it difficult to gather similar data in women, blacks, Hispanics, and Asians. Such data are critical to complete our understanding and to provide appropriate, more targeted intervention efforts. Despite the dose-response relation observed for physical activity and physical fitness in relation to CVD and CHD, these data are largely gathered from observations among white men. Further study in other ethnic groups and in women may reveal different patterns to the association, such as a threshold or nonlinear relation. Although there is little physiologic rationale to support that differences in the association of physical inactivity and CVD would exist between women and men or among different ethnic groups, it is important to quantify these relationships.

References

1. Morris JN, Heady JA, Raffle PAB, Roberts CG, Parks JW. Coronary heart disease and physical activity of work. *Lancet.* 1953;265:1053-1057, 1111-1120.

2. Bijnen FC, Caspersen CJ, Mosterd WL. Physical inactivity as a risk factor for coronary heart disease: A WHO and International Society and Federation of Cardiology position statement. *Bull WHO.* 1994; 72(1):1-4.

3. Fletcher GF, Blair SN, Blumenthal J, Caspersen C, Chaitman B, Epstein S, Falls H, Froelicher ES, Froelicher VF, Pina IL. Statement on exercise. Benefits and recommendations for physical activity programs for all Americans. A statement for health professionals by the Committee on Exercise and Cardiac Rehabilitation of the Council on Clinical Cardiology, American Heart Association. *Circulation.* 1992; 86(1):340-344.

4. Berlin JA, Colditz GA. A meta-analysis of physical activity in the prevention of coronary heart disease. *Am J Epidemiol.* 1990;132:612-628.

5. Kohl HW, McKenzie JD. Physical activity, physical fitness, and stroke. In Bouchard C, Shephard RJ, Stevens T (Eds): *Physical activity, fitness, and health: International proceedings and consensus statement.* Champaign, IL: Human Kinetics, 1994: pp. 609-621.

6. Blair SN, Kohl HW, Barlow CE. Physical activity, physical fitness, and all-cause mortality in women: Do women need to be active? *J Am Coll Nutr.* 1993;12(4):368-371.

7. Paffenbarger RS Jr, Wing AL, Hyde, RT. Physical activity as an index of heart attack risk in college alumni. *Am J Epidemiol.* 1978;108:161-175.

8. Ekelund LG, Haskell WL, Johnson JL, Whaley FL, Criqui MH, Sheps DS. Physical fitness as a predictor of cardiovascular disease mortality in asymptomatic North American men. *N Engl J Med.* 1988;319:1379-1384.

9. Blair SN, Kohl HW III, Paffenbarger RS Jr, Clark DG, Cooper KH, Gibbons LW. Physical fitness and all-cause mortality: A prospective study of healthy men and women. *JAMA.* 1989;262:2395-2401.

10. Blair SN, Kohl HW III, Barlow CE, Paffenbarger RS Jr, Gibbons LW, Macera CA. Changes in physical fitness and all-cause mortality. *JAMA.* 1995;273:1093-1098.

The Prevalence of Physical Inactivity in the United States

Carl J. Caspersen and Matthew M. Zack

Centers for Disease Control and Prevention, Atlanta, Georgia, USA

Physical activity can have a significant effect on public health because of its influence on coronary heart disease (Powell, Thompson, Caspersen, & Kendrick, 1987). National health objectives specifically call for a decrease in physical inactivity and an increase in regular patterns of physical activity for the express purpose of reducing coronary heart disease deaths (Public Health Service, 1991; Caspersen, 1994). Surveillance estimates from existing physical activity data sources identify progress in meeting objectives and also provide an understanding of physical activity levels in the United States. This paper covers selected Year 2000 physical activity objectives, physical activity data sources in the United States, adult and youth physical activity levels according to demographic factors, physical activity trends, and research recommendations.

Physical Activity Objectives and Data Sources

Three Year 2000 objectives (Figure 1), linked specifically to coronary heart disease (CHD) prevention, are reducing leisure-time physical inactivity; increasing regular, sustained activity; and increasing regular, vigorous activity (Public Health Service, 1991; Caspersen, 1994). The five major data sources providing national or state-based estimates to monitor these three physical activity objectives are the 1986-1994 Behavioral Risk Factor Surveillance System (BRFSS), the 1988-1991 National Health and Nutrition Examination Survey (NHANES), the 1985/1990/ 1991 National Health Interview Survey-Health Promotion/Disease Prevention (NHIS-HPDP) supplements, the 1992 National Health Interview Survey-Youth Risk Behavior (NHIS-YRB) supplement, and the 1991/1993/1995 Youth Risk Behavior Survey (YRBS). The BRFSS and YRBS sources provide state-based data.

Three sources assess physical activity among adults. The BRFSS asked 10 open-ended questions representing the two most frequent activities performed during leisure time in the past month and assessed the type, frequency, duration, and the usual distance covered (for walking, running, and swimming only). The 1985 and 1990 NHIS-HPDP assessed participation during the past two weeks of 22 common activities (13 for adults aged 65 years and older), probing for frequency, duration, and reported increases in breathing or heart rate to grade perceived intensity for each activity. For all age groups, the 1991 NHIS-HPDP assessed participation of 19 activities (excluding duration or intensity for bowling, golf, downhill or water

Number	Objective
1.3	Increase to at least 30% the proportion of people aged 6 and older who engage regularly, preferably daily, in light to moderate physical activity for at least 30 minutes per day. (Baseline: 22% of people aged 18 and older were active for at least 30 minutes five or more times per week, and 12% were active seven or more times per week in 1985.)
1.4	Increase to at least 20% the proportion of people aged 18 and older and to at least 75% the proportion of children and adolescents aged 6 through 17 who engage in vigorous physical activity that promotes the development and maintenance of cardiorespiratory fitness three or more days per week for 20 or more minutes per occasion. (Baseline: 12% for people aged 18 and older in 1985; 66% for youth aged 10 through 17 in 1984.)
1.5	Reduce to no more than 15% the proportion of people aged 6 and older who engage in no leisure-time physical activity. (Baseline: 24% for people aged 18 and older in 1985.)

Figure 1. Three Year 2000 objectives pertaining to coronary heart disease risk reduction (Public Health Service, 1991).

skiing, and perceived intensity for weight lifting). Each NHIS-HPDP survey allowed for the reporting of two other activities. The 1988-1991 NHANES probed for the frequency of walking a mile or more without stopping in the past month under any circumstances. For leisure time, NHANES probed for the frequency but not the duration in the past month of eight common activities and allowed for the reporting of four other activities.

Two sources assess physical activity among youth. In eight questions, the YRBS assesses participation during the past seven days in vigorous physical activity lasting 20 minutes or more, walking or bicycling lasting 30 minutes or more, and the frequency of strengthening or toning exercises as well as stretching exercises. The YRBS also assesses enrollment in physical education (PE), time spent being active during PE (if enrolled), and participation in a team sport as part of school or other organization offerings. The NHIS-YRB assesses the frequency of participation during the past seven days of 11 activity groupings ranging from vigorous activity (irrespective of duration) and walking or bicycling lasting 30 minutes or more to housecleaning or yard work lasting 30 minutes or more.

Estimates from the data sources are largely restricted to leisure-time physical activity, in part because the sources do not completely or uniformly assess household chores, transportation-related behaviors, and occupational activity. For example, the YRBS ascertained housecleaning or yard work lasting 30 minutes or more; NHIS-HPDP gardening or yard work; and BRFSS carpentry, gardening, painting or papering a house, raking, and snow shoveling or snow blowing. For transportation-related behaviors, the YRBS and NHIS-YRB ascertained walking or bicycling lasting 30 minutes or more; NHIS-HPDP walking for exercise, and biking; BRFSS bicycling for pleasure and walking; NHANES walking a mile or more without stopping and riding a bicycle or an exercise bicycle. The YRBS and NHIS-YRB did not assess occupational activity for all ages of youth under investigation. Technically, young adults aged 18 to 21 years who completed the YRB supplement could also be linked to occupational status on the NHIS core questionnaire. As well, it would be possible to link adults of any age to occupational status for the NHIS-HPDP. The 1985 and 1990 NHIS-HPDP surveys include two questions about "hard" work and "hard" main daily tasks, which were dropped from the 1991 survey because of their limited utility. The NHANES survey solicits information on type of occupation and job duties, whereas the BRFSS does not ascertain work-related behavior (aside from employment status). The inconsistent quality of work-related activity questions among the five surveys precludes any consistent or meaningful use of such information. In addition, occupational data are plagued with many problems, including within-job classification variability, job intensity misclassification, and seasonal as well as secular changes in job requirements (Caspersen, 1989).

Unlike blood pressure or blood lipids, physical activity measures are unstandardized (Caspersen, 1989). As a result, including inconsistent information about household chores, transportation-related behaviors, and occupational activities only confuses the issue. Also, it is difficult to precisely compare estimates when different surveys vary by the number of survey items, the methods of survey solicitation, the modes of survey administration, and the formulation of a summary index. Despite these concerns, many similarities exist between data sources regarding certain behavioral patterns among adults and youth.

Patterns Among Adults

Recent national estimates of leisure-time physical inactivity, available through the 1991 NHIS-HPDP, help reflect the prevalence of this important CHD risk factor (Caspersen, 1994). The 1992 BRFSS and the 1988-1991 NHANES data yield many results similar to the 1991 NHIS-HPDP (although the latter are reported herein; see also US Department of Health and Human Services, 1996). Reducing leisure-time physical inactivity to 15% is a Year 2000 objective (Figure 1; number 1.5); however, about one in four adults reported being physically inactive (24%). Women reported significantly higher amounts of inactivity (27%) than men (21%), and important variations occur by race/ethnicity. Hispanic men had significantly higher rates of physical inactivity (30%) than did black, non-Hispanic men (23%) or white, non-Hispanic men (20%). Black, non-Hispanic women (33%), Hispanic women (37%), and women of other race/ethnic origin (31%) reported significantly higher amounts of inactivity than did white, non-Hispanic women (25%).

The prevalence of physical inactivity increased with age from about one in five (21%) adults, aged 18 to 29 years, to almost one in three (33%) adults aged 75 years and older. Men aged 18 to 29 years had significantly lower levels of physical inactivity (18%) than men at any older age, whereas only women aged 75 years and older had significantly higher levels of physical inactivity (38%) than women at any younger age.

Physical inactivity uniformly decreased as education level increased, from 37% for adults having less than a high school education to 14% for adults having a college education or more. The prevalence of physical inactivity among adults with household income of less than $10,000 was about 30%, decreasing progressively to 14% at incomes of $50,000 or greater.

By geographic region, physical inactivity was highest in the Northeast and the South (each around 26% to 27%) than in the Midwest (21%). Physical inactivity peaked in December (34%) and bottomed-out in June (18%).

Increasing regular, sustained physical activity to 30% is a Year 2000 objective (Figure 1; number 1.3) intended to prevent coronary heart disease deaths and to promote weight loss and control (Caspersen, 1994). The 1991 NHIS-HPDP data reveal that 24% of adults participated in regular, sustained activity of 30 or more minutes, five or more times per week.

Women (22%) reported less regular, sustained activity than did men (27%). Regular, sustained activity declined nearly continuously with age in men, from 32% at ages 18 to 29 years, to 25% at ages 75 years and older. Among women, however, this pattern remained the same (20% to 23%) up to age 74 years and only decreased to 14% with further increasing age.

Regular sustained activity did not vary by race/ethnicity among men. However, black, non-Hispanic women and Hispanic women reported significantly lower amounts of regular, sustained activity (almost 17% each) than did white, non-Hispanic women (22%).

Regular, sustained activity was highest among adults having a college education or more (29%) and increased slightly from 24% among adults with household income of less than $10,000 to 28% for adults with income of $50,000 or more. Regular, sustained activity was lowest in the South (21%) than in the other three geographic regions and was highest in June (31%) and lowest in December (17%).

Patterns Among Youth

Among youth, the concept of leisure time is somewhat tenuous, given their large amounts of discretionary time. As a result, estimates of physical inactivity can be inordinately small, necessitating the use of reported levels of regular physical activity patterns to represent CHD risk. For example, increasing regular, vigorous physical activity patterns among youth to 75% is a Year 2000 objective (Figure 1; number 1.4). This pattern can be estimated from the 1992 NHIS-YRB, which offers a broader age span (i.e., 12 to 21 years) and more sociodemographic contrasts than the 1995 YRBS, which generally corroborates NHIS-YRB results (US Department of Health and Human Services, 1996).

In 1992, 60% of all male youth, but only 47% of all female youth, reported vigorous activity, three or more times per week. This large discrepancy is age-dependent. At 12 years of age, males and females had nearly identical levels of vigorous physical activity (68%); however, by age 21, levels declined to 42% for males and to 30% for females. White, non-Hispanic females had higher levels of vigorous physical activity (49%) than did black, non-Hispanic or Hispanic females (about 42% each), whereas males had similar levels regardless of race/ethnicity status.

The prevalence of vigorous physical activity among youth increased from about 47% within households of less than $10,000 income to 60% within households of $50,000 income or greater. Vigorous physical activity participation did not vary by geographic region; however, prevalence levels from March through June (59%) were significantly higher than levels during November and December (48%).

Sustained walking and bicycling of 30 or more minutes, five or more days per week reflect the Year 2000 target among youth to increase to 30% the prevalence of regular, sustained activity (Figure 1; number 1.3). The 1992 NHIS-YRB data reveal that about 3 in 10 males (29%) and one in four females (24%) reported walking or bicycling for 30 or more minutes, five or more days per week. This was significantly higher for males than for females overall, but did not hold among specific age groups. For example, at age 12, males (39%) reported a somewhat higher prevalence of regular walking and bicycling than did females (32%), although the difference was not statistically significant. At age 21, the prevalence was virtually identical for males (23%) and females (22%).

Hispanic males reported greater amounts (36%) of walking and bicycling than did white, non-Hispanic males (28%); likewise, Hispanic females (29%) reported greater amounts of these activities than did white, non-Hispanic females (23%).

Sustained walking and bicycling were lower (but not statistically significantly lower) among youth having household income of $50,000 or more than in other income groups. The prevalence was statistically lower in the Midwest (23%) and South (25%), than in the Northeast (29%) and the West (31%). Walking and bicycling prevalence was lowest during January and February (23%) and highest during September and October (28%).

Trends

Only three sources provided enough consistent data to help estimate time trends: the BRFSS, the NHIS-HPDP (for 1985 and 1990 only), and the YRBS. The 1986-1990 BRFSS data suggested a decrease in leisure-time physical inactivity (−2.3%) among adults from 26 states (Caspersen and Merritt, 1995), whereas 1985 to 1990 NHIS-HPDP data suggested an increase (US Department of Health and Human Services, 1996). Efforts are underway to clarify this discrepancy. The 1991 to 1995

YRBS data suggested no significant change among youth in walking and bicycling or vigorous physical activity.

Research Recommendations

It is possible that the assessment of leisure-time physical activity among minority populations might miss substantial amounts of work, household chores, transportation, and caregiving, or even cultural ceremonies involving considerable activity such as dance. However, the evidence needed to demonstrate misclassification is lacking, and the contribution of such forms of activity to health status outcomes must be established. Future analytical epidemiologic research should determine if health outcomes in these subgroups are associated with present-day patterns of work, household chores, transportation, caregiving, and so on. Additional methodological research should identify and quantify the error from activity classifications that differ by sociodemographic groups. Because such rudimentary information about the nature and extent of misclassification between subgroups and the contribution to health status outcomes is absent, it is not possible to justify including these types of physical activity into surveillance systems.

It is also necessary to establish the reliability and validity for data systems monitoring Year 2000 objectives for the general population and population subgroups (Haskell, Leon, Caspersen et al., 1992). Studies of questionnaire reliability and validity, protocols for survey administration, quality control information, data scoring issues, and interpretation of summary scores should be published.

The Year 2000 objective focusing on regular, sustained physical activity lasting 30 minutes is clearly distinct from the concept of accumulating 30 minutes throughout a day (Caspersen, 1994). Relevant epidemiological studies assessing accumulated bouts of physical activity during a day do not exist (Caspersen, 1994). Because surveillance efforts can only follow epidemiological studies, a guide to create a valid surveillance estimate does not exist. Therefore, new physical activity assessment batteries should be developed that reflect specific health-related dimensions of physical activity and dose-response concerns (Haskell, Leon, Caspersen et al., 1992) and that evaluate the benefits of accumulated daily activity. Quick, concise modules that reflect these larger batteries should be developed for use in other surveys to generate hypotheses, to control for confounding, or to evaluate interventions.

Summary and Conclusions

About one in four adults reported being physically inactive in leisure time, almost 10% more than the Year 2000 target. About one in five adults reported regular, sustained physical activity of 30 or more minutes, five or more times in the past week, almost 6% less than the Year 2000 target.

Among youth, only about half reported vigorous physical activity of three or more days per week in the past week, almost 20% less than the Year 2000 target. Only about one in four youth reported 30 or more minutes of walking and bicycling for five or more days in the past week, almost 6% less than the Year 2000 target.

Because so many adults are physically inactive in leisure time and are not meeting the recommended target for regular, sustained activity (Public Health Service, 1991; Caspersen, 1994) and because so many youth fail to engage in regular patterns of vigorous physical activity, or walking and bicycling, efforts to promote physical activity should be vigorously pursued. However, such promotional efforts should take into account the many sociodemographic differences associated with specific physical activity patterns and should focus special efforts on women, minority populations, and older adults.

Acknowledgments

Special acknowledgment goes to the National Center for Health Statistics for providing national estimates of physical activity, especially to Charlotte A. Schoenborn and Christine M. Plepys, and to Drs. Laura Kann and Wick C. Warren for providing YRBS estimates.

References

1. Caspersen CJ. Physical activity epidemiology: Concepts, methods and applications to exercise science. *Exercise Sport Sci Rev*, 1989;17:423-473.

2. Caspersen CJ. What are the lessons from the US approach to setting targets? In Killoran AJ, Fentem P, & Caspersen CJ (Eds.): *Moving on: International perspectives on promoting physical activity*. London, England: Health Education Authority, 1994:35-55.

3. Caspersen CJ, Merritt RK. Trends in physical activity participation among 26 states, 1986-1990. *Med Sci Sports Exercise*, 1995;27(5):713-720.

4. Haskell WL, Leon AS, Caspersen CJ, Froelicher VF, Hagberg JM, Harlan W, Holloszy JO, Regensteiner JG, Thompson PD, Washburn RA, Wilson PWF. Cardiovascular benefits and assessment of physical activity and physical fitness in adults. *Med Sci Sports Exercise*, 1992;24(6):S201-S220.

5. Powell KE, Thompson PD, Caspersen CJ, Kendrick JS. Physical activity and the incidence of coronary heart disease. *Annu Rev Public Health*, 1987; 8:253-287.

6. Public Health Service. *Healthy People 2000: National health promotion and disease prevention objectives—Full report with commentary*. DHHS publication no. (PHS) 91-50212. Washington, DC: US Department of Health and Human Services, 1991.

7. US Department of Health and Human Services. *Physical Activity and Health: A Report of the Surgeon General.* Atlanta, GA: US Department of Health and Human Services, Centers for Disease Control and Prevention, National Center for Health Promotion and Disease Prevention, 1996.

Population Attributable Risk of Physical Inactivity

Kenneth E. Powell

Centers for Disease Control and Prevention, Atlanta, Georgia, USA

In 1992, cardiovascular diseases accounted for 42% of all deaths in the United States, with coronary heart disease (CHD) alone being responsible for 22% of all deaths. The risk of CHD is known to be higher among those who are sedentary.[1] The purpose of this report is to estimate the proportion of CHD deaths that occur because US citizens are not physically active. This proportion, referred to as the population attributable risk (PAR), is about 34%, representing 163 000 deaths in 1992.

The data in this report pertain to CHD. Although research is sparse, one would expect similar findings for other atheromatous cardiovascular disease. It is worth noting that regular physical activity also is associated with reduced rates of several noncardiovascular diseases, such as colon cancer, non-insulin-dependent diabetes mellitus, and depression.[1] The physical activity-associated PARs for colon cancer and non-insulin-dependent diabetes mellitus are reported elsewhere.[2]

Population Attributable Risk

The PAR is an estimate of the percent of deaths that would not occur if a particular risk factor were absent. The excess number of deaths is the difference between the total deaths that did occur and the estimated number of deaths that would have occurred if a given risk factor (e.g., inactivity) were absent. The excess, divided by the total number of cases and multiplied by 100, gives the percent of cases that are extra and attributable to the presence of the risk factor (Table 1, Formula 1). Even if every American were optimally active, the rate would not fall to zero because there are other causes of CHD. The CHD mortality rate would fall to a value determined by the prevalence of cigarette smoking, the distributions of blood pressure and blood cholesterol concentration, and other causal factors.

The number of cases of CHD that would occur if everyone were active is not directly measurable, but can be estimated using the relative risk (RR) of inactive individuals with respect to active individuals, and the prevalence of physical inactivity (Table 1, Formula 2).

For complex variables, such as physical activity, the accuracy of the PAR can be improved by separating the population into more than two levels of exposure (activity). The PAR can be calculated when there are multiple levels of exposure (Table 1, Formula 3) and for each individual level of exposure (Table 1, Formula 4). This method not only estimates the overall PAR, but also identifies the activity pattern(s) associated with the largest number of excess deaths.

Table 1.   Formulas for Calculating Overall and Stratum-Specific Population Attributable Risk

Formula 1.   Conceptual Formula

$$PAR = \frac{Cases_{total} - Cases_{if\,all\,active}}{Cases_{total}} \times 100$$

Formula 2.   Most commonly used formula, two levels of exposure

$$PAR = \frac{P_{exp} * (RR - 1)}{1 + P_{exp} * (RR - 1)} \times 100$$

Formula 3.   Formula for more than one level of exposure

$$PAR = \frac{\Sigma P_{exp\,(i)} * (RR_i - 1)}{1 + \Sigma P_{exp\,(i)} * (RR_i - 1)} \times 100$$

Formula 4.   Formula for one level exposure, if there are several levels

$$PAR_i = \frac{P_{exp\,(i)} * (RR_i - 1)}{1 + \Sigma P_{exp\,(i)} * (RR_i - 1)} \times 100$$

PAR = population attributable risk

P_{exp} = prevalence of the exposure

RR = relative risk

$P_{exp\,(i)}$ = prevalence of one level exposure, if there are several (i) levels

RR_i = relative risk for one level of exposure, if there are several levels

Prevalence of Physical Inactivity

Estimates of levels of physical activity in this report are based on categories of physical activity developed for the national public health goals described in *Healthy People 2000*.[3] This scheme categorizes the population on the basis of leisure-time activity patterns. The prevalence estimates derive from the 1992 Behavioral Risk Factor Surveillance System (BRFSS). (Personal communication, Michael Pratt, December 1995.) The BRFSS surveys are described in detail elsewhere.[4,5] Briefly, state health departments conduct telephone surveys of persons aged 18 and older each month to learn about health-related behaviors, such as smoking, alcohol use, or physical activity. Respondents are selected using random-digit dialing, and one adult per household is interviewed.

Respondents are told that the physical activity questions do not pertain to activity on the job. They are asked if, during the past month, they have participated "in any physical activities or exercises, such as running, calisthenics, golf, gardening, or walking for exercise." If they respond positively, they are asked what activity they did, how many times per month they did it, and the time for one session. If the activity is walking, running, or swimming, they are asked the average distance traversed. Information is obtained for up to two activities.

Based upon their responses, respondents are categorized into four groups. The *sedentary* (29% of respondents in 1992) are those who engage in no leisure-time physical activity; the *irregularly active* (44%) engage in some light-to-moderate physical activities, but for fewer than 30 minutes per day or fewer than five days per week; the *regularly active* (13%) engage in light-to-moderate leisure-time physical activity for 30 minutes or more at least five days per week but are not vigorously active; and the *vigorously active* (14%) engage in vigorous (>50% of capacity) physical activity three or more days per week for 20 or more minutes per session.

Relative Risks

Empirically determined RRs for these categories of physical activity do not exist. For most calculations in this report, an RR of 2.0 for sedentary individuals with respect to vigorously active individuals is assumed. Reviews of the relationship between CHD and physical activity report the median or summary RR to be about 1.9.[6,7] The slightly higher value of 2.0 is selected because better studies generally have reported RRs higher than 2.0;[6] because studies with more than two exposure groups generally have reported higher RRs for the least active group compared with the most active group, than have studies with two exposure groups;[7] and also for the sake of simplicity. The RR of irregularly active individuals with respect to vigorously active people is assumed to be 1.5, because much of the benefit of regular physical activity appears to accrue with modest increases in activity.[1] The RR of the regularly active with respect to the vigorously active is assumed to be 1.1, because vigorous activity appears to provide some additional benefit over that of regular moderate activity.[8]

Quantitative Estimates

Based on the above estimates, approximately 34% of the deaths from CHD are attributable to physical inactivity (Table 2). Thus, in 1992, an estimated 163 000 of the 480 000 CHD deaths would not have occurred if everyone had been optimally physically active. Those who were sedentary (29% of the population) accounted for about 56% of the excess deaths (19%-34%), and those who were irregularly active (44% of the population) accounted for about 41% of the excess deaths (14%-34%).

Of course, not everyone will become vigorously physically active. If we assume that the physical activity goals from *Healthy People 2000* are achieved,[3] the PAR would decline to 28% (Table 2). If we assume that one-half of each activity group moves to the next more active category, the PAR would decline to 26%. These

Table 2.   Population Attributable Risk of Physical Inactivity*

Exposure level groups	RR	1992 BRFSS activity level estimates		Year 2000 objectives achieved		50% of each move to next level	
		P_{exp}	PAR	P_{exp}	PAR	P_{exp}	PAR
Sedentary	2.0	29%	19%	15%	11%	14%	10%
Irregular	1.5	44%	14%	45%	16%	37%	14%
Regular	1.1	13%	1%	20%	1%	28%	2%
Vigorous	1.0	14%	0%	20%	0%	21%	0%
			34%		28%		26%

RR = relative risk

P_{exp} = prevalence of the exposure in the population

PAR = population attributable risk

*These data are based on 1992 Behavioral Risk Factor Surveillance System activity estimates and assuming Year 2000 objectives are achieved, and assuming that 50% of each activity group becomes more active.

achievements would reduce the number of CHD deaths by about 40,000 and 52,000, respectively.

PAR With Refined Exposure Estimates

Recalculating the PAR using exposure estimates for specific population subgroups does not appreciably change the PAR. Population surveys of physical activity patterns indicate that, in general, younger people are more active than older people, and men are more active than women.[9] Using the same RR estimates (i.e., 2.0, 1.5, and 1.1 for the sedentary, irregularly active, and the regularly active, respectively), substituting the age- or sex-specific activity estimates from the 1992 BRFSS make very little difference in the calculated PAR. The calculated PARs for men and for women are 34% and 35%, respectively; and the PARs for those 18 to 64 and 65+ years of age are 34% and 36%, respectively.

PAR With Different Relative Risks

Recalculating the PAR with different RRs indicates that the PAR estimate is quite sensitive to changes in the relative risk. For example, if the maximum RR is estimated at 1.5 instead of 2.0, and the intermediate RRs are spaced at the same relative positions between the poles (i.e., 1.25 and 1.05 instead of 1.5 and 1.1), the PAR is 21% (Figure 1). If the maximum RR is estimated at 3.0, and the intermediate RRs are again similarly spaced (i.e., 2.0 and 1.2), the PAR is 51% (Figure 1).

This exercise demonstrates two points. First, the PAR is substantially less, although still quite large (21%), if one assumes a maximum RR of only 1.5. It is substantially larger (51%) if the RR is as high as 3.0. Second, an accurate estimate of the relative risk is necessary for an accurate assessment of the population burden of inactivity. This emphasizes the importance of determining the RRs specifically associated with behavioral patterns commonly used in population surveys, such as the BRFSS.

PAR for Physical Activity Compared With Other Risk Factors

Based on the assumptions in this report, among commonly recognized risk factors for CHD, the PAR for inactivity is exceeded by blood cholesterol >200 mg/dl, but is greater than those for blood pressure >140/90 mmHg, cigarette smoking, obesity, and diabetes (fasting blood sugar >140 mg/dl[10]) (Figure 2).

Summary

Assuming RRs of 2.0, 1.5, and 1.1 for those who are sedentary, irregularly active, and regularly active, respectively, approximately 34% of all deaths and new clinical cases of CHD would not occur if all Americans were optimally active. More than half (about 56%) of the excess CHD events occur among those who are sedentary. It is not likely that everyone will become optimally active. If the nation's

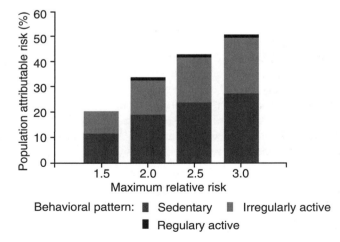

Figure 1.   Population attributable risk by maximum relative risk and behavioral pattern.

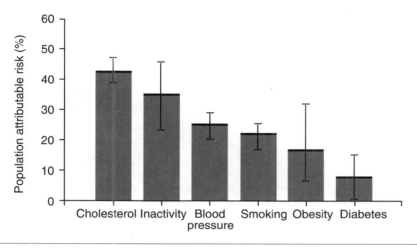

Figure 2.   Population attributable risk by risk factor.

Source: Chronic Disease Epidemiology and Control (reference 10).

goals for the year 2000 are met, the number of deaths and new cases of CHD would still decline about 8%. The PAR is sensitive to different estimates of RR, ranging from 21% to 51% as the maximum RR ranges from 1.5 to 3.0. Physical inactivity is responsible for a large portion of deaths and new cases of CHD and is among the most important risk factors for CHD in the United States.

References

1. Pate RR, Pratt M, Blair SN, Haskell WL, Macera CA, Bouchard C et al. Physical activity and public health: A recommendation from the Centers for Disease Control and American College of Sports Medicine. *JAMA*, 1995;273:402-407.

2. Powell KE, Blair SN. The public health burdens of sedentary living habits: Theoretical but realistic estimates. *Medicine Sci Sports Exercise*, 1994;26:851-856.

3. US Public Health Service. *Healthy People 2000: National health promotion and disease prevention objectives*. US Department of Health and Human Services. DHHS publication no. (PHS)91-50212. Washington, DC: Department of Health and Human Services, 1991.

4. Frazier EL, Franks AL, Sanderson LM. Using behavioral risk factor surveillance data. In: *Using chronic disease data: A handbook for public health practitioners*. Atlanta, GA: Centers for Disease Control and Prevention, 1992.

5. Siegal PZ, Frazier EL, Mariolis P, Brackbill RM, Smith C. Behavioral risk factor surveillance, 1991: Monitoring progress toward the nation's Year 2000 objectives. *CDC Surveill Summ*, 1993;42(No. SS-4): 1-21.

6. Powell KE, Thompson PD, Caspersen CJ, Kendrick JS. Physical activity and the incidence of coronary heart disease. *Ann Rev Public Health*, 1987;8:253-287.

7. Berlin JA, Colditz GA. A meta-analysis for physical activity in the prevention of coronary heart disease. *Am J Epidemiol*, 1990;132:612-628.

8. Morris JN, Clayton DG, Everitt MG, Semmence AM, Burgess EH. Exercise in leisure time: Coronary attack and death rates. *Br Heart J*, 1990;63:325-334.

9. Caspersen CJ, Merritt RK. Physical activity trends among 26 states, 1986-1990. *Med Sci Sports Exercise*, 1995;27:713-720.

10. Smith CA, Pratt M. Cardiovascular disease. In Brownson RC, Remington PL, Davis JR (Eds.): *Chronic disease epidemiology and control*. Washington, DC: American Public Health Association, 1993:83-107.

Part III

CURRENT ISSUES RELATED TO THE NATURE OF PHYSICAL ACTIVITY AND CARDIOVASCULAR DISEASE

Physical Activity and Prevention of Cardiovascular Diseases: Potential Mechanisms

Claude Bouchard
Laval University, Sainte Foy, Quebec, Canada

Based on a variety of experimental and epidemiological studies, it appears that a sedentary lifestyle is a risk factor for a number of atherosclerotic, metabolic, and hypertensive diseases which become more prevalent with advancing age in both genders. On the other hand, a physically active lifestyle offers some protection against the same diseases with the association generally suggestive of a dose-dependent relationship. The biological mechanisms responsible for these preventive effects of regular physical activity are not well understood. However, the effects of regular physical activity on relevant morphological, physiological, and metabolic variables and related risk factors may provide a basis for the definition of some of the mechanisms responsible for these benefits. These effects of regular physical activity were extensively reviewed in two recent conferences which provide the basis for the present summary (Bouchard et al., 1994; Fletcher, 1994).

Common Effects of Regular Physical Activity

Body Weight and Body Fat

Being overweight (BMI > 27) or obese (BMI > 30) augments the risk of coronary heart disease (CHD) and other vascular diseases. Some studies have even suggested that the lowest risk of CHD is observed among the leanest individuals, that is, those with a BMI of about 20 to 22 (Rich-Edwards et al., 1995). Because physical activity accounts, on average, for only about 20% of the daily energy expended in sedentary individuals, a slight increase in habitual physical activity is unlikely to have a substantial impact on total daily energy expenditure and thus on energy balance. However, with a more substantial energy expenditure resulting from a higher level of habitual physical activity, greater influences are likely to be seen on energy balance and thus on body fat content (Bouchard et al., 1993).

Upper Body Fat and Abdominal Visceral Fat

Upper body fat and abdominal visceral fat are better predictors of metabolic anomalies and diseases than are body weight and total body fat. In particular, the amount of abdominal fat, and especially the size of the visceral fat depot, are well correlated with undesirable alterations in glucose, lipid and lipoprotein, and insulin

48

metabolism (Després et al., 1990). The loss of abdominal fat is well correlated with the improvement in insulin, glucose, and lipid metabolism observed with regular aerobic exercise. Visceral fat can be greatly diminished by regular exercise when it is not associated with caloric intake compensation (Bouchard et al., 1994a).

Insulin Metabolism

The impairment of in vivo glucose disposal rate in the presence of insulin is the consequence of an insulin-resistant state in peripheral tissues, particularly the skeletal muscle. A diminished insulin-mediated inhibition of hepatic glucose output also occurs when the liver becomes resistant to the action of insulin. The vascular complications of diabetes are numerous and include not only coronary heart disease, which is the most frequent cause of death in diabetic patients, but also peripheral vascular disease, nephropathy, retinopathy, and other conditions.

In middle-aged individuals, regular exercise tends to improve glucose tolerance and to modify favorably several recognized risk factors for cardiovascular disease. One apparent consequence of regular exercise is an improvement in the sensitivity of liver, skeletal muscle, and adipose tissues to insulin action, a decrease in the basal level of plasma glucose in hyperglycemic subjects, a decrease in fasting insulin levels, a reduction of the insulin response to a glucose load, and an increase in the glucose disposal rate assessed under various conditions during euglycemic-hyperinsulinemic clamp procedures (Gudat et al., 1994).

Such changes are observed with programs of walking and other low-intensity, long-duration exercise sessions that do not necessarily cause an increase in maximal oxygen intake. It is not fully established whether the insulin-lowering effect of regular physical activity and the apparent improvement of an insulin-resistant state result from an acute or a persistent increase in the insulin sensitivity of skeletal muscle and other peripheral tissues, because of a reduction in insulin secretion, an increased rate of hepatic removal of insulin, or a combination of these mechanisms.

Blood Pressure

Many epidemiological studies have reported an inverse relationship between level of habitual physical activity and resting blood pressure. Intervention studies have shown that regular physical activity in essential hypertensives can reduce systolic and diastolic blood pressures by approximately 10 mmHg, a reduction which is, in several instances, of clinical significance (Fagard & Tipton, 1994). This favorable effect has not been noted in all cases, and increased physical activity alone may not always be sufficient to normalize blood pressure. The currently available data suggest that regular endurance exercise at an intensity of 40% to 60% of $\dot{V}O_2$max is sufficient to induce these effects.

Studies indicate that, relative to controls, endurance training is associated with a mean reduction of systolic and diastolic blood pressure of 3 mmHg in subjects with a normal pressure and of 6 mmHg in borderline hypertensives. The mechanism and the significance of such observations for prevention of CHD are not known. The hemodynamic mechanism underlying the hypotensive effect of endurance training remains controversial.

Lipid Oxidation

In acute response to physical activity, fat is oxidized in progressively increasing amounts as the total energy expenditure increases, so that lipids may cover up to 90% of oxidative metabolism in prolonged bouts of exercise at moderate intensity. Endurance training increases the capability for fat oxidation. The absolute mass of the skeletal muscle mitochondria increases with training, resulting in an increased capacity to oxidize fats. There is a greater reliance on fat as a source of energy during submaximal exercise at the same absolute work rate in trained individuals. Endurance training results in an increased lipolytic responsiveness to beta-adrenergic stimulation, concomitant with lower plasma catecholamine concentrations. Training increases the activity of both skeletal muscle and adipose tissue lipoprotein lipase, thereby facilitating the use of circulating triglycerides as a fuel source in trained muscles and promoting the clearance of circulating triglycerides even at rest. The net effect is an improved capacity to remain in fat balance despite a relatively high dietary fat intake (Tremblay et al., 1994).

Lipid and Lipoprotein Metabolism

Regular physical activity lowers plasma triglycerides in subjects with initially high levels but has little impact on those with normal concentrations (Stefanick & Wood, 1994). On the average, regular physical activity increases HDL cholesterol, particularly the cholesterol content of the HDL_2 subfraction, and may also increase apolipoprotein A-I, the main apolipoprotein of HDL. Among subjects with elevated cholesterol levels, regular physical activity is occasionally associated with decreases in total cholesterol and LDL cholesterol. However, regular physical activity may also reduce LDL particle number without concomitant decrease in LDL-cholesterol levels.

An increase in lipoprotein lipase activity, the key enzyme in the conversion of VLDL to HDL, associated with regular exercise may contribute to the augmentation of the HDL cholesterol level particularly the HDL_2 subfraction. The reduction in hepatic lipase activity observed with regular exercise may be one of the mechanisms favoring the high levels of HDL_2 cholesterol observed in active individuals. Another mechanism of importance is the role of regular physical activity on insulin action, as activity tends to increase insulin sensitivity and reduce plasma insulin levels, a phenomenon that may also favorably alter plasma lipoprotein-lipid levels (Bouchard & Després, 1995).

Coagulation and Hemostatic Factors

Blood coagulation, fibrinolysis, and platelet aggregation are intimately involved with stages of atherosclerosis. Heavy exercise transiently increases in vitro blood coagulation, whereas moderate intensity effort is sufficient to activate fibrinolysis. Data suggest decreased plasma fibrinogen concentration, increased fibrinolytic and diminished antifibrinolytic activity after intensive exercise training in clinically healthy older men (Rauramaa & Salonen, 1994). In addition, limited data in middle-aged, overweight, mildly hypertensive men suggest that regular moderate-intensity exercise training inhibits platelet aggregability.

Cardiac Performance

Regular endurance exercise leads to an increase in maximal oxygen uptake, due to an enhanced ability to increase stroke volume and to widen the total body arteriovenous oxygen difference. The ability to deliver a greater peak stroke volume may reflect an eccentric hypertrophy of the left ventricle, and increases in total blood volume, vascular capacitance, and venous compliance among other factors (Mitchell & Raven, 1994).

Aerobic training increases the vascular transport capacity in both cardiac and skeletal muscle by augmenting both the peak blood flow and capillary exchange capacity. The increases in transport capacity result from both structural adaptations and altered control of vascular resistance. Structural vascular adaptations take at least two forms: increases in the cross-sectional area and length of the large and small arteries and veins, and increased numbers of capillaries and other microvessels per gram of muscle (Laughlin et al., 1994). Regular endurance exercise causes moderate cardiac hypertrophy, while maintaining or increasing the capillary density and increasing the arteriolar density, and alters coronary vascular control.

Potential Mechanisms for the Cardiovascular Benefits

This brief overview indicates that regular physical activity has favorable impact on common risk factors for atherosclerotic diseases. The mechanisms associated with the beneficial effects of regular physical activity identified in prospective epidemiological studies and described in experimental intervention studies can be grouped in three categories: those pertaining to the cardiac muscle; those affecting blood flow and myocardial vascularization; and those related to the metabolic environment.

Favorable changes in the heart muscle, cardiac blood vessels, coronary blood flow, and myocardial metabolic characteristics as a result of sustained exposure to exercise have been described (Saltin, 1990; Mitchell & Raven, 1994; Laughlin et al., 1994, 1994a). Common adaptive responses include an increase in heart size and left ventricular mass, an augmented blood volume, an increase in stroke volume at rest and during exercise, a higher maximal cardiac output, a decreased heart rate at rest, and for a given submaximal power output. Other alterations that have been described primarily from research based on animal models include changes in myocardial contractile and structural proteins as a result of differential gene expression caused by the demands imposed on the heart muscle (Brand & Schneider, 1994; Ianuzzo et al., 1994). Animal research and some observations based on human subjects also reveal that the size of existing cardiac vessels can be increased, that capillary density augments even in the presence of cardiac hypertrophy, that coronary blood flow capacity can be improved, and that neuro-humoral control over the myocardial vascular bed is also improved (Laughlin et al., 1994, 1994a).

The metabolic effects of regular physical activity are complex and numerous. Here we are concerned by the primary or fundamental metabolic mechanisms that may be responsible for the benefits of regular physical activity commonly noted in morbidity and mortality data. Figure 1 lists the four factors that, in my judgment, emerge as the most fundamental mechanisms. They are the hypothalamic-pituitary-adrenal axis activity and associated cortisol levels, the insulin action and related insulin levels, the capacity to oxidize fatty acids in various tissues but particularly in the skeletal muscle, and the growth hormone status. All are intimately interrelated in metabolic regulation. They are also all favorably affected by regular physical activity as they progressively evolve in the direction of a metabolic environment characterized by an increased insulin sensitivity, lower insulin and cortisol levels or excursions, improved growth hormone status, and an augmented fatty acid oxidation rate in the presence of a high glucose disposal rate.

In contrast, a sedentary lifestyle, particularly in the presence of other adverse behaviors such as a high fat diet and smoking or failure to cope with stress, is altering these fundamental metabolic determinants in opposite directions. For instance, a decrease in insulin action is met by an increase in circulating insulin. Hyperinsulinemia is in turn promoting increases in counter-regulatory factors such as cortisol and fatty acids (Brindley, 1995). The balance between insulin and cortisol and fatty acids will over time be restored but at higher levels. Figure 2 illustrates these relationships as proposed by Brindley. The basic theorem here is that elevated levels of insulin or of cortisol will promote a counter-regulatory response of the other axis to restore balance. Hence, hyperinsulinemia accompanied by elevated levels of cortisol and fatty acids provide a metabolic environment which represents a strong risk for vascular diseases (Brindley, 1995).

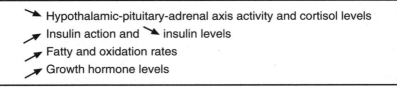

Figure 1.   A hypothesis about fundamental metabolic mechanisms responsible for the favorable relationships between physical activity and vascular diseases.

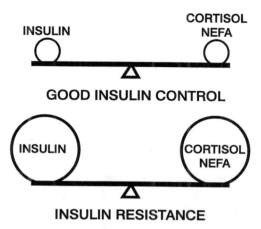

Figure 2. Modified balance between insulin and cortisol plus fatty acid levels in regulating metabolism when insulin resistance occurs. NEFA = non-esterified fatty acids. From Brindley, 1995.

Regular physical activity is a powerful agent to influence favorably the trilogy of the cardiac muscle, the blood flow and myocardial vascularization, and, perhaps even more importantly, the metabolic environment. Indeed, regular physical activity promotes an improved insulin action and lower circulating insulin levels (Sutton et al., 1990; Richter & Sutton, 1994; Gudat et al., 1994). Regular physical activity is also a powerful stimulant for lipid oxidation during the activity period and in the post-exercise recovery as a result of repeated exposure (Bouchard et al., 1993). Indeed, trained individuals oxidize more lipids than do sedentary controls in a variety of circumstances. Although we still need more research on the influence of regular physical activity on the hypothalamic-pituitary-adrenal axis and growth hormone levels, it is known that they are affected by acute and chronic exposure to exercise (Sutton et al., 1990; Richter & Sutton, 1994). Greater excursions of glucocorticoid levels are observed in sedentary persons compared to active individuals when challenged by a similar stress. Normal growth hormone levels may also be promoted by regular physical activity in growth hormone deficient individuals. A metabolic environment characterized by normal insulin action, normal growth hormone and cortisol levels, and high fatty acid oxidative capacity would also impact favorably on other metabolic traits, including the plasma lipid and lipoprotein profile, thereby contributing to a lower risk level for vascular diseases.

Figure 3 displays some of the complex relationships that may exist among a variety of behaviors, including the level of habitual physical activity, and some of the mechanisms and risk factors for vascular diseases identified in this brief review.

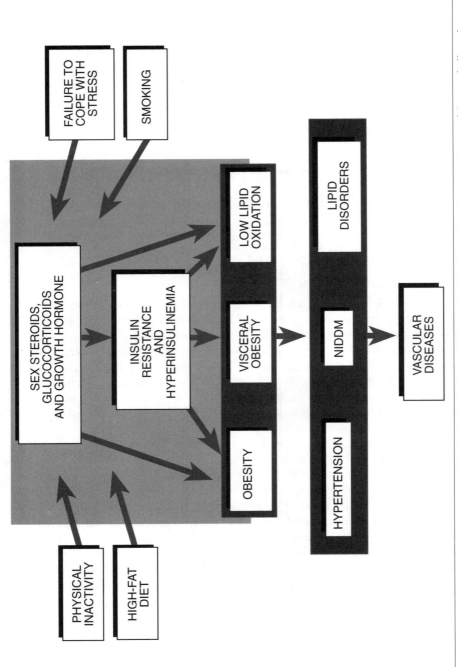

Figure 3. Interrelationships among some of the behaviors known to influence the risk of vascular diseases and some of the metabolic and morphological factors altered by these behaviors. The level of risk may vary considerably depending on the genetic susceptibility of the individuals.

References

1. Bouchard C, Després JP. Physical activity and health: Atherosclerotic, metabolic, and hypertensive diseases. *Res Q Exercise Sport*, 1995;66:1-8.

2. Bouchard C, Després JP, Tremblay A. Exercise and obesity. *Obes Res*, 1993;1: 133-47.

3. Bouchard C, Shephard RJ, Stephens T, eds. *Physical activity, fitness, and health: International proceedings and consensus statement*. Champaign, IL: Human Kinetics, 1994.

4. Bouchard C, Tremblay A, Després JP, Thériault G, Nadeau A, Lupien PJ, Moorjani S, Prud'homme D, Fournier G. The response to exercise with constant energy intake in identical twins. *Obes Res*, 1994a;2:400-10.

5. Brand T, Schneider MD. Peptide growth factors as determinants of myocardial development and hypertrophy. In Fletcher GF, ed.: *Cardiovascular response to exercise*. Mount Kisco, NY: Futura, 1994, pp. 59-99.

6. Brindley DN. Role of glucocorticoids and fatty acids in the impairment of lipid metabolism observed in the metabolic syndrome. *Int J Obesity*, 1995;19:S69-S75.

7. Després JP, Moorjani S, Lupien PJ, Tremblay A, Nadeau A, Bouchard C. Regional distribution of body fat, plasma lipoproteins and cardiovascular disease. *Arteriosclerosis*, 1990;10:497-511.

8. Fagard RH, Tipton CM. Physical activity, fitness, and hypertension. In Bouchard C, Shephard RJ, Stephens T, eds.: *Physical activity, fitness, and health: International proceedings and consensus statement*. Champaign, IL: Human Kinetics, 1994, pp. 633-55.

9. Fletcher GF, ed. *Cardiovascular response to exercise*. Mount Kisco, NY: Futura, 1994.

10. Gudat U, Berger M, Lefèbvre PJ. Physical activity, fitness, and non-insulin-dependent (Type II) diabetes mellitus. In Bouchard C, Shephard RJ, Stephens T, eds.: *Physical activity, fitness, and health: International proceedings and consensus statement*. Champaign, IL: Human Kinetics, 1994, pp. 669-83.

11. Ianuzzo CD, O'Brien PJ, Salerno TA, Laughlin MH. Effects of chronic tachycardia on the myocardium. In Fletcher GF, ed.: *Cardiovascular response to exercise*. Mount Kisco, NY: Futura, 1994, pp. 111-40.

12. Laughlin MH, McAllister RM, Delp MD. Physical activity and the microcirculation in cardiac and skeletal muscle. In Bouchard C, Shephard RJ, Stephens T, eds.: *Physical activity, fitness, and health: International proceedings and consensus statement*. Champaign, IL: Human Kinetics, 1994, pp. 302-19.

13. Laughlin MH, Oltman CL, Muller JM, Myers PR, Parker JL. Adaptation of coronary circulation to exercise training. In Fletcher GF, ed.: *Cardiovascular response to exercise*. Mount Kisco, NY: Futura, 1994a, pp. 175-205.

14. Mitchell JH, Raven PB. Cardiovascular adaptation to physical activity. In Bouchard C, Shephard RJ, Stephens T, eds.: *Physical activity, fitness, and health: International proceedings and consensus statement*. Champaign, IL: Human Kinetics, 1994, pp. 286-301.

15. Rauramaa R, Salonen JT. Physical activity, fibrinolysis, and platelet aggregability. In Bouchard C, Shephard RJ, Stephens T, eds.: *Physical activity, fitness, and health: International proceedings and consensus statement*. Champaign, IL: Human Kinetics, 1994, pp. 471-79.

16. Rich-Edwards JW, Manson JE, Hennekens CH, Buring JE. The primary prevention of coronary heart disease in women. *N Engl J Med*, 1995;332:1758-66.

17. Richter EA, Sutton JR. Hormonal adaptation to physical activity. In Bouchard C, Shephard RJ, Stephens T, eds.: *Physical activity, fitness, and health: International proceedings and consensus statement*. Champaign, IL: Human Kinetics, 1994, pp. 331-42.

18. Saltin B. Cardiovascular and pulmonary adaptation to physical activity. In Bouchard C, Shephard RJ, Stephens T, Sutton JR, McPherson B, eds.: *Exercise, fitness, and health. A consensus of current knowledge*. Champaign, IL: Human Kinetics, 1990, pp. 187-204.

19. Stefanick ML, Wood PD. Physical activity, lipid and lipoprotein metabolism, and lipid transport. In Bouchard C, Shephard RJ, Stephens T, eds.: *Physical activity, fitness, and health: International proceedings and consensus statement*. Champaign, IL: Human Kinetics, 1994, pp. 417-31.

20. Sutton JR, Farrell PA, Harber VJ. Hormonal adaptation to physical activity. In Bouchard C, Shephard RJ, Stephens T, Sutton JR, McPherson B, eds.: *Exercise, fitness, and health. A consensus of current knowledge*. Champaign, IL: Human Kinetics, 1990, pp. 217-58.

21. Tremblay A, Alméras N, Boer J, Kranenbarg EK, Després JP. Diet composition and post-exercise energy balance. *Am J Clin Nutr*, 1994;59:975-79.

Contributions of Regular Moderate-Intensity Physical Activity to Reduced Risk of Coronary Heart Disease

Arthur S Leon

University of Minnesota, Minneapolis, Minnesota, USA

Despite a progressive decline in the age-adjusted death rate from cardiovascular disease (CVD) over the past 25 years, it remains the leading cause of death in the United States, responsible in 1992 for 42.5% of all deaths. Coronary heart disease (CHD) is the principal contributor to these deaths from CVD in both men and women and is the leading cause of overall mortality, while strokes are the third leading contributor. CHD is a disease of multifactorial etiology. Both modifiable factors and immutable biological factors, such as heredity, advancing age, and sex differences contribute to its pathophysiology. Major modifiable physiological and biochemical risk factors include levels of blood pressure; blood lipid and lipoproteins, particularly elevated low density (LDL) and reduced high density lipoprotein (HDL) cholesterol levels; glucose-insulin dynamics; and obesity (especially when there is an excess deposition of upper body, abdominal, and/or visceral adipose tissue). Contributing behavioral risk factors include cigarette smoking, a diet high in saturated fat and energy intake, and low levels of habitual physical activity (PA)—the latter being the focus of this manuscript.

It now is generally recognized that a marked reduction in PA on the job and during leisure time (LTPA), associated with the modern mode of living, is a major contributing factor to the pathophysiology of the underlying atherthrombotic process of CHD. National surveys of PA status during the past 20 years have consistently reported a high prevalence of physical inactivity in American adults.[1] About 24% to 40% are reported to be completely sedentary; about 40% to 54% do some PA, but not enough to improve cardiorespiratory fitness; and only about 20% to 22% report a sufficient intensity and quantity of PA or exercise to improve cardiorespiratory fitness (i.e., rhythmic PA involving large muscle groups, such as brisk walking, jogging, cycling, or swimming for 15 to 60 minutes continuously or intermittently, 3 to 5 times a week, at an intensity of 40% to 85% of maximal oxygen uptake (VO_2max) or 50% to 90% of maximal heart rate).[2] These data suggest that a low level of PA is the most prevalent risk factor for CHD in the United States. It has been estimated that as many as 250,000 deaths per year in the United States (approximately 12% of the total death rate) are attributable to lack of regular PA.[3]

Contribution of Physical Activity to Risk of CHD

The primary basis of the postulated inverse relationship of PA to risk of CHD is 40 years of epidemiologic observational studies. Extensive reviews and critiques have been published of the more than 100 reported studies on this topic.[4,5] Although the emphasis in the earlier observational studies was on occupational PA, most of the studies during the past decade have emphasized LTPA as assessed by a variety of questionnaires. Less commonly cardiorespiratory fitness, as assessed by exercise testing, has been compared with incidence of CHD. The populations in these studies have consisted predominately of middle-aged and older white men. Only a small number of studies (fewer than 10) have included white women. There is a paucity of studies looking at this association in African Americans and other racial and ethnic minority groups.

About two-thirds of the observational studies between 1950 and 1990 support an inverse relationship of PA or cardiorespiratory fitness to risk of CHD, which generally persists after statistical adjustments for age and other potential confounding variables. Meta-analysis of those first 4 decades of studies judged to be of "better" quality in terms of methodology, indicates that the risk of CHD death is about doubled in those who are physically inactive as compared to those who are more active.[4,5] Further, Whaley and Blair[6] recently reviewed 18 additional studies published since 1990, and 17 of them showed an inverse association between PA or fitness and risk of CHD or fatal CVD (the only negative study being a 16-year follow-up of over 1 400 middle-aged and older women in the Framingham Heart Study cohort). The results from these more recent studies remain consistent with the previously reported twofold increased risk for CHD, when the least physically active men are compared with those who were more active.

However, the relatively few studies involving women have yielded mixed results. This may reflect both the lower incidence of CHD in women, at least until late in life, and the focus of most PA survey instruments on types of activities (such as sports and formal exercise programs) more commonly performed by men than women. These questionnaires also generally do not include homemaking and child care activities, traditionally pursued predominately by women. Failure to assess such activities has been shown in our laboratory to result in a gross under estimation of PA status in most women.[7]

The dozen or so studies which assessed cardiorespiratory fitness by exercise testing have noted almost unanimously in both men and women an inverse relationship of fitness and risk of CHD with a risk ratio generally greater than 5 for CHD or CVD death between the least fit and most fit men or women.[6] However, one recent study that assessed both PA and fitness showed that sedentary men with high aerobic capacities had a higher risk of CVD than did men with lower levels of fitness, who performed at least four hours per week of light to moderate PA (e.g., walking, light gardening, or bowling).[8] It should be noted that although cardiorespiratory fitness is related to exercise habits, it also is strongly influenced by genetic factors and by life habits, and therefore should not be viewed simply as a more accurate measure or a surrogate of habitual high intensity PA. For example, in a sample of healthy middle-aged men screened in Minnesota for the Multiple Risk Factor Intervention Trial (MRFIT), the total quantity of LTPA and of high intensity LTPA accounted for only 17% and 19%, respectively, of the variability in exercise test performance.[9]

Type and Quantity of PA to Reduce Risk of CHD

Haskell[10,11] has extensively analyzed data from epidemiologic studies to determine the characteristics and dose of PA related to health consequences, including reduced risk of CHD. He observed that in the majority of these studies, reduced risk of CHD mortality has been associated with predominately light to moderate PA (i.e, < 6 METs [1 MET is the resting metabolic rate and is approximately equal to 3.5 ml of oxygen uptake per kg of body weight per minute] or < 7.5 kcal per minute in intensity for an average-sized man), performed generally at an intermittent, rather than at a continuous, basis. These included such PAs as walking, stair climbing, gardening, and household chores, which in adults are generally performed more frequently than strenuous conditioning exercises or sports. The estimated difference in energy expenditure between the least active participants at increased risk of CHD mortality and moderately-active participants with a lower CHD mortality rate in these studies was about 150 to 400 kcal/day or 1,050 to 2,800 kcal/wk for an average-sized person, with most of the PA classified as moderate intensity (3-6 METs or 4-7 kcal/min for an average-sized man).

In some of the recent studies reviewed by Whaley and Blair[6] and Haskell,[10,11] the inverse association between PA or fitness and CHD mortality rate existed across the full range of PA or fitness. An example is an 8-year prospective study by Shaper et al.,[12] involving middle-aged British men. Other studies, such as the MRFIT[13,14] and the Harvard College Alumni Health study,[15-17] have demonstrated that most of the association is accounted for by the difference in CHD mortality rate between the least-active or fit and the moderately-active or fit individuals, with little or no additional reduction in CHD mortality rate between the moderately and highly active or fit categories.

In the MRFIT, middle-aged men at high risk for CHD were classified by tertiles of LTPA. Those in the middle tertile, who averaged 48 minutes per day of continuous or intermittent PA at an estimated energy cost of 224 kcal/day (about 22 kcal per kg per week), had a 5% and 25% lower risk of CHD mortality at the 7 and 10.5 year follow-ups, respectively, as compared to those in the least active tertile who averaged about 10 minutes of PA per day at an approximate energy cost of 74 kcal/day.[13,14] An additional volume of similar types of PA in the most active tertile was not associated with a further reduction in risk of CHD mortality. However, it is important to note that less than 5% of the MRFIT cohort performed a sufficient volume and intensity of PA as would be expected to improve their aerobic power, that is, one hour per week of strenuous PA. Further, the men in both tertiles 2 and

3 were only average in cardiorespiratory fitness, while those in the least active tertile were below average in fitness for men of their age. Findings such as these are the basis for the current public health focus on persuading the least active (and fit) adults in the United States to perform moderate intensity PA for 30 minutes or more on a nearly daily basis.

On the other hand, some studies, such as the British Civil Servants Study[18] and a recent study in Finland by Lakka et al.,[19] suggest that only regular, high-intensity PA (i.e., >6 METs or 7.5 kcal/min or higher for an average-sized man) is required to reduce risk of CHD mortality. At least part of this controversy may be due to a PA classification problem. For example, some of the activities classified in the British Civil Servants Study[18] as high-intensity are classified by the Minnesota LTPA[1] questionnaire used in MRFIT as moderate-intensity. Furthermore, validation studies of PA survey questionnaires indicate that high-intensity activities are better remembered and more often exaggerated than are more moderate activities, such as walking, which is usually underreported.[20]

In addition, as one's cardiorespiratory fitness level progressively declines during aging, the relative intensity of an activity, as a percentage of $\dot{V}O_2$max, increases so that what was a relative moderate intensity activity in youth becomes more vigorous later in life. Thus, in middle-aged and older individuals a PA classified as moderate in terms of peak METs or energy cost may actually be quite vigorous in terms of percent of $\dot{V}O_2$max required for its performance and would have a conditioning effect in sedentary, deconditioned older individuals. Limited evidence recently reviewed by Whaley and Blair[6] also shows that sedentary middle-aged men and women who adopt a more physically active lifestyle, especially if this improves their level of physical fitness, substantially decrease their risk of CHD, CVD mortality, and age-adjusted all-cause mortality.

Biological Mechanisms for the Protective Effects of PA

Cross-sectional epidemiologic comparison of physically active or athletic people versus sedentary controls, and short-term animal and human experimental studies have identified multiple plausible biologic mechanisms, which help explain how PA and cardiorespiratory fitness reduce risk of CHD and improve survival after a heart attack. These mechanisms previously have been reviewed[21] and are briefly categorized in Table 1. Each of these apparent biologic protective mechanisms appears to have a different dose-response relationship.[10,11] In addition, there is a great deal of variability between individuals in their responses to a similar dose of exercise, as well as gender differences in some responses. Further, some of these exercise effects occur acutely during exercise and persist for hours or days following each single exercise session, that is, increases in insulin sensitivity and glucose uptake, and reductions in blood pressure and plasma triglyceride levels. Other effects result from adaptations to a sufficient volume of regular moderate intensity activity, while still others require a high enough intensity and volume of PA/exercise to improve cardiorespiratory fitness (e.g., the anti-ischemic effects).

Table 1.   Multiple Biologic Mechanisms Proposed for the Reduced Risk of Coronary Heart Disease by Regular Physical Activity

I. Anti-atherosclerotic effects
   A. Direct
   B. Indirect through attenuation of other risk factors
      1. Weight control and reduction of adiposity
      2. Blood pressure lowering
      3. Reduced plasma triglycerides and increased high density lipoprotein levels
      4. Improved cell insulin sensitivity and glucose disposal

II. Anti-thrombotic effects
   A. Reduced hemostatic factors contributing to clot formation
   B. Increased fibrinolytic activity

III. Anti-ischemic effects
   A. Reduced myocardial oxygen demands
   B. Increased myocardial oxygen supply
   C. Increased myocardial metabolic capacity and contractile function

IV. Anti-arrhythmic effect
   A. Decreased sympathoadrenalmeduallary activity during submaximal work
   B. Increased ventricular fibrillation threshold

The available epidemiologic and experimental data suggest that moderate-intensity PA acts primarily to reduce vulnerability to fatal ventricular arrhythmias and sudden death and perhaps also risk of coronary thrombosis.[22] A formal endurance exercise program sufficient to enhance and maintain cardiorespiratory fitness appears to be required to promote most of the additional biologic protective effects elucidated in Table 1. The ideal PA program would be a combination of moderate-intensity PA as part of one's daily routine and LTPA to total at least 30 to 60 minutes duration nearly every day, plus participation in a formal exercise program three to five times a week to improve aerobic power and also strength and flexibility.

Physical Activity Pyramid

Figure 1 shows The Activity Pyramid (Park Nicollet Medical Foundation, St. Louis Park, MN) analogous to the USDA's Food Guide Pyramid, which has been proposed as a model to facilitate public and patient education for adoption of a progressively more active lifestyle.[23] This pyramid reflects the stepwise weekly set of goals for promotion of PA and physical fitness, in place of time spent sitting and other sedentary activities, in order to reduce risk of CVD and other health

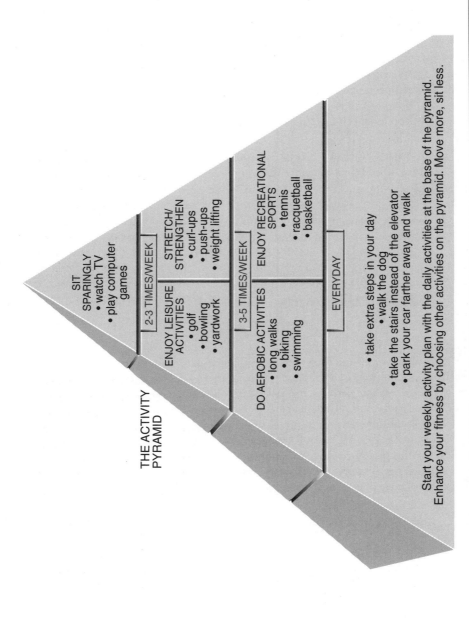

Figure 1. The Activity Pyramid.

problems related to a sedentary lifestyle. The base of the pyramid reflects the important public health goal of having sedentary people accumulate at least 30 minutes a day of moderate-intensity routine lifestyle activities. These include walking more for transportation and stair climbing. The middle panels show that the next step would be to encourage regular physically active recreational and leisure-time pursuits in place of sedentary activities. These could include yard and garden work, dancing, cycling, or swimming. The ideal next step would be to add a formal exercise program to promote physical fitness to obtain the optimal cardiovascular and general health benefits from PA.

Safety Considerations

In terms of safety of PA, it appears that both risk of orthopedic injuries and of sudden death in middle-aged people with latent coronary artery disease are closely linked primarily to high-intensity exercise or strenuous exertion, such as jogging.[11,24] A trade-off for similar health benefits may be a larger volume of moderate-intensity PA (i.e., for a longer duration and greater frequency of sessions). Moderate-intensity PA results in a lower release of catecholamines and requires lower heart rate, blood pressure, and myocardial oxygen requirements than does high-intensity PA, and is therefore less likely to precipitate a fatal ventricular arrhythmia or exceed the ischemic threshold or damage an atherosclerotic plaque initiating coronary thrombosis in middle-aged people with advanced, but asymptomatic, coronary atherosclerosis.

Recommendations

1. A controlled, randomized trial would be the ideal reference standard for testing the PA-CHD hypothesis; however, this does not appear to be feasible using CHD morbidity/mortality as end points. A unifactorial exercise trial also would be unethical, and multiple risk factor intervention with randomization to an exercise or nonexercise group would require a study too large in terms of sample size, duration, logistical difficulty, and cost to achieve funding. An alternative approach would be primary and secondary intervention trials in men and women using new markers of coronary artery disease progression, such as ultrasonography of the carotid artery as a surrogate for coronary vessels. The feasibility of such studies have already been demonstrated.
2. Additional prospective epidemiologic studies on the association of PA to CVD are needed in women (especially older women in the age group most susceptible to CHD) and in ethnic and racial minority groups. These will require better survey instruments for assessing specific gender and ethnic group preferred activities.
3. Randomized trials should be conducted in men and women, including

relevant population subgroups (i.e., older men and women, African Americans, Hispanics, Asian Americans, etc.) to better define the dose-response relationship of PA to the various risk factors and biologic mechanisms for CHD believed to be favorably impacted by PA/exercise.

4. National studies on PA and physical fitness need to be conducted on an ongoing basis, using a representative sample of Americans, including relevant population subgroups. The National Health and Nutrition Examination Survey (NHANES) could serve as the vehicle for performing such studies. The resulting data would provide normative standards and help monitor national patterns of PA and fitness, which could in turn be compared with trends in chronic diseases, including CHD.

5. A National PA/Exercise Educational/Promotion Campaign should be initiated analogous to the National Hypertension and Adult Cholesterol Screening and Education Programs.

6. More studies need to be conducted on how to motivate people of all ages and ethnic/racial origins to initiate and sustain regular PA/exercise, including determination of psychological and social factors involved, the possibility of incentive payments via reduced health and life insurance premiums, the use of work-site exercise programs, and environmental manipulations to make PA more user-friendly.

References

1. Pate RR, Pratt M, Blair SN, Haskell WL, Macera AA, Bouchard C, Buchner D, Ettinger W, Health GW, King A, Kriska A, Leon AS, Marcus BH, Morris J, Paffenbarger RS Jr, Patrick K, Pollock ML, Rippe JM, Sallis J, Wilmore JH. Physical activity and public health. A recommendation from the Centers for Disease Control and Prevention and the American College of Sports Medicine. *JAMA*, 1995;273:402-407.

2. American College of Sports Medicine. *Guidelines for Exercise Testing and Prescription. Fifth Edition.* Philadelphia: Lea & Febiger, 1995:151-176.

3. Siegel PZ, Brackbill RM, Frazier EL. Behavioral risk factor surveillance 1986-1990. *Weekly Reports*, 1991: 40 (No. 55-4): 1-23.

4. Powell KE, Thompson PA, Caspersen CJ, Kendrick JS. Physical activity and coronary heart disease. *Ann Rev Public Health*, 1987:8:253-287.

5. Berlin JA, Colditz A. A meta-analysis of physical activity in the prevention of coronary heart disease. *Am J Epidemiol*, 1990;132:612-627.

6. Whaley MH, Blair SN. Epidemiology of physical activity, physical fitness, and coronary heart disease. *Am Coll Sports Med Certified News*, 1995;5:1-7.

7. Ainsworth BE, Richardson M, Jacobs DR Jr, Leon AS. Gender differences in physical activity. *Women in Sports & Physical Activity*, 1993;2(1):1-14.

8. Hein HO, Suadicani P, Gyntelberg F. Physical fitness or physical activity as a predictor of ischaemic heart disease. A 17-year follow-up in the Copenhagen Male Study. *J Intern Med*, 1992;232:471-479.

9. Leon AS, Jacobs DR Jr, DeBacker G, Taylor HL. Relationship of physical characteristics and life habits to treadmill exercise capacity. *Am J Epidemiol*, 1981;113:653-660.

10. Haskell WL. Dose-response of physical activity and disease risk factors. In Pekka O, Telma R (Eds.): *Sport for All*. Amsterdam: Elsevier Science, 1991:125-134.

11. Haskell WL. Health consequences of physical activity: Understanding and challenges regarding dose-response. *Med Sci Sports Exercise*, 1994;26:649-660.

12. Shaper AG, Wannamethee G. Physical activity, hypertension and risk of heart attacks in men without evidence of ischaemic heart disease. *Br Heart J*, 1991;66:384-394.

13. Leon AS, Connett J, Jacobs DR Jr, Rauramaa R. Leisure-time physical activity and risk of coronary heart disease and death: The Multiple Risk Factor Intervention Trial. *JAMA*, 1987;285:2388-2395.

14. Leon AS, Connett J. Physical activity and 10.5 year mortality in the Multiple Risk Factor Intervention Trial. *Int J Epidemiol*, 1991;20:690-697.

15. Paffenbarger RS Jr, Wing AL, Hyde RT. PA as an index of heart attack risk in college alumni. *Am J Epidemiol*, 1978;108:161-175.

16. Paffenbarger RS Jr, Wing AL, Steinmetz CH. A natural history of athleticism and cardiovascular health. *JAMA*, 1984;52:491-495.

17. Paffenbarger RS Jr, Hyde RT, Wing AL, Lee I-M, Jung DL, Kampert JB. The association of changes in PA level and other lifestyle characteristics with mortality among men. *N Engl J Med*, 1993;328:538-545.

18. Morris JN, Clayton DG, Everitt M, Semmence AA, Burgess EH. Exercise in leisure time: Coronary attack and death rates. *Br Heart J*, 1990;63:325-334.

19. Lakka TA, Venalinen JM, Rauramaa R, Salonen R, Tuomilehto J, Salonen JT. Relation of leisure-time physical activity and cardiorespiratory fitness to the risk of acute myocardial infarction. *N Engl J Med*, 1994;330:1549-1554.

20. Ainsworth BE, Leon AS, Richardson MT, Jacobs DR, Paffenbarger RS Jr. Accuracy of the College Alumni Physical Activity Questionnaire. *J Clin Epidemiol*, 1993;46:1403-1411.

21. Leon AS. Physical activity and risk of ischemic heart disease—an update 1990. In Pekka O, Telma R (Eds.): *Sport for All*. Amsterdam: Elsevier Scientific, 1991:251-264.

22. Leon AS. Effects of exercise conditioning on physiological precursors of coronary heart disease. *J Cardiopulmonary Rehabil*, 1991:11:46-57.

23. Leon AS, Norstrom J. Evidence of the role of physical activity and cardiorespiratory fitness in the prevention of coronary heart disease. *Quest*, 1995:47:311-319.

24. Mittleman MA, Maclure M, Tofler GHJ, Sherwood JB, Goldberg RJ, Muller JE. Triggering of acute myocardial infarction by heavy physical exertion. Protection by regular exertion. *N Engl J Med*, 1993:329:1677-1681.

Is Vigorous Physical Activity Necessary to Reduce the Risk of Cardiovascular Disease?

I-Min Lee and Ralph S. Paffenbarger, Jr.
Harvard Medical School, Boston, Massachusetts; and Stanford University School of Medicine, Stanford, California, USA

Observational epidemiologic studies consistently have shown that persons with higher levels of physical activity experience lower risk of coronary heart disease.[1,2] While the data for stroke have been less consistent, the available evidence suggests that increased physical activity also is likely to be associated with lower risk of stroke occurrence.[3,4] Because persons who accumulate high levels of energy expenditure in physical activity tend to engage in vigorous kinds of physical activity as well, this begs the question: Is it the total *quantity* of physical activity, or is it the *intensity* of the activity carried out that is necessary for a reduced risk of cardiovascular disease?

The lack of clarity around this issue is reflected by the different recommendations that we have for physical activity. Previously, a commonly prescribed regimen advocated exercise that was vigorous enough to produce sweating or hard breathing (60%-90% of maximum heart rate), for at least 20 minutes, three times per week.[5] This recommendation was developed based on physiologic data showing that such a regimen was sufficient to induce cardiorespiratory fitness in untrained individuals. Recently, however, the US Centers for Disease Control and the American College of Sports Medicine issued a new, less formidable recommendation, stating instead that: "Every US adult should accumulate 30 minutes or more of moderate-intensity physical activity on most, preferably all, days of the week."[6] In part, this less stringent recommendation was meant to minimize barriers to physical activity among the almost 60% of US adults who engage in little or no leisure-time activity.[7]

Is one exercise recommendation more beneficial for cardiovascular health than the other? Or do the available data support both recommendations equally? In this chapter, we examine data from the few studies that have tried to disentangle the relative merits of physical activity of different intensities with respect to cardiovascular health, in an attempt to answer the question: Is vigorous physical activity necessary to reduce the risk of cardiovascular disease?

Studies of British Civil Servants

Morris and colleagues were among the first investigators to examine the relative importance of vigorous versus nonvigorous physical activity in preventing coronary heart disease (CHD). Between 1968 and 1970, they assembled a cohort of 17,944 male British civil servants who were aged 40 to 65 years and free of CHD.[8]

When these men showed up for work on a Monday morning, they were asked, without prior warning, to report their physical activities in five-minute blocks for the preceding Friday and Saturday. Investigators then categorized men as engaging in vigorous exercise (physical activities apt to require at least 7.5 kcal/min or 6 METs) or not. Investigators followed the men for an average of 8.5 years, during which 1 138 first attacks of CHD occurred. The age-standardized cumulative incidence of CHD was 3.1% among men reporting vigorous exercise, and 6.9% among those who did not. This differential was observed within strata of height, body mass index, cigarette smoking, and parental history of early cardiovascular disease death.

In a later report published in 1990, Morris et al. extended their study to another cohort of 9 376 male British civil servants who were aged 45 to 64 years and free of cardiovascular disease at study entry.[9] In the fall of 1976, these men reported on questionnaires their leisure-time physical activities during the preceding four weeks. Vigorous exercise was defined as in the earlier study, that is, any physical activity apt to require at least 7.5 kcal/min or 6 METs. Men then were classified according to the frequency of participation in vigorous and nonvigorous exercise. During follow-up that averaged 9.3 years, 474 first attacks of CHD ensued.

In age-standardized analyses, investigators observed a trend of decreasing CHD incidence rates with increasing frequency of participation in vigorous exercise. When comparing extreme groups, men who reported >8 episodes of vigorous exercise in the previous four weeks experienced an age-standardized CHD rate of 2.1 per 1,000 person-years, as contrasted to 5.8 per 1,000 person-years among those with no episodes of vigorous exercise. This contrast was seen within different strata defined by height, body mass index, cigarette smoking, and parental history of early cardiovascular disease death. However, no such trend was noted with increasing frequency of participation in nonvigorous exercise: Men reporting >12 episodes of nonvigorous exercise during the preceding four weeks experienced a CHD rate of 6.8 per 1,000 person-years, while among those reporting no episodes of nonvigorous exercise the rate was 5.4 per 1,000 person-years. Investigators further examined the relation between energy expended in nonvigorous exercise and CHD incidence. They found no association; the age-standardized CHD incidence rates did not differ among men expending <2,000, 2,000-2,999, and >3,000 kcal/week in nonvigorous exercise (5.7, 5.2, and 5.3 per 1,000 person-years, respectively).

The US Railroad Study

The relative contributions of vigorous and nonvigorous physical activity also were examined in the US Railroad Study and published by Slattery et al. in 1989.[10] Between 1957 and 1960, investigators assessed leisure-time physical activity, using the Minnesota Leisure-Time Physical Activity (LTPA) questionnaire, in 2,458 white, middle-aged men who were free of cardiovascular disease. The Minnesota

LTPA questionnaire provides a detailed list of activities (in the version used for this study, over 50 different activities were specified) and queries subjects regarding frequency and duration of participation. Based on the physical activity information provided, investigators classified men as engaging in "intense" (>6 METs) or "light-to-moderate" (<6 METs) activities. The men were followed for 17 to 20 years; during this time, 280 CHD deaths occurred. In multivariate analyses that adjusted for age, cigarette smoking, serum cholesterol, and systolic blood pressure, as well as intense activity (no, yes) and light-to-moderate activity (four levels: ≤160, 161-750, 751-1 700, >1 700 kcal/week) simultaneously, the relative risks for CHD mortality associated with intense and light-to-moderate activities were 0.75 (p = 0.034) and 0.95 (p = 0.051), respectively.

British Regional Heart Study

In 1991, Shaper et al. published their findings from an investigation of physical activity in preventing ischemic heart disease (IHD). They enrolled a cohort of 7,735 men who were aged 40 to 59 years and drawn from 24 general practices in Britain.[11] Investigators queried men regarding the frequency and duration of their participation in regular walking, cycling, recreational activity, and sporting activity. They then scored men based on these data, categorizing men into six groups labelled "inactive," "occasional," "light," "moderate," "moderately vigorous," or "vigorous." However, it is unclear whether intensity of physical activity is adequately addressed with this scheme. For example, golf may be considered a sporting activity. Thus, a man who frequently golfs would be given a high score in this study and perhaps be classified as vigorous, although golfing is not considered a vigorous activity. Over an average follow-up of eight years, 488 IHD events occurred. Among the 5,714 men who were free of IHD at baseline, the relative risks for developing IHD associated with the six activity levels were 1.0 (referent), 0.9 (95% confidence interval, 0.5-1.3), 0.9 (0.6-1.4), 0.5 (0.2-0.8), 0.5 (0.3-0.9), and 0.9 (0.5-1.8), respectively, after taking into account differences in age, cigarette smoking, body mass index, and social class.

The Multiple Risk Factor Intervention Trial

The Multiple Risk Factor Intervention Trial was a multicenter, primary-prevention trial designed to investigate whether multifactor risk intervention could reduce CHD mortality among men at high risk. Between 1973 and 1976, 12,866 men aged 35 to 57 years were enrolled into the trial. Of these, 12,138 provided physical activity information at study entry.[12,13] Leon et al. assessed physical activity in these men using the Minnesota Leisure-Time Physical Activity questionnaire; this questionnaire had been updated since the US Railroad Study and now listed 62 different activities. Investigators then calculated the time spent on the activities queried. Seventy percent of all activities reported were light or moderate, requiring <6 kcal/min. In 1991, investigators published the findings for an average follow-up of 10.5 years, during which 518 deaths from cardiovascular disease ensued. The relative risks for cardiovascular disease mortality, adjusted for age, cigarette smoking, plasma cholesterol level, diastolic blood pressure, and treatment assignment, associated with 0 to 29, 30 to 69, and 70 to 359 min/day of leisure-time physical activity were 1.00 (referent), 0.81 (0.66-1.01), and 0.89 (0.72-1.09), respectively. Because few men reported any vigorous physical activity, investigators did not separate out the time spent in vigorous and nonvigorous activities.

Study of Finnish Men

Another study to investigate the relevance of vigorous and nonvigorous physical activity was conducted by Lakka et al. between 1984 and 1989, and published in 1994.[14] Investigators enrolled a small cohort of 1,453 Finnish men who were aged 42 to 60 years and who were free of cardiovascular disease and cancer. Subjects then were followed for an average of 4.9 years. At baseline, a modified version of the Minnesota Leisure-Time Physical Activity questionnaire, including activities commonly carried out in Finland, was used to assess physical activity. Investigators divided these leisure-time physical activities into three kinds: conditioning physical activity (mean intensity, 6.0 METs), nonconditioning physical activity (3.6 METs), and walking or bicycling to work (4.0 METs). Among the 1,166 men with normal electrocardiograms at baseline, 42 experienced a first myocardial infarction during follow-up. The relative risks for myocardial infarction associated with <0.7, 0.7-2.2, and >2.2 hr/week of conditioning physical activity were 1.0 (referent), 1.19 (0.61-2.31), and 0.34 (0.12-0.94), respectively, after adjusting for multiple potential confounders including age, cigarette smoking, history of diabetes mellitus, and family history of coronary heart disease. However, increasing time spent either on nonconditioning physical activity, or walking or bicycling to work was not associated with significantly lower risk of myocardial infarction.

The Harvard Alumni Health Study

We recently examined the associations of vigorous ($\geq$6 METs) and nonvigorous (<6 METs) physical activity with all-cause mortality in the Harvard Alumni Health Study.[15] Only vigorous but not nonvigorous physical activity predicted lower all-cause mortality rates. Further, the inverse trend observed across categories of vigorous energy expenditure differed significantly from the trend across categories of nonvigorous energy expenditure.

Here, we include observations that are specific for CHD mortality (unpublished). Briefly, 17,321 men who were aged 30 to 79 years and free of cardiovascular disease, cancer, and chronic obstructive pulmonary disease, provided information, via questionnaires, on walking, stair climbing, and participation in sports or recreational activities. Men reported their physical activity twice: once in either 1962 or

1966 (1962/1966) and again in 1977. At each time, we estimated the energy expended in vigorous and nonvigorous physical activity, separately, using the cutpoint of >6 METs to define vigorous activity. (Because we did not ascertain walking speed, all walking was deemed nonvigorous.) Men were followed from 1962/1966 through 1988 for mortality. In multivariate analyses, we used physical activity assessed initially in 1962/1966 and updated in 1977, and adjusted for age, cigarette smoking, body mass index, hypertension, diabetes mellitus, and early parental death (Table 1). These analyses also mutually adjusted for vigorous and nonvigorous energy expenditure. In order to minimize potential bias from men who may have decreased their physical activity level because of preclinical illness, we excluded the first five years of follow-up after either activity assessment. With increasing energy expended in vigorous physical activity, CHD mortality rates declined (p, trend = 0.02). For nonvigorous energy expenditure, no such trend was apparent (p, trend = 0.24). The relative risk estimates for the two kinds of energy expenditure, however, did not differ significantly from one another (e.g., when comparing >1,500 with <150 kcal/week, the relative risk estimate of 0.68 for vigorous energy expenditure was not significantly different from 0.89, the relative risk estimate for nonvigorous energy expenditure).

Discussion

Data regarding the relative merits of vigorous and nonvigorous physical activity for cardiovascular health have been sparse, with only seven studies attempting to address this issue. Of these, the British Regional Heart Study did not adequately separate out physical activity by intensity alone, as investigators classified subjects using a composite scheme based on frequency, duration, and intensity of physical activity. In the Multiple Risk Factor Intervention Trial, because few men reported any vigorous physical activity, investigators did not examine the separate relations of vigorous and nonvigorous physical activity with cardiovascular disease risk. Of the remaining five studies, the two studies of British civil servants, the study of Finnish men, and the Harvard Alumni Health Study all observed that vigorous but not nonvigorous physical activity predicted lower risk of this disease. In the last study, the US Railroad Study, vigorous physical activity significantly predicted lower risk of cardiovascular disease, while the association with light-to-moderate physical activity was of borderline significance.

   It is conceivable that only vigorous physical activity is associated with lower cardiovascular disease risk, since such kinds of activity are more efficient for inducing physical fitness, and other studies have shown that physical fitness independently predicts lower cardiovascular disease risk.[16] However, before we conclude that vigorous physical activity is necessary to reduce the risk of this disease, several issues need consideration. First, because vigorous kinds of physical activity tend to be carried out on a routine basis (e.g., running), such kinds of activity may be recalled more precisely than other nonvigorous activities (e.g., miscella-

Table 1. Relative Risks of Coronary Heart Disease (CHD) Mortality Among Harvard Alumni, 1962 or 1966 Through 1988, According to Vigorous and Nonvigorous Physical Activity, Assessed in 1962/1966 and Updated in 1977*

Kind of activity	Energy expenditure (kcal/week)					p, trend
	<150	150-399	400-749	750-1,499	≥1,500	
Vigorous activity						
No. of CHD deaths	180	151	52	41	41	
RR	1.00	0.94	0.77	0.89	0.68	0.02
95% confidence interval	referent	0.76-1.17	0.56-1.06	0.63-1.26	0.48-0.96	
Nonvigorous activity						
No. of CHD deaths	56	89	95	110	115	
RR	1.00	1.15	1.10	1.12	0.89	0.24
95% confidence interval	referent	0.82-1.61	0.79-1.53	0.81-1.54	0.64-1.23	

* The first five years of follow-up after either physical activity assessment is discarded. Relative risks are adjusted for age, cigarette smoking, body mass index, hypertension, diabetes mellitus, and early parental death. Relative risks for vigorous and nonvigorous energy expenditure are mutually adjusted. Vigorous activities are those requiring ≥6 MET; nonvigorous activities, those requiring <6 METs.

neous chores around the home and yard). Thus, the imprecision with which nonvigorous physical activity may have been assessed in the above studies could have obscured a true inverse relation between nonvigorous activity and cardiovascular disease risk.

Second, the studies generally used 6 METs (as is conventional[17]) to dichotomize physical activities into those considered vigorous versus those considered nonvigorous. In the recent physical activity recommendation from the US Centers for Disease Control and the American College of Sports Medicine, moderate-intensity physical activity—requiring between 3 or 4 METs and 6 METs—was encouraged. There are no epidemiologic data specifically examining whether physical activities within this range of intensity is predictive of decreased cardiovascular disease risk, although other studies clearly have shown that such physical activity can improve intermediate variables associated with cardiovascular health, such as blood lipoprotein profile,[18] blood pressure,[19] and glucose tolerance.[20]

A further issue to consider is whether there are risks associated with vigorous physical activity. Mittleman et al.[21] and Willich et al.[22] have shown that physical activity of intensity >6 METs can trigger the onset of an acute myocardial infarction, with the likelihood of such an occurrence being far greater among those habitually inactive. In the former study, among the most inactive (i.e., reporting physical activity of >6 METs less than once a week), the risk of developing myocardial infarction in the hour after vigorous activity, as compared with the hour after nonvigorous activity, was 107 times greater. However, among those active (physical activity of >6 METs at least five times per week), the relative risk was 2.4. These two studies suggest that discrete episodes of physical exertion can increase the short-term risk of myocardial infarction; however, over the long term, habitual physical activity is associated with a decreased risk of coronary events.[1,2]

Conclusion and Recommendations

In conclusion, based on the available data, it remains unclear whether it is the total quantity or the intensity of physical activity that is important for a reduced risk of cardiovascular disease. Where vigorous, but not nonvigorous, physical activity has been shown to be associated with reduced cardiovascular risk in previous studies, this may have resulted from imprecise assessment of the latter kinds of activities. For the purpose of future research, methods of physical activity assessment that utilize a list of physical activities probably are less susceptible to such imprecise assessment. Additionally, studies that separate out physical activities by three different intensity levels—light, moderate, or vigorous—in order to examine their separate relations with cardiovascular disease are needed, since current physical activity recommendations emphasize moderate intensity activity. Finally, no data among women and specifically among minorities are available; this shortcoming has to be addressed.

References

1. Powell, KE, PD Thompson, CJ Caspersen, & JS Kendrick. Physical activity and the incidence of coronary heart disease. *Ann Rev Public Health*. 8:253-87, 1987.

2. Berlin, JA & GA Colditz. A meta-analysis of physical activity in the prevention of coronary heart disease. *Am J Epidemiol*. 132:612-28, 1990.

3. Kohl, HW III & JD McKenzie. Physical activity, fitness, and stroke. In Bouchard, C, RJ Shephard, T Stephens, eds.: *Physical activity, fitness, and health: International proceedings and consensus statement*. Champaign, IL: Human Kinetics, pp. 609-21, 1994.

4. Bronner, LL, DS Kanter, & JE Manson. Primary prevention of stroke. *N Engl J Med*. 333:1392-1400, 1995.

5. American College of Sports Medicine. *Guidelines for graded exercise testing and exercise prescription*. 3d ed. Philadelphia: Lea & Febiger, 1985.

6. Pate, RR, M Pratt, SN Blair et al. Physical activity and public health: A recommendation from the Centers for Disease Control and Prevention and the American College of Sports Medicine. *JAMA*. 273:402-7, 1995.

7. Siegel, PZ, RM Brackbill, EL Frazier et al. Behavioral Risk Factor Surveillance, 1986-1990. *MMWR*. 40(no. SS-4):1-23, 1991.

8. Morris, JN, MG Everitt, R Pollard, SPW Chave, & AM Semmence. Vigorous exercise in leisure-time: Protection against coronary heart disease. *Lancet*. 2:1207-10, 1980.

9. Morris, JN, DG Clayton, MG Everitt, AM Semmence, & EH Burgess. Exercise in leisure-time: Coronary attack and death rates. *Br Heart J*. 63:325-34, 1990.

10. Slattery, ML, DR Jacobs Jr, & MZ Nichaman. Leisure time physical activity and coronary heart disease death: The US Railroad Study. *Circulation*. 79:304-11, 1989.

11. Shaper, AG, G Wannamethee, & R Weatherall. Physical activity and ischaemic heart disease in middle-aged British men. *Br Heart J*. 66:384-94, 1991.

12. Leon, AS, J Connett, DR Jacobs, & R Rauramaa. Leisure-time physical activity levels and risk of coronary heart disease and death: The Multiple Risk Factor Intervention Trial. *JAMA*. 258:2388-95, 1987.

13. Leon, AS & J Connett for the MRFIT research group. Physical activity and 10.5 year mortality in the Multiple Risk Factor Intervention Trial (MRFIT). *Int J Epidemiol*. 20:690-7, 1991.

14. Lakka, TA, JM Venalainen, R Rauramaa, R Salonen, J Tuomilehto, & JT Salonen. Relation of leisure-time physical activity and cardiorespiratory fitness to the risk of acute myocardial infarction in men. *N Engl J Med*. 330:1549-54, 1994.

15. Lee, I-M, C-C Hsieh, & RS Paffenbarger Jr. Exercise intensity and longevity in men: The Harvard Alumni Health Study. *JAMA*. 273:1179-84, 1995.

16. Blair, SN, HW Kohl III, RS Paffenbarger Jr, DG Clark, KH Cooper, & LW Gibbons. Physical fitness and all-cause mortality: A prospective study of healthy men and women. *JAMA*. 262:2395-401, 1989.

17. Taylor, HL, DR Jacobs Jr, B Schucker, J Knudsen, AS Leon, & G Debacker. A questionnaire for the assessment of leisure time physical activities. *J Chron Dis*. 31:741-55, 1978.

18. Hagberg, JM. Exercise, fitness, and hypertension. In Bouchard, C, RJ Shephard, T Stephens, JR Sutton, & BD McPherson (eds): *Exercise, fitness, and health: A consensus of current knowledge*. Champaign, IL: Human Kinetics, pp. 455-66, 1990.

19. King, AC, WL Haskell, DR Young, RK Oka, & ML Stefanick. Long-term effects of varying intensities and formats of physical activity on participation rates, fitness, and lipoproteins in men and women aged 50 to 65 years. *Circulation*. 91:2596-604, 1995.

20. Horton, ES. Exercise and diabetes mellitus. *Med Clin North Am*. 72:1301-21, 1988.

21. Mittleman, MA, M Maclure, GH Tofler, JB Sherwood, RJ Goldberg, & JE Muller. Triggering of acute myocardial infarction by heavy physical exertion: Protection against triggering by regular exertion. *N Engl J Med*. 329:1677-83, 1993.

22. Willich, SN, M Lewis, H Löwel, H-R Arntz, F Schubert, & R Schröder. Physical exertion as a trigger of acute myocardial infarction. *N Engl J Med*. 329:1684-90, 1993.

Physiological Responses to Structured Versus Lifestyle Activities

Roy J. Shephard
University of Toronto, Toronto, Ontario, Canada

A variety of data[1,2] now suggest that the largest improvement in cardiovascular health is associated with progression from the lowest to the next lowest level of fitness. This, in turn, has encouraged the hope that public health might be enhanced by encouraging everyday lifestyle activities such as walking, cycling, and gardening rather than enrollment in costly, structured programs of aerobic exercise.

The present chapter thus examines the physiological effectiveness of lifestyle versus structured exercise, leaving to other contributors such issues as relative costs, recruitment, and adherence patterns. Several questions may be posed from the physiological standpoint:

1. Is an active lifestyle favorably correlated with health-related variables? If so, can issues of selection be excluded by longitudinal experiments?
2. How much physical activity is needed to achieve the desired health benefits? Are there differences in the required dose between different types of physical activity, or between population groups?
3. How much physical activity can be generated by occupation or by the encouragement of an active lifestyle?
4. How do gains in cardiovascular health compare between lifestyle activities and structured exercise programs?

An Active Lifestyle and Cardiovascular Health

Occupational studies have, almost without exception, shown an association between physically demanding employment and protection against ischemic heart disease.[3] However, employment in heavy manual work commonly depends on physique, selection being made by either the individual or management.[4] Brunner and Manelis[5] argued that there was little choice of duties in an Israeli Kibbutzim, but even in such a situation it is difficult to believe that physique did not influence the allocation of duties.

The association between cardiovascular health and self-reported patterns of leisure activity can be illustrated (Figure 1) by some recent data from Quebec.[6] We questioned subjects about the frequency in which they engaged in demanding activity, the intensity of their active leisure pursuits, their perceived level of fitness, and their perceived level of physical activity relative to their peers. On each of

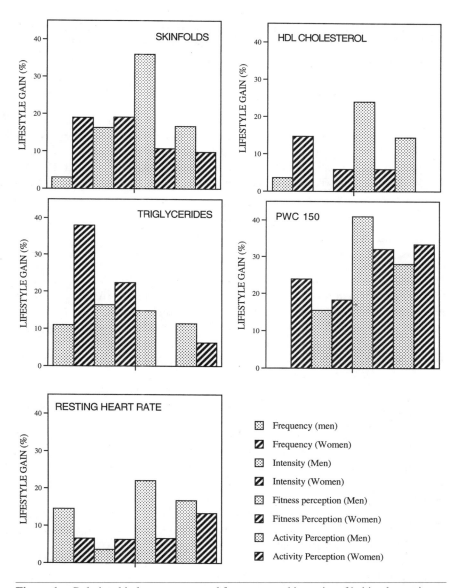

Figure 1.   Relationship between reported frequency and intensity of habitual exercise, perceived fitness, and perceived habitual activity and fitness variables. All data expressed as percent difference between most active and least active group. Based on data of Shephard and Bouchard[6] for healthy adults.

these measures, there were substantial difference of skinfold thickness, HDL cholesterol, serum triglycerides, physical work capacity at a heart rate of 150 beats per minute (PWC 150), and resting heart rate between the least active and the most active quartiles of our sample; indeed, differences were larger than would have been anticipated with most structured exercise programs. However, the problem remains that participation in leisure activities was self-selected.

Longitudinal experiments[7] (Blair and associates, personal communication) are somewhat less vulnerable to selection effects, although the results can still be distorted by a high drop-out rate of unfit subjects from the experimental group, and/or a defection of fit individuals from the control group. Oja et al.[7] found a 3% increase of aerobic power in those assigned to an active commuting program, as compared with a 1% decrease in controls.

Required Amount of Physical Activity

A review of occupational studies suggested that cardiovascular health was enhanced if job demands increased energy expenditures by 1.6 to 3.6 MJ or 400-900 kcal per day.[8] If distributed over an entire working day, such activity would boost energy expenditures by 4 to 8 kJ/min, 1 to 2 kcal/min. In some jobs, periods of relatively high intensity effort are interspersed with rest, but in other occupations conducive to good cardiovascular health (for example, postal carrier), the benefit is associated with several hours per day of moderate activity (gross intensities of 20 kJ/min, 5 kcal/min or less).

A higher intensity of active leisure might be needed to enhance cardiovascular health, because most leisure pursuits are of relatively short duration. Traditionally, physiologists have called for an intensity of effort near the ventilatory threshold, 60% to 70% of peak aerobic power. However, recent research has suggested that cardiovascular health is improved at much lower intensities of effort, possibly without any increase in aerobic power.[1] Blair[2] plotted fitness or physical activity in relation to mortality in five major prospective studies. With the exception of the Morris study,[4] the gain in prognosis was greatest on moving from the lowest to the next highest activity or fitness category. If the intensity of exercise was increased further, benefit soon plateaued, and the added health derived from such intense effort was disappointingly small.

Benefit seemed greater in studies where changes in aerobic fitness were measured. This could reflect a need to increase aerobic fitness, but it could also be because changes in fitness were measured more precisely than changes in physical activity. These observations led the American College of Sports Medicine (ACSM) to reduce the minimum recommended intensity of an aerobic exercise prescription to 50% of maximal oxygen intake, practiced for one hour three to five times per week,[1] and the NIH Consensus Conference on Physical Activity and Cardiovascular Health of December 1995 to advocate 30 minutes of moderate intensity activity such as brisk walking on most, and preferably all, days of the week. In an average, 75-kg, middle-aged man with an aerobic power of 35 ml/(kg · min), the new standard implies a gross energy expenditure of 5 METs, 27 kJ/min or 6.5 kcal/min, although in an elderly or unfit individual, the minimum intensity could drop to around 3.5 METs, 19 kJ/min, or 4.5 kcal/min.

Energy Costs of an Active Lifestyle

Even the new minimum intensity of exercise is fairly demanding, relative to the energy cost of many common leisure pursuits. The most frequently reported activity is walking. Making the charitable assumption that the average pace is 4.8 km/h (3 mph), the gross energy cost is 3.5 METs, or around 19 kJ/min, 4.6 kcal/min in a man of 75 kg.[9-11] This would meet the new ACSM prescriptive standard for the elderly,[1] but not for the young or the middle-aged. In order to attain the 5 MET standard, a person would need to engage in jogging, race walking, or walking uphill with a load. Cycling at 16 km/h (10 mph) has a net cost of 29 kJ/min, and other activities of adequate intensity are skiing at 4.0 km/h, swimming at 25 meters/min, walking up stairs, the heaviest forms of gardening, sawing hardwood, and chopping wood.[9,12] However, the majority of recreational activities and domestic chores fall below the theoretical requirement.

Duncan et al.[13] compared the physiological effects of strolling at 4.8 km/h, brisk walking at 6.4 km/h, and aerobic walking at 8 km/h. The subjects, women aged 20 to 40 years, were followed for 24 weeks. Gains of aerobic power increased with walking speed, but the decreases in body fat and total cholesterol were as large with moderate as with brisk exercise (Figure 2). Likewise, Hopkins et al.[14] found that in adult New Zealanders, hard activity (as assessed by either the CORE or the Stanford questionnaire) was correlated with aerobic power, a decrease of skinfolds, vital capacity, and protection against exercise-induced myocardial ischemia; however, there was no improvement of health-related variables with low-intensity activity (Figure 3). DiPietro et al.[15] found that in adults aged 60 to 86 years, vigorous leisure activity was correlated with aerobic power; however, leisure walking and total leisure activity showed a modest correlation with body fat, but not with aerobic power (Figure 4).

Can commuting generate the sense of urgency needed to reach an appropriate intensity of walking or cycling? Oja et al.[7] asked a small group of middle-aged Tampere citizens who normally drove to work to adopt either walking or cycling for a 10-week trial. Commuting demanded 30 minutes or more of physical activity in each direction every working day. The pace chosen by the cyclists corresponded to an oxygen consumption of 23 to 24 ml/(kg · min), 65% to 70% of aerobic power. The walking speed (5.7 km/h) was relatively brisk, but commanded an oxygen consumption of only 13 ml/(kg · min), about 37% of aerobic power. The average heart rates were 131 and 121 beats/min, respectively, corresponding to 65% and 55% of aerobic power. Presumably, the heart rates of the walkers were augmented by a combination of heat, hills, and the carrying of a briefcase. Habitual walkers

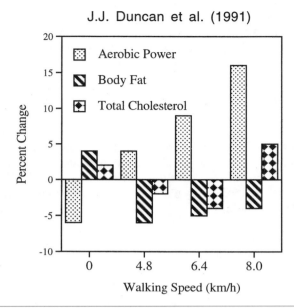

Figure 2.   Changes in aerobic power, body fat, and total cholesterol; response to three different walking speeds compared with control findings. Based on data of Duncan et al.[13]

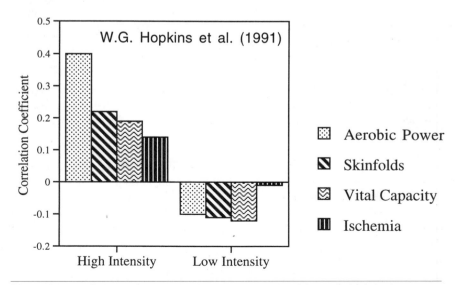

Figure 3.   Coefficients of correlation between reported activity and physiologic variables; findings for measures of high-intensity and low-intensity activity. Based on data of Hopkins et al. [14]

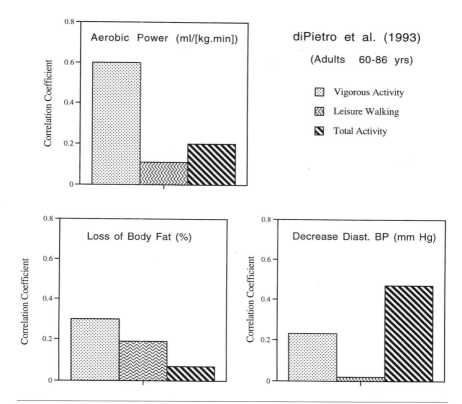

Figure 4.   Correlations of vigorous physical activity, leisure walking, and total reported physical activity with physiological measures in subjects aged 60-86 years. Based on data of DiPietro et al. [15]

may adopt a somewhat higher speed; Spelman et al.[16] found an average of 6.4 km/h (52% of aerobic power) in 22 women and 7 men with a mean age of 35 years ± 9 SD.

Comparison of Structured and Unstructured Programs

The Behavioral Risk Factor Surveillance System Survey of 1989 provides data on the effectiveness of various types of activity in subjects who were attempting to lose weight.[17] Unfortunately, data on structured aerobics programs were included only for women. The loss of weight from running was as great, and that from cycling was almost as great, as that for the aerobics program; however, walking and gardening induced weight loss only in older members of the group (Figure 5).

Industrial fitness programs are a second potential source of information on structured programs (Figure 6). Unfortunately, most studies have included interventions other than exercise, and many have been uncontrolled, focusing on the ben-

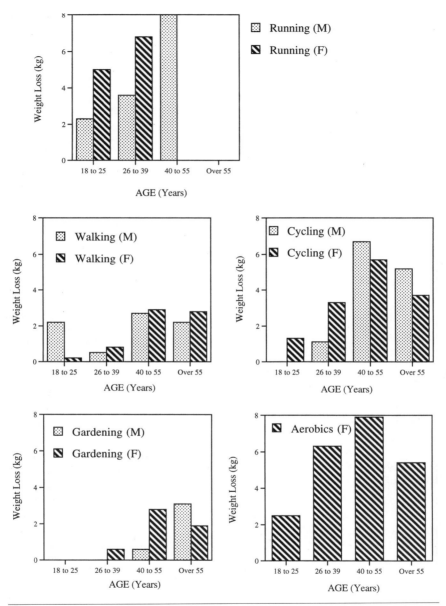

Figure 5.   Weight loss achieved by subjects desiring to decrease their body mass in relation to the type of activity undertaken. Based on the data of DiPietro et al. [17]

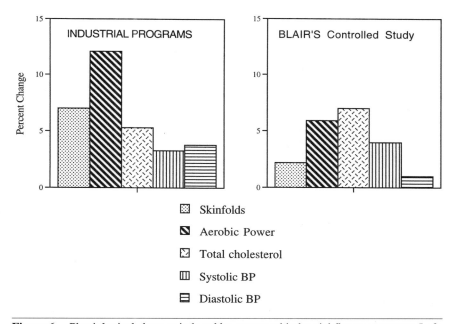

Skinfolds

Aerobic Power

Total cholesterol

Systolic BP

Diastolic BP

Figure 6. Physiological changes induced by structured industrial fitness programs. Left panel, average response; right panel, difference between experimental and control work sites in study of Blair et al. [18]

efits seen in small residues of high adherents. Perhaps the best of such studies[18] suggested that the likely impact of such a program was a 2% decrease in body fat, a 6% increase of aerobic power, a 7% decrease in serum cholesterol, a 4 mmHg decrease of systolic, and a 1 mmHg decrease of diastolic blood pressure. Such benefits are smaller than those seen with self-selection of an active lifestyle, but at least in terms of aerobic power are somewhat greater than can be achieved by walking or cycling to work. King et al.[19] compared a structured versus a supervised home-based program in women and men aged 50 through 65 years; over a one-year period, adherence was better for home-based than for structured exercise, and perhaps for this reason the women achieved larger gains of aerobic power with the home-based program. Changes of body mass and lipids were not significant for either group (Figure 7).

Are these conclusions modified by age, gender, or ethnic group? The primary determinant of response is initial fitness: To the extent that the elderly, women, and minority groups have a low level of fitness, they will show greater susceptibility to benefit from light activities, whether structured or unstructured. Against this potential advantage, there are age, gender, and ethnic-group related differences in the manner of participation in both structured and unstructured activities; for example, a young person will, on average, walk or cycle at a higher speed than an older adult. The Behavioral Risk Factor Surveillance System Survey data[15,17] fur-

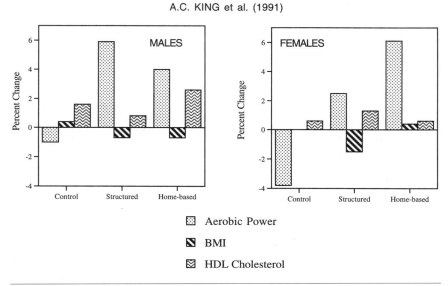

Figure 7.   Percentage changes in physiological variables in response to structured and home-based programs compared with control findings. Based on data of King et al. [19]

ther suggests that unstructured activities are on the increase in women and in the elderly, but are decreasing in the poorly educated and minority groups.[20,21]

Areas for Further Research

1. Suggestions that structured programs may have a greater effect upon cardio-vascular health than do unstructured leisure activity require further testing by a well-designed and sustained prospective trial.
2. Further information is needed on how responses to unstructured activity differ among young men, women, older adults, and children.

References

1. American College of Sports Medicine. The recommended quantity and quality of exercise for developing and maintaining fitness in healthy adults. *Med Sci Sports Exercise*, 1991; 22:265-274.

2. Blair SN. Physical activity, fitness and coronary heart disease. In C Bouchard, RJ Shephard, T Stephens (Eds.): *Physical Activity, Fitness and Health*, Champaign, IL: Human Kinetics, 1994; 579-590.

3. Powell KE, PD Thompson, CJ Caspersen, JS Kendrick. Physical activity and the incidence of coronary heart disease. *Ann Rev Public Health: International Proceedings and Concensus Statement.* 1987; 8:253-287.

4. Morris JN, J Heady, P Raffle. Physique of London busmen. *Lancet*, 1956; (ii):569-570.

5. Brunner D, G Manelis. Physical activity at work and ischemic heart disease. In OA Larsen & RO Malmborg (Eds.): *Coronary Heart Disease and Physical Fitness*. Baltimore: University Park Press, 1971.

6. Shephard RJ, C Bouchard. Population evaluations of health related fitness from perceptions of physical activity and fitness. *Can J Appl Physiol*, 1994; 19:151-173.

7. Oja P, A Mänttäri, R Nieminen, K Kukkonen-Harjular, I Vuori, M Pasanen. Effects of walking and cycling to and from work on physical fitness. In: *International Conference on Exercise, Fitness and Health*. Toronto: Ontario Ministry of Culture and Recreation, 1988: Poster Session.

8. Fox SM, JS Skinner. Physical activity and cardiovascular health. *Am J Cardiol*, 1964; 14:731-746.

9. Ainsworth BE, WL Haskell, AS Leon et al. Compendium of physical activities: Classification of energy costs of human activities. *Med Sci Sports Exercise*, 1993; 25:71-80.

10. Goodman J, L Goodman. Exercise prescription for the sedentary adult. In P Welsh, RJ Shephard (Eds.), *Current Therapy in Sports Medicine 1985-1986*. Burlington, ON: BC Decker, 1985; 17-23.

11. Mahadeva K, R Passmore, B Woolf. Individual variations in the metabolic cost of standardized exercises: The effects of food, age, sex and race. *J Physiol*, 1953; 121:225-231.

12. Wynder EL. *The Book of Health. American Health Foundation*. New York: Franklin Watts, 1981.

13. Duncan JJ, NF Gordon, CB Scott. Women walking for health and fitness: How much is enough? *JAMA*, 1991; 266:3295-3299.

14. Hopkins WG, NC Wilson, DG Russell. Validation of the physical activity instrument for the life in New Zealand National Survey. *Am J Epidemiol*, 1991; 133:73-82.

15. DiPietro L, CJ Caspersen, A Ostfeld et al. A survey for assessing physical activity among older adults. *Med Sci Sports Exercise*, 1993; 25:628-642.

16. Spelman CC, RR Pate, CA Macera et al. Self-selected exercise intensity of habitual walkers. *Med Sci Sports Exercise*, 1993; 25:1174-1179.

17. DiPietro L, DF Williamson, CJ Caspersen et al.The descriptive epidemiology of selected physical activities and body weight among adults trying to lose weight: The Behavioral Risk Factor Surveillance System Survey, 1989. *Int J Obesity*, 1993; 17:69-76.

18. Blair SN, PV Piserchia, CS Wilbur et al. A public health intervention model for work site health promotion: Impact on exercise and physical fitness in a health promotion plan after 24 months. *JAMA*, 1986; 255:921-926.

19. King A, WL Haskell, B Taylor et al. Group- vs home-based exercise training in healthy older men and women. A community-based clinical trial. *JAMA*, 1991; 266:1535-1542.

20. Caspersen CJ, RK Merrit. Physical activity trends among 26 states, 1986-1990. *Med Sci Sports Exercise*, 1995; 27:713-720.

21. Heath GW, JD Smith. Physical activity patterns among adults in Georgia: Results from the 1990 Behavioral Risk Factor Surveillance System. *Southern Med J*, 1994; 87:435-440.

Part IV

PHYSICAL ACTIVITY IN THE PREVENTION OF CARDIOVASCULAR DISEASE AND OTHER CVD RISK FACTORS

Physical Activity, Body Weight, and Body Fat Distribution

James O. Hill
University of Colorado Health Sciences Center, Denver, Colorado, USA

Physical activity may affect the risk of cardiovascular disease (CVD) directly or indirectly via its effects on the amount and location of body fat. Excess body fat (i.e., obesity), particularly if located in the intra-abdominal region, carries increased risk for diabetes and CVD.[1] While researchers recognize that both dietary patterns and level of physical activity influence body weight, there is still a lack of consensus about the importance of physical activity in prevention and treatment of obesity. This has led to inconsistent recommendations to the public about how to use physical activity to prevent or reduce obesity.

This chapter will address the role of physical activity in body weight regulation. Other chapters in this book will address the nature of the link between body fatness and CVD. In particular, I will discuss physical activity in the theoretical framework of energy balance, the relationship between physical activity and body fatness, and how physical activity impacts upon weight loss in the overweight.

Physical Activity in the Theoretical Framework of Energy Balance

An individual maintaining a constant body weight and body composition must be in a steady-state where the amount of total energy ingested is equal to the amount of total energy expended. In addition, over some period of time, the composition of the energy ingested must equal the composition of substrate oxidized.[2] Conditions necessary for energy and nutrient balance are illustrated in Figure 1. Any disruption of energy and nutrient balance elicits compensatory responses to restore these balances. Physical activity directly affects the right side of Figure 1.

There are clear theoretical reasons why level of physical activity should be important in body weight regulation. First, physical activity is a major factor determining total level of energy expenditure. Increases in physical activity will increase total energy expenditure, and decreases in physical activity will reduce total energy expenditure. Unless such changes are accompanied by compensatory changes in energy intake, body weight will change.

Physical activity is also a major determinant of fat balance, and obesity is a result of positive fat balance. Protein and carbohydrate balances appear to be well-maintained acutely, even following challenges to body weight regulation (e.g., diet and exercise alterations). Fat oxidation and intake, however, are not acutely responsive to changes in each other. Because total fat oxidation varies directly

$$E_{IN} = E_{EXPEND}$$

$$PRO_{IN} = PRO_{OX}$$

$$CHO_{IN} = CHO_{OX}$$

$$FAT_{IN} = FAT_{OX}$$

Figure 1.   Energy and nutrient balance.

with body fat mass,[3] increases or decreases in the body fat mass may be required to reestablish fat balance. Changes in physical activity provide another means of altering fat oxidation, so that the higher one's level of physical activity, the less body fat mass is required to maintain fat balance at any given fat intake. Similarly, increasing physical activity without a change in fat intake will increase fat oxidation above fat intake and produce negative fat balance and loss of body fat mass.

The Relationship Between Physical Activity and Body Fatness

In this section, evidence for a link between physical activity and the amount and location of body fat will be examined. Particular attention will be given to characteristics of the physical activity that may be important for body weight regulation.

Is a Low Level of Physical Activity a Risk Factor for Development of Obesity?

The recent report from NHANES III shows that the prevalence of obesity has increased over the past eight years in US adults from about 25% to 33%.[4] A similar increase in pediatric obesity was also found.[5] A reduction in physical activity is certainly one factor that could have contributed to the increased prevalence of obesity.

Negative relationships between measures of physical activity (usually self-reports) and indices of obesity (usually body mass index [BMI]) are seen in most data sets obtained from the general US population.[6,7] The relationship appears to be similar in men and women, and across all ages.[8-11] Further, there is evidence for a similar relationship in African Americans,[12] Hispanics,[13] and Native Americans.[14]

While BMI is a reproducible measure, self-reports of physical activity have been criticized as potentially unreliable. At least two studies using doubly labeled water to measure the energy expended in physical activity have shown a significant negative relationship between physical activity and BMI.[15,16]

Further, studies in which subjects are followed over time suggest that changes in physical activity are associated with changes in body fatness. This can be illustrated in the three studies shown in Table 1. In each study, self-reported physical activity and BMI were recorded at baseline and at follow-up (2-10 years later). In all studies, the level of physical activity was negatively related to BMI at baseline, and level of physical activity at follow-up was negatively related to change in BMI from baseline to follow-up. In two of the three studies, the level of physical activity at baseline was negatively related to change in BMI from baseline to follow-up. Finally, all studies suggest a negative relationship between change in level of physical activity and change in BMI.

Does Type of Physical Activity Relate to BMI?

It is not clear which characteristics of physical activity influence body weight regulation. In most of the studies discussed above, the self-reports of physical activity capture total dose of physical activity. There is scant data about how other characteristics of physical activity, such as type, intensity, duration, and frequency, affect body weight regulation independently of total dose of physical activity.

Both aerobic and resistance exercise have been used successfully in weight reduction programs, and although the latter may preserve or increase fat-free mass, both seem to reduce body fat similarly when total dose of activity is considered.[17] Further, a variety of aerobic activities have been successfully used in weight-reduction studies.[18]

While moderate-intensity exercise uses proportionally more fat than does high-intensity, there is some suggestion that exercise of greater intensity is associated with lower BMI than is exercise of moderate intensity.[19] It should be realized that moderate-intensity aerobic exercise must be performed for a longer period of time to produce as much fat oxidation as would high-intensity aerobic exercise. It is not possible with the available data to conclusively separate effects of intensity from effects of total amount of physical activity.

A great deal of new information suggests that short bouts of activity may be just as effective for body weight regulation as would longer bouts. Jakicic et al.[20] demonstrated similar weight loss in overweight subjects given an exercise program consisting of the same dose of activity either as 30-minute or 10-minute bouts of exercise.

Little data are available regarding how frequency of physical activity impacts upon body weight regulation. Most experts recommend that people exercise 3 to 5 days per week, and while such recommendations are reasonable, we have no data at present to allow determination of optimum frequency of exercise for body weight regulation.

Finally, many obesity experts are recommending decreases in sedentary activities and increases in lifestyle activities in addition to increases in planned exercise. Many Americans spend a great deal of time in sedentary activities, such as sitting at a desk and watching television, where energy expenditure is very low. By reducing time spent in sedentary activity (even without specifying a specific alternative), total energy expenditure can be increased. Epstein[21] has shown the effectiveness of such a strategy on weight loss and maintenance in children. Total energy

Table 1. Are Changes in Physical Activity Associated With Changes in BMI?

	Healthy Worker study French et al.[11] (2 years)	Healthy Women study Owens et al.[10] (3 years)	NHANES I Follow-up study Williamson et al.[7] (10 years)
Baseline physical activity negatively related to BMI	Yes	Yes	Yes
Baseline physical activity negatively related to change in BMI	Yes	Yes	No
Follow-up physical activity negatively related to change in BMI	Yes	Yes	Yes
Change in physical activity negatively related to change in BMI	Yes	Yes	Small effect

expenditure can also be greatly increased by increasing lifestyle activities, such as taking the stairs and parking farther away from one's destination.

Physical Activity and Body Fat Distribution

Only a few studies have examined the relationship between physical activity and body fat distribution (usually assessed as waist-to-hip ratio [WHR]). The CARDIA study[12] found a negative relationship between levels of physical activity and WHR in African American men and women and in Caucasian men. The relationship was not found in Caucasian women. Physical activity was negatively related with WHR and to waist circumference in the European Fat Distribution Study.[22] Few studies have examined this relationship, and much more information is needed. It may be that visceral adipose tissue is preferentially lost during negative energy balance, regardless of how it is produced. Alternatively, negative energy balance produced by physical activity may lead to preferential reduction in visceral adipose tissue as compared to negative energy balance produced by energy restriction.

Do Changes in Physical Activity Lead to Changes in Body Fatness in the Overweight?

In this section, we will consider how increases in physical activity can impact upon overall fatness. In particular, we will consider how physical activity can affect amount of weight loss, composition of weight loss, change in body fat distribution, and maintenance of weight loss.

Substantial weight loss can be produced by exercise alone. This is illustrated in the study by Lee et al.[23] where overweight men were drafted into the Singapore army and subjected to 20 weeks of supervised vigorous exercise. The average loss of body weight in this study was 12.5 kg in 20 weeks. Subjects were free to consume as much food as they desired. While this study represents an extreme physical activity program, it does illustrate that physical activity alone can produce weight loss. Less-intense physical activity programs will produce slower weight loss and may require much longer time periods to observe significant changes in body weight.

Increases in physical activity will increase the right side of the energy balance equation shown in Figure 1. This will produce negative energy balance, negative fat balance, and weight loss unless subjects increase the left side of the equation (i.e., energy intake). While we can accurately estimate the effects of a given increase in physical activity on energy expenditure, we know little about effects of such changes on energy intake. Thus, we still do not have a good ability to predict the effects of a given increase in physical activity on weight loss. Table 2 illustrates some estimated effects of increasing physical activity on body weight, depending on how the increase in physical activity affects energy intake.

Studies from Wood and colleagues[24,25] show that adding physical activity to caloric restriction programs can increase the amount of weight and fat loss. Table 3

Table 2.   Potential Impact on Body Weight of Adding 5 hr/wk of Moderate Exercise

Length of program	Caloric deficit	Weight loss
No compensation		
12 weeks	16,800 kcal	1.9-2.2 kg
20 weeks	28,000 kcal	3.1-3.7 kg
52 weeks	72,800 kcal	8.1-9.7 kg
25% compensation		
12 weeks	12,600 kcal	1.4-1.7 kg
20 weeks	21,000 kcal	2.3-2.8 kg
52 weeks	54,600 kcal	6.1-7.3 kg
50% compensation		
12 weeks	8,400 kcal	0.9-1.1 kg
20 weeks	14,000 kcal	1.5-1.9 kg
52 weeks	36,400 kcal	4.0-4.8 kg

[1]Assumes the energy expended in exercise is 280 cal/hour above resting and that weight loss comes entirely from body fat.

shows results of one such study, which was one year in duration. Men and women were randomly assigned to a control group, a group receiving food restriction alone (diet only), or a group receiving diet and physical activity (diet and exercise). After one year, men in the diet and exercise group lost about 4 kg more of body fat and body weight than did subjects in the diet-only group. This suggests that energy intake compensation may have been in the order of 50% of total calories expended in physical activity. For women, the differences were less and were only about 1 kg of total body weight and 1.5 kg of body fat. This could suggest that caloric compensation was greater in women than men.

Many studies have reported that the combination of physical activity and energy restriction do not lead to any greater weight loss than does energy restriction alone. However, a close examination of such studies shows them to be of short duration and of questionable power to detect the expected additional effects of physical activity on body weight.

There are reports in the literature that adding physical activity to energy restriction minimizes loss of fat-free mass and maximizes loss of body fat.[26-28] Unfortunately, most such studies are short in duration and involve small numbers of subjects.

Weight loss produced by physical activity includes substantial reduction of visceral adipose tissue.[29] However, it is not clear whether weight loss produced by exercise alone or exercise combined with energy restriction includes a greater proportion of visceral adipose tissue reduction than weight loss produced by energy

Table 3.   One-Year Weight Loss With Diet and Exercise

	Control	Diet only	Diet & exercise
Men	n = 40	n = 40	n = 39
Total wt (kg)	1.7± 4.8	-5.1 ± 5.8	-8.7 ± 5.7
Total fat (kg)	1.2± 3.8	-4.3 ± 5.2	-7.8 ± 4.6
WHR	0.0 ± 0.02	-0.02 ± 0.02	-0.04 ± 0.03
Women	n = 39	n = 31	n = 42
Total wt (kg)	1.3 ± 5.2	-4.1 ± 5.5	-5.1 ± 5.3
Total fat (kg)	0.5 ± 4.9	-4.0 ± 4.7	-5.5 ± 5.1
WHR	0.00 ± 0.06	-0.01 ± 0.06	-0.03 ± 0.05

From Wood et al.[24]

restriction alone. While loss of visceral adipose may be affected by physical activity, it may also vary due to gender and age.

It is also unclear whether men and women show a similar reduction in visceral adipose tissue with weight loss and particularly with exercise. Wing and Jeffery[30] assessed waist-to-hip ratio (WHR) in men and women participating in a six-month behavioral weight-loss program. They found a greater reduction in WHR in men versus women at the end of the program and at the 12-month follow-up period. However, at the 18-month follow-up period, the results were reversed, with women showing a greater reduction in WHR than did men. Schwartz et al.[31] examined body fat loss due to endurance exercise training in young and elderly men. They found greater loss of visceral adipose tissue in younger versus older men.

Despite the relatively small effects of exercise on acute loss of body weight and body fat mass, the benefits of physical activity for body weight and body fat regulation become apparent when long-term maintenance of body weight losses is examined. Subjects who are most successful in maintaining a body weight reduction are those who engage in regular physical activity.[32]

Summary

While it has not been definitively shown that a low level of physical activity causes obesity, the two are closely linked with a strong theoretical basis for suspecting that a low level of physical activity is a risk factor for obesity. Highly active populations have a lower prevalence of obesity than do sedentary populations, and the higher one's level of physical activity, the less likely that BMI will increase over time.

Maintaining a high level of physical activity helps to reduce body fatness and to avoid future increases in body fatness. Increases in physical activity, either alone or in combination with dietary modification, can reduce body fat content. How-

ever, the public needs to have reasonable expectations regarding the
and rapidity with which increases in physical activity can reduce body fatness.
With moderate increases in physical activity, this is likely in the range of 2 to 6 kg/
year, with 60% to 80% of the weight loss coming from body fat. Whether or not
increases in physical activity preferentially reduce visceral adipose tissue is unclear.

At present the most important characteristic of physical activity for body weight
regulation is how much you do—or total dose. The best advice to the public is to
find enjoyable physical activities in which to participate on a lifelong basis. Time
spent in sedentary activities should be minimized, and efforts should be made to
increase physical activity in daily living. Maintaining an active lifestyle is a major
benefit in maintaining a healthy body weight, and maintaining a healthy body
weight is one way to lower risk of cardiovascular disease.

References

1. Pi-Sunyer FX. Medical hazards of obesity. *Ann Intern Med*, 1993; 119:655-660.

2. Hill JO, Pagliassotti MJ, Peters JC. Nongenetic determinants of obesity and
fat topography. In Bouchard C (Ed.): *Genetic determinants of obesity*. Boca Raton:
CRC Press, 1994; 35-48.

3. Astrup A, Buemann B, Western P, Toubro S, Raben A, Christensen NJ. Obesity
as an adaptation to a high-fat diet: Evidence from a cross-sectional study. *Am J
Clin Nutr*, 1994; 59:350-355.

4. Kuczmarski RJ, Flegal KM, Campbell SM et al. Increasing prevalence of
overweight among US adults. *J Am Med Assoc*, 1994; 272:205-211.

5. Troiano RP, Flegal KM, Kuczmarski RJ, Campbell SM, Johnson CL.
Overweight prevalence and trends for children and adolescents—The National
Health and Nutrition Examination Surveys, 1963 to 1991. *Arch Pediatr Adolesc
Med*, 1995; 149:1085-1091.

6. Eck LH, Hackett-Renner C, Klesges LM. Impact of diabetic status, dietary
intake, physical activity, and smoking status on body mass index in NHANES II.
Am J Clin Nutr, 1992; 56:329-333.

7. Williamson DF, Madans J, Anda RF et al. Recreational physical activity and
ten-year weight change in a US national cohort. *Int J Obesity*, 1993; 17:279-286.

8. Obarzanek E, Schreiber GB, Crawford PB et al. Energy intake and physical
activity in relation to indexes of body fat: The National Heart, Lung, and Blood
Institute Growth and Health Study. *Am J Clin Nutr*, 1994; 60:15-22.

9. Reaven PD, Barrett-Connor E, Edelstein S. Relation between leisure-time
physical activity and blood pressure in older women. *Circulation*, 1991; 83:559-565.

10. Owens JF, Matthews KA, Wing RR et al. Can physical activity mitigate the
effects of aging in middle-aged women? *Circulation*, 1992; 85:1265-1270.

11. French SA, Jeffery RW, Forster JL et al. Predictors of weight change over two years among a population of working adults: The healthy worker project. *Int J Obesity*, 1994; 18:145-154.

12. Slattery ML, McDonald A, Bild DE et al. Associations of body fat and its distribution with dietary intake, physical activity, alcohol, and smoking in blacks and whites. *Am J Clin Nutr*, 1992; 55:943-949.

13. Mayer EJ, Burchfiel CM, Eckel RH et al. The role of insulin and body fat in associations of physical activity with lipids and lipoproteins in a biethnic population: The San Luis Valley Diabetes Study. *Arterioscler Thromb*, 1991; 11:973-984.

14. Fontvieille AM, Kriska A, Ravussin E. Decreased physical activity in Pima Indian compared with Caucasian children. *Int J Obesity*, 1993; 17:445-452.

15. Davies, PSW, Gregory J, White A. Physical activity and body fatness in pre-school children. *Inter J Obesity*, 1995; 19:6-10.

16. Schulz LO, Schoeller DA. A compilation of total daily energy expenditures and body weights in healthy adults. *Am J Clin Nutr*, 1994; 60:676-681.

17. Ballor DL, Keesey RE. A meta-analysis of the factors affecting exercise-induced changes in body mass, fat mass and fat-free mass in males and females. *Int J Obesity*, 1991; 15:717-726.

18. Ballor DL, Poehlman ET. Exercise-training enhances fat-free mass preservation during diet-induced weight loss: A meta-analytical finding. *Int J Obesity*, 1994; 18:35-40.

19. Tremblay A, Després JP, Leblanc C et al. Effect of intensity of physical activity on body fatness and fat distribution. *Am J Clin Nutr*, 1990; 51:153-157.

20. Jakicic JM, Wing RR, Butler et al. Prescribing exercise in multiple short bouts versus one continuous bout: Effects on adherence, cardiorespiratory fitness, and weight loss in overweight women. *Int J Obesity*, 1995; 19:893-901.

21. Epstein LH, Valoski AM, Vara LS et al. Effects of decreasing sedentary behavior and increasing activity on weight change in obese children. *Health Psych*, 1995; 14:109-115.

22. Seidell JC, Cigolini M, Deslypere JP et al. Body fat distribution in relation to serum lipids and blood pressure in 38-year-old European men: The European fat distribution study. *Atherosclerosis*, 1991; 86:251-260.

23. Lee L, Kumar S, Chin Leong L. The impact of five-month basic military training on the body weight and body fat of 197 moderately to severely obese Singaporean males aged 17 to 19 years. *Int J Obesity*, 1994; 18:105-109.

24. Wood PD, Stefanick ML, Williams PT et al. The effects on plasma lipoproteins of a prudent weight-reducing diet, with or without exercise, in overweight men and women. *N Engl J Med*, 1991; 325:461-466.

25. Stefanick ML. Exercise and weight control. *Exercise Sport Sci Rev*, 1993; 21:363-396.

26. Hill JO, Drougas H, Peters JC. Physical activity and moderate obesity. In C Bouchard, R Shephard, & T Stephens (Eds.): *Physical activity, fitness & health: International proceedings and concensus statement.* Champaign, IL: Human Kinetics, 1993.

27. Donnelly JE, Pronk NP, Jacobsen DJ et al. Effects of a very low-calorie diet and physical-training regimens on body composition and resting metabolic rate in obese females. *Am J Clin Nutr*, 1991; 54:56-61.

28. Donnelly JE, Sharp T, Houmard J et al. Muscle hypertrophy with large-scale weight loss and resistance training. *Am J Clin Nutr*, 1993; 58:561-565.

29. Després JP, Pouliot MC, Moorjani S et al. Loss of abdominal fat and metabolic response to exercise in obese women. *Am J Physiol*, 1991; 261:E159-E167.

30. Wing RR, Jeffery RW. Effect of modest weight loss on changes in cardiovascular risk factors: Are there differences between men and women or between weight loss and maintenance? *Int J Obesity*, 1995; 19:67-73.

31. Schwartz RS, Shuman WP, Larson V et al. The effect of intensive endurance exercise training on body fat distribution in young and older men. *Metab*, 1991; 40:545-551.

32. Kayman S, Bruvold W, Stern JS. Maintenance and relapse after weight loss in women: Behavioral aspects. *Am J Clin Nutr*, 1990; 52:800-807.

Physical Activity and Lipid Metabolism

Marcia L. Stefanick
Stanford University School of Medicine, Stanford, California, USA

An NIH Consensus Development Conference on lipoproteins in the early 1980s resulted in strong statements regarding the independent risk of elevated, low-density lipoprotein cholesterol (LDL-C) for coronary heart disease (CHD).[1] In the early 1990s, an NIH Consensus Development Conference on triglycerides, high-density lipoprotein cholesterol (HDL-C), and CHD resulted in a similar consensus that HDL-C is an independent CHD risk factor, with low levels being associated with greater risk, and high levels demonstrating a protective effect.[2] In contrast, there was disagreement regarding an independent role of elevated triglycerides (TG) in CHD, despite substantial evidence of such a relationship, due in part to the strong, inverse relationship of TG to HDL-C, as well as the association of TG with other CHD risk factors, including impaired glucose tolerance.[2]

Cross-Sectional Studies

In the mid 1970s, Wood, Haskell, and colleagues reported that active women and men (defined as running more than 24 km/week) had higher HDL-C, lower LDL-C and total cholesterol, lower triglycerides, and lower body fat weight than age-matched, predominantly sedentary, men and women randomly selected from three California communities.[3] Since that report, cross-sectional studies have repeatedly shown that middle-aged and older men and women who report engaging in regular physical activity, by a wide variety of questionnaires and surveys, have HDL-C levels that are typically 20% to 30% higher than do their sedentary counterparts.[4-7] These studies also report lower TG and very-low-density lipoprotein-cholesterol (VLDL-C) levels in active versus inactive adults; however, this is less consistently seen in women, who tend to have lower TG and VLDL-C levels than do their male counterparts, regardless of activity level. These studies also consistently report lower obesity levels in men and women who report greater physical activity, and they report an inverse association between body fat and HDL-C and a positive association between body fat and TG levels.

Findings of higher HDL-C have been reported for many different types of aerobic activities (e.g., running, brisk walking, tennis, swimming, cross-country skiing).[7] In contrast, individuals who engage primarily in anaerobic-type activities (e.g., sprinting) or resistance exercise involving few repetitions have generally not been shown to have higher HDL-C or lower TG.

Recently, cross-sectional studies have focused on how the amount of exercise achieved by individuals relates to lipid changes. Kokkinos and colleagues reported lipid values in 2 906 men, aged 30 to 64 (70% of whom were military officers, the rest being civilians) by distance of running per week, as well as by frequency and duration of exercise bouts, and showed that as mileage increased (with both greater frequency and duration of exercise sessions), HDL-C increased in what would appear to be a "dose-response" relationship.[8] Similar findings were reported by Williams and Moussa at the November 1995 AHA meetings in 1 833 women.[9] In both studies, HDL-C was significantly elevated in individuals who achieved about 10 miles of running per week versus no activity or lower mileage, but higher levels were seen in those who achieved greater mileage.[8,9]

A significant relationship between endurance activity and total and low-density lipoprotein-cholesterol (TC; LDL-C) levels has not been consistently reported in men or women, although some studies have found lower TC and LDL-C levels in active versus inactive people.[5-7] Furthermore, lower levels of small, dense LDL particles, the purportedly more atherogenic component of LDL, have been reported in male runners versus nonrunners.[10]

It is well understood that cross-sectional data cannot provide evidence of causality. Clearly, genetic differences can account for these associations. Endurance athletes have higher proportions of red (slow-twitch) muscle fibers, which are known to have higher levels of lipoprotein lipase activity (LPLA), which in turn is associated with higher HDL-C and lower TG.[11] Such muscle is specifically affected by endurance training also. Using a single-leg (knee extension) endurance-training model, in which one leg serves as the untrained control (for the same person), Kiens and Lithell showed increases in LPLA of 70% in the trained leg, relative to the untrained leg, which were accompanied by markedly greater VLDL triglyceride uptake and HDL production by the trained versus untrained leg during an exercise bout.[12]

Other confounding associations in cross-sectional data include the lower obesity status and lower amounts of visceral fat in active individuals, both of which are associated with higher HDL-C in individuals regardless of activity or fitness level.[13] Other factors may also differ between active and inactive individuals which relate to HDL-C and TG, including smoking status, alcohol consumption, diet composition, and hormonal status. Unfortunately, most cross-sectional data on lipoprotein levels in physically active versus inactive individuals do not include large numbers of minority individuals, so it is unclear whether relationships reported for predominantly white populations are also found in other ethnic groups.

Exercise Training Studies

Training studies have generally failed to show changes in TC or LDL-C in men or women, or in small or large LDL particles. Endurance-exercise training studies of initially sedentary individuals have shown either an increase in HDL-C and/or decrease in TG, or no change in HDL-C or TG.[5-7] Training studies of premenopausal women should be designed to accommodate lipoprotein variations through the menstrual cycle[5] or with menopause; however, it is unclear whether training responses differ more in pre- versus postmenopausal women than in young versus older men, or in early versus late postmenopausal women more than in men of similar age differences. Although few comparable data are available for children, physically fit and active youth have been reported to have lower TG levels than unfit and inactive children, whereas levels of total and LDL-C and HDL-C are generally not found to differ by activity level in children.[5] Large training studies have failed to attract adequate numbers of minority individuals to allow comparisons. These factors that confound cross-sectional comparisons, described above, can also confound results from training studies. To assess the independent role of increased physical activity, it may be necessary to hold each of these constant. Furthermore, there are important measurement issues, including laboratory standardization, controlling for the menstrual cycle and menopausal status, seasonal variations, and so on that may be particularly important in interpreting results from training studies.

When beneficial HDL-C or TG changes are reported, the training period is usually at least 12 weeks in length and is often accompanied by significant fat weight loss.[5-7] The evidence that adoption of a more active lifestyle will increase HDL-C and/or reduce TG is much weaker in women than in men[5-7] and in older than in younger adult populations;[6] however, positive effects in older populations may require a longer training period. Whereas one year of exercise training, at either moderate and higher intensity levels, failed to show significant lipoprotein improvements in men or women aged 50 to 65,[14] significant HDL-C increases were reported in men and women (combined) after an additional year of training.[15] These increases were particularly pronounced for subjects in the lower-intensity condition (assigned to five 30-minute sessions at 60% to 75% of peak treadmill heart rate), compared to higher intensity groups (assigned to three 40-minute sessions at 73% to 80% of maximal heart rate), possibly due to more frequent exercise sessions per week.

Controversy exists about the optimal exercise intensity for HDL-C increases. Similar HDL-C increases were reported by Duncan and colleagues in middle-aged women after 24 weeks of training consisting of 24 km/week of strolling (4.8 km/hr), brisk walking (6.4 km/hr), or aerobic walking (8.0 km/hr), when women were compared to their pretraining levels (although no differences were seen in any training group versus control), suggesting that greater HDL-C increases are not seen with higher- versus lower-intensity exercise;[16] however, it may be that even higher-intensity exercise (jogging) is necessary to demonstrate a dose-response.

One possible explanation for the more consistent finding of HDL-C increases in training studies of men versus women is that men seem to be more likely to lose weight with aerobic exercise than do women; in fact, the majority of training studies of women have failed to show significant changes in body weight.[5,13] There is increasing evidence that loss of body fat is a major factor in the HDL-C increases seen with exercise.[13] HDL-C was increased equally, relative to controls, in a large group of initially overweight men who were randomly assigned to lose weight by either calorie restriction, with no change in diet composition or exercise level, or by increased aerobic exercise, with no change in diet,[17] suggesting that weight loss is the essential component of exercise-induced HDL-C improvements. There is emerging evidence, however, that physiological differences between exercise-induced weight loss and diet-induced weight loss result in different effects on lipoproteins.

The role of intra-abdominal fat loss may underlie some of these differences and be particularly important for the HDL-C increases associated with weight loss.[13] Because men generally have a larger proportion of excess fat distributed in visceral stores than do women, the effect of exercise on this fat store may play a major role in the differences reported between men and women with respect to the effects of exercise on lipoproteins. Differences in lean body mass are also likely to contribute to these sex differences. The interrelationships of obesity, regional adiposity, and activity level with the lipoprotein profile are clearly important areas to explore in both men and women.

Although loss of body fat may be a chief contributor to increases in HDL-C levels in population studies, which are likely to include many individuals who are initially overweight, it is not the only explanation for HDL-C increases that accompany endurance training. Diet composition also appears to be an important confounding variable regarding the effects of increasing physical activity on the lipoprotein profile. HDL-C was not increased in men who were assigned to lose weight by caloric reduction achieved primarily by reducing dietary fat,[18] even though the amount of weight lost (including fat mass loss) was similar to that previously shown to increase HDL-C, when diet composition was not altered simultaneously with caloric reduction.[17] However, when aerobic exercise was added to the hypocaloric, reduced-fat diet, significant HDL-C improvements resulted versus both control and the diet-only condition.[18] An important note is the fact that the addition of exercise was accompanied by greater weight loss in the men. This latter study included premenopausal, moderately overweight women who showed HDL-C reductions with the hypocaloric, low-fat diet, despite an average 4.1 kg weight loss. The addition of approximately 16 km/week of brisk walking and/or jogging prevented the HDL-C- effect of this diet, without leading to greater weight loss (which averaged 5.1 kg) compared to diet alone.[18] Thus, the addition of aerobic exercise to a weight-reducing, low-fat diet resulted in HDL-C increases relative to diet alone in men and women; however, HDL-C levels were raised, relative to controls, only in the men.

Diet and Exercise for Elevated Risk Trial

In terms of public health benefits, a clinically relevant group to consider are those individuals who have initially low HDL-C. This is likely to be a heterogeneous group of overweight people, smokers, individuals consuming a low-fat diet, and, among many other possibilities, individuals with genetic factors that predispose them to low HDL-C levels. We have recently completed the Diet and Exercise for Elevated Risk (DEER) trial of 197 men and 180 postmenopausal women with initial HDL-C levels below the sex-specific mean of the population, combined with moderately elevated LDL-C for which a low-fat diet is likely to be recommended. These men and women were randomized to one year of: National Cholesterol Education Program (NCEP) Step II diet;[19] aerobic exercise; NCEP Step II diet plus aerobic exercise; or delayed intervention (control). The primary results were presented at a recent national meeting.[20] HDL-C was not elevated in men or women assigned to either exercise alone or to exercise combined with diet; however, strong associations were seen in the exercise-only men between weight loss, particularly fat-mass loss, and HDL-C increases. The most interesting result, however, was the finding in both men and women that the diet-only groups did not improve LDL-C versus control, whereas both the male and female diet-plus-exercise groups showed highly significant LDL-C reductions versus control. These findings support revised NCEP guidelines to incorporate physical activity (and weight loss) into dietary management of high-risk lipoproteins.[19]

As in a previous trial of premenopausal women,[19] differences between weight loss in diet-only and diet-plus-exercise postmenopausal women were not seen in the DEER trial. Furthermore, neither men nor women assigned to exercise only lost significant fat weight versus control. While other investigators have reported HDL-C increases in individuals who have initially low HDL-C, these are generally relative to each individual's pretraining level rather than to randomly assigned controls. The DEER trial would suggest that men with low HDL-C may need to do enough exercise to lose weight (particularly fat weight) to produce significant HDL-C increases. It may be that women need to lose enough body fat to reduce visceral fat stores to achieve HDL-C increases. These speculations deserve further investigation. It is worth noting, however, that both men and women in the DEER study accumulated a volume of exercise recommended by the Centers for Disease Control and Prevention and the American College of Sports Medicine.[21]

Considerable work is needed to determine who can benefit the most from aerobic exercise, in terms of the lipoprotein profile, and what the optimal training program should be for men and women across various age groups and among ethnic groups. Particular emphasis should be given to particular clinical subpopulations who have high-risk lipoprotein profiles and who are at risk for coronary heart disease.

Summary

1. There is considerable evidence that endurance exercise may increase HDL-cholesterol and reduce triglycerides in both young and older men and women, particularly if accompanied by body fat loss. (Visceral fat loss may be particularly important in the exercise-induced benefits on HDL-C.)

2. Initially sedentary, overweight adults are likely to improve their lipoprotein profiles with modest levels of exercise. Individuals who can achieve a greater volume of activity may have greater lipoprotein improvements.

3. The optimal "dose" of endurance exercise required to bring about clinically significant HDL-cholesterol and other lipid improvements in a large proportion of men and women remains to be determined.

4. Data on lipoprotein effects of endurance training are particularly sparse in non-white populations, groups of low socioeconomic status, and clinically relevant subsamples (such as individuals with low HDL-C, elevated LDL-C, high triglycerides, glucose intolerance or diabetes, etc.).

References

1. Consensus Development Conference: Lowering blood cholesterol to prevent heart disease. *JAMA*, 1985; 253:2080-2086.

2. NIH Consensus Conference: Triglyceride, high-density lipoprotein, and coronary heart disease. *JAMA*, 1993; 269:505-510.

3. Wood PD, Haskell WL. Plasma lipoprotein distributions in male and female runners. *Acad Sci*, 1977; 301:748-763.

4. Wood PD, Williams PT, Haskell WL. Physical activity and high-density lipoproteins. In Miller NE, Miller GT (Eds.): *Clinical and metabolic aspects of high-density lipoproteins*. Amsterdam: Elsevier Science, 1984, pp. 133-165.

5. Krummel D, Etherton TD, Peterson S, Kris-Etherton PM. Effects of exercise on plasma lipids and lipoproteins of women. *PSEBM*, 1993; 240:123-137.

6. Durstine JL, Haskell WL. Effect of exercise training on plasma lipids and lipoproteins. In Holloszy JO (Ed.): *Exercise and sport sciences reviews: 44*. Boston, MA: Williams & Wilkins, 1994, pp. 477-521.

7. Stefanick, ML. Exercise, lipoproteins, and cardiovascular disease. In Fletcher GF (Ed.): *Cardiovascular response to exercise*. Mount Kisco, NY: Futura, 1994, pp. 325-345.

8. Kokkinos PF, Holland JC, Narayan P, Colleran JA, Dotson CO, Papdemetriou V. Miles run per week and high-density lipoprotein cholesterol levels in healthy, middle-aged men. *Arch Int Med*, 1995; 155:415-420.

9. Williams PT, Moussa DK. Women runners show improvements in plasma HDL-cholesterol and adiposity at higher exercise levels than currently recommended. *Circulation*, 1995; 92 (Suppl.), Abstract #2956.

10. Williams PT, Krauss RM, Wood PD et al. Lipoprotein subfractions of runners and sedentary men. *Metabolism*, 1986; 35:45-52.

11. Stefanick ML, Wood PD. Physical activity, lipid and lipoprotein metabolism, and lipid transport. In Bouchard C, Shephard RJ, Stephens T (Eds): *Physical activity, fitness and health*: *International proceedings and consensus statement*. Champaign, IL: Human Kinetics, 1994, pp. 417-431.

12. Kiens B, Lithell H. Lipoprotein metabolism influenced by training-induced changes in human skeletal muscle. *J Clin Invest*, 1989; 83:558-564.

13. Stefanick ML. Exercise and weight control. In Holloszy JO (Ed): *Exercise and sport sciences reviews 1993*. American College of Sports Medicine Series, no. 21. Baltimore: Williams & Wilkins, pp. 363-396.

14. King AC, Haskell WL, Taylor CB, Kraemer HC, DeBusk RF. Group- vs. home-based exercise training in healthy older men and women: A community-based clinical trial. *JAMA*, 1991; 266:1535-1542.

15. King AC, Haskell WL, Young DR, Oka RK, Stefanick ML. Long-term effects of varying intensities and formats of physical activity on participation rates, fitness, and lipoproteins in men and women aged 50-65 years. *Circulation*, 1995; 91:2596-2604.

16. Duncan JJ, Gordon NF, Scott CB. Women walking for health and fitness: How much is enough? *JAMA*, 1991; 266:3295-3299.

17. Wood PD, Stefanick ML, Dreon DM et al. Changes in plasma lipids and lipoproteins in overweight men during weight loss through dieting as compared with exercise. *N Engl J Med*, 1988; 319:1173-1179.

18. Wood PD, Stefanick ML, Williams PT, Haskell WL. The effects on plasma lipoproteins of a prudent weight-reducing diet, with or without exercise, in overweight men and women. *N Engl J Med*, 1991; 325:461-466.

19. National Cholesterol Education Program: Second Report of the Expert Panel on Detection, Evaluation, and Treatment of High Blood Cholesterol in Adults. *Summary of the second report of the expert panel on detection, evaluation and treatment of high blood cholesterol in adults (adult treatment panel ii)*. NIH Publication No. 93-3095, September 1993 (and *JAMA* 1993; 269: 3015-3023).

20. Stefanick ML, Wood PD. The effects of the NCEP step II diet versus aerobic exercise on plasma lipoproteins in postmenopausal women and men with low-HDL and elevated-LDL cholesterol. *Circulation*, 1996.

21. Pate RR, Pratt M, Blair SN et al. Physical activity and public health: A recommendation from the Centers for Disease Control and Prevention and the American College of Sports Medicine. *JAMA*, 1995; 273:402-407.

Physical Activity, Insulin Resistance, and Diabetes

Robert S. Schwartz
University of Washington, Seattle, Washington, USA

Non-insulin-dependent diabetes mellitus (NIDDM) is a common disorder, especially in middle-aged and older individuals. The prevalence of NIDDM varies from 6% in Caucasian Americans, 10% in African Americans, and 13% in Hispanic Americans to about 20% in Native and Japanese Americans. Diabetes has a profound effect not only on the afflicted individuals but also on the health-care system, accounting for one-seventh of all health-care dollars spent.[1] The development of the disease seems to occur as a progression from normal to impaired glucose tolerance (IGT) and finally to NIDDM. There is now convincing evidence that insulin resistance plays a major role in the pathogenesis of NIDDM, as well as in several other important risk factors for coronary artery disease.[2] While the etiology of this syndrome of insulin resistance is unclear, it probably involves genetic factors as well as environmental or lifestyle factors, such as central obesity, inactivity, and diet.

This review will concentrate on the importance of physical activity in mitigating against the development of insulin resistance and the subsequent development of IGT and NIDDM. It will also address the role of physical activity in the treatment of diabetes once it has developed. Lastly, it will address the risks and benefits of exercise in diabetics or prediabetics and make recommendations about implementation of an exercise prescription in these populations.

Acute Effects of Exercise on Glucose and Insulin Homeostasis

Although the effects of exercise as an adjunct to treat diabetes mellitus were described in India around 500 B.C., its effect on glucose concentration and tolerance was first clearly demonstrated in 1919.[3] In recent years numerous peripheral responses to exercise have been described that might potentially improve glucose homeostasis, including changes in the muscle fiber types, muscle hypertrophy, increased muscle capillary density, increments in enzyme systems associated with both storage and oxidation of glucose, enhanced lipid oxidation, increased concentrations of the mRNA and protein for the insulin-responsive glucose transporter (GLUT4), and augmented translocation of GLUT4 from the cytosol to the active state at the plasma membrane.[4] These acute exercise changes, in concert with numerous other changes in counter-regulatory hormones, work together under normal circumstances to insure adequate delivery of fuel to exercising muscle while maintaining plasma levels of glucose.

The regulation of fuel homeostasis has been thoroughly reviewed.[5] Of importance to this review is how abnormalities in regulation of this complex system associated with either insulin-dependent diabetes mellitus (IDDM) or non-insulin-dependent diabetes mellitus (NIDDM) can produce difficulties in exercising diabetics. In the patient with IDDM who remains insulin deficient, hepatic glucose production is enhanced while peripheral glucose utilization (oxidation) is impaired, resulting in a further elevation of plasma glucose. In addition, this group of patients frequently has exaggerated glucagon and catecholamine responses to exercise, causing elevations in lipolysis, free fatty acids, and ketones.

In the over-insulinized state, which can occur in either IDDM or NIDDM patients who are treated with insulin, exercise-induced hypoglycemia is the major concern. This occurs because the significant reduction in plasma insulin that normally begins with the initiation of exercise cannot take place. In addition, the absorption of insulin from the subcutaneous depot above working muscle may be accelerated with exercise. The relatively excessive plasma insulin, in association with the exercise-induced enhancement in insulin action, impairs both hepatic glucose production and lipolysis while promoting peripheral glucose utilization. This can result in disastrously low plasma glucose levels. The improvement in insulin action after moderate to heavy exercise can be sustained for many hours after a single bout, thus extending the period of risk for hypoglycemia well beyond the time of the exercise itself.

The Effect of Increasing Physical Activity on Insulin and Glucose Homeostasis in NIDDM

While most reviewers feel that exercise is useful in the treatment of diabetes mellitus and is associated with improvements in both plasma glucose level, and insulin sensitivity and action,[6-11] not all agree.[12] Some of the disagreement reflects differences in the population of diabetics trained in various studies (insulin resistant vs insulin deficient) and when determinations of glucose tolerance and insulin sensitivity were measured with respect to the last bout of exercise.[10] In almost all of the studies, exercise training was associated with improved insulin action, while in only some were there also improvements in oral glucose tolerance and/or glycosylated hemoglobin. Whether or not exercise training improves plasma glucose levels, it would be expected to impact on the risk for coronary artery disease in other ways, such as a reduction in hyperinsulinemia.[13] These positive effects of exercise on glucose and insulin homeostasis in NIDDM have more recently been extended to older subjects, as well as the use of resistance training.[14,15]

It is not entirely clear whether improvements in glucose and insulin homeostasis following exercise training require losses in weight or adiposity. However, this is a moot point since in most studies in which exercising subjects are free to eat ad libitum, they lose a small amount of weight, most of which is fat. Furthermore, this fat loss appears to come preferentially from the metabolically active intra-abdominal fat stores.[16] In addition, exercise seems to be an important adjunct in the maintenance of weight loss that is attained by dieting.[17]

Physical Activity and Prevention of Diabetes Mellitus

Probably the clearest evidence for the use of exercise is in an effort to prevent the development of NIDDM.[18] There are now several large prospective studies in both men and women that strongly suggest that regular physical activity reduces the risk of developing NIDDM. In one study, the protective effect of leisure-time exercise was strongest in subjects at greatest risk for developing NIDDM, that is, those with a body mass index (BMI) >25, hypertension, and a parental history of NIDDM.[19] The age-adjusted relative risk for developing NIDDM in subjects who exercised at least once per week was .64 and .67 in men and women, respectively.[20,21] Of interest, there was no marked dose-response relationship noted between the number of exercise bouts per week and protection from developing NIDDM. In Pima Indians, historical activity was inversely related to the future development of NIDDM, while current activity was inversely associated to both fasting and two-hour postprandial glucose.[22]

While these studies potentially suffer from the usual selection bias associated with epidemiological research, an additional problem must be noted. In these studies, the presence of NIDDM is determined by history and since nearly 50% of NIDDM cases are undiagnosed, a substantial number of true cases may be missed. One important strength of these studies is that they can be used to assess the effects of long-term physical activity. This is preferable to the short-term training that is most common in the more well-controlled prospective intervention trials. It may be that the extended duration of the exercise training in the epidemiological studies accounts for the impressive effects despite low frequency and intensity. While the exact mechanisms producing this protection are not known, it is likely that they involve less age-related weight gain[23] and reduced central adiposity,[16] and therefore enhanced insulin sensitivity.[24] Although there is little data in humans, available data in animal models suggest that exercise does not mitigate or even postpone the development of IDDM.[25]

At present, there are no published, randomized, controlled trials that have investigated the possibility of preventing NIDDM. However, an important community-based study has been completed. While the study involved some diet instruction as well as an exercise prescription, it appears that much of the benefit stemmed from the exercise. In this six-year Malmo study, 181 subjects with IGT and 41 with early NIDDM were entered into the study and compared to 79 IGT subjects who did not enter (nonrandomized). There was a 3-kg loss of weight and a 10% to 24% increment in fitness in the treated subjects.[26] This was associated with conversion of 50% of the IGT patients to normal glucose tolerance and 50% of the NIDDM patients to nondiabetic status. In addition, the conversion rate from IGT to NIDDM was only 10.6% as compared to 28.6% in the control group. A prospective, randomized, controlled, multicentered study (Diabetes Prevention Program [DPP]) to assess whether drug therapy or lifestyle change can reduce the conversion of IGT to NIDDM, sponsored by the National Institutes of Health, is just beginning patient recruitment.

Recommendations

Screening.   Prior to initiating an exercise program, all diabetics should have a complete screening evaluation. This examination should be aimed at detecting both vascular (macro- and microvascular) as well as neurological complications. In addition, other contraindications for participating in an exercise program should be excluded. Patients should have had a retinal examination within the year. A symptom-limited, graded exercise test should be performed in all subjects with known or suspected coronary artery disease (CAD), IDDM patients over age 30 or with IDDM for more than 15 years, or NIDDM patients over age 35.[27] The exercise stress test should only be performed after adequate glucose control is attained and documented by home glucose monitoring.

Exercise prescription.   Despite the recent evidence that resistance exercise is also associated with improvements in glucose and insulin homeostasis, endurance training should remain the major recommendation. This is because only endurance training has also been demonstrated to improve both blood pressure and lipoprotein profiles. However, unlike power lifting, which increases ocular pressure due to valsalva, resistance training is not necessarily contraindicated in diabetics.

Exercise should be prescribed on a regular basis, 2 to 5 times per week—but, as noted above, it appears that any chronic activity level may be helpful. The duration of exercise should be between 20 and 60 minutes for each bout and at an intensity between 50% and 80% of maximal capacity or heart-rate reserve (as determined by exercise testing). It should be noted that recent studies suggest benefit from multiple exercise bouts as short as 10 minutes each, but this requires further confirmation. As with all participants, exercise should be preceded by an adequate warm-up period. Exercise in diabetics might be most beneficial during the period of morning insulin resistance, but must be convenient for the individual in order to promote compliance.

Avoiding complications.   The most important complication to exercise in diabetics is hypoglycemia. This can be avoided by appropriately reducing insulin or oral hypoglycemic therapy. Because of the myriad of factors that might affect glycemia, it is not possible to make specific recommendations, but a reduction in dose of 30% to 50% is reasonable. This recommendation will need to be individualized to each patient depending upon their exercise schedule, intensity, duration, and other factors. This process may require frequent home blood-glucose monitoring. Insulin should not be injected over actively exercising muscles. To assist further in avoiding hypoglycemia, patients should be instructed to eat 10 to 15 gm of carbohydrate for each 30 min of expected exercise. Patients should carry additional carbohydrates while they exercise and information identifying them as being diabetic. Because of the prolonged improvement in insulin action, insulin/oral agent therapy and calories may need to be adjusted even on the next (nonexercise) day. It is preferable that exercise begin as part of a monitored program but should at least include an exercise partner who, like the patient, should be knowledgeable about the signs and symptoms of hypoglycemia. If possible, use of beta-blockers should be avoided, and alcohol consumption kept to a minimum.

Diabetics who exercise should have appropriate footwear and take meticulous care of their feet. Patients with peripheral neuropathy must be especially careful to avoid foot ulcers or other orthopedic injuries. In addition, all diabetics should be concerned about maintaining adequate hydration and need to be aware of postexercise orthostatic hypotension.

Summary

There is now adequate data from a combination of different types of exercise studies to strongly support an effect in improving both glucose and insulin homeostasis. The most convincing data, and probably the most critical role for exercise, is in the prevention of NIDDM in at-risk populations. There is at present no data to suggest that exercise can delay or mitigate the onset of IDDM but, like patients with NIDDM, patients with IDDM can safely exercise and may benefit from other advantages of exercise in reducing cardiac risk factors.

It is imperative that all diabetics be screened prior to initiating an exercise program. While formal exercise testing is commonly warranted, it must be noted that the presence of CAD does not itself contraindicate the initiation of a carefully monitored exercise program in patients with diabetes. Any diabetic involved in an exercise program must be aware of the possibility of hypoglycemia both at the time of exercise, as well as for about 24 hours thereafter. In addition, meticulous foot care is necessary to insure against foot sores, ulcers, and infections, especially in those with peripheral neuropathy.

References

1. Rubin RJ, Altman WM, Mendelson DN. Health care expenditures for people with diabetes mellitus. *J Clin Endo Metab*, 1992; 78:809A-809F.

2. DeFronzo RA, Ferrannini E. Insulin resistance. A multifaceted syndrome responsible for NIDDM, obesity, hypertension, dyslipidemia, and atherosclerotic cardiovascular disease. *Diabetes Care*, 1991; 14:173-94.

3. Allen FM, Stillman E, Fitz R. Total dietary regulation in the treatment of diabetes. *Exercise* (Monograph 11). New York: Rockefeller Institute of Medical Research, 1919.

4. Ivy JL. Exercise physiology and adaptations to training. In Ruderman N, Devlin JT (Eds): *Health professional's guide to diabetes and exercise*. Alexandria, VA: American Diabetes Association, 1995; 5-26.

5. Wasserman DH, Zinman B. Fuel homeostasis. In Ruderman N, Devlin JT (Eds): *Health professional's guide to diabetes and exercise*. Alexandria, VA: American Diabetes Association, 1995; 27-48.

6. Krotkiewski M, Lonnroth P, Mandroukas K et al. The effects of physical training on insulin secretion and effectiveness and on glucose metabolism in obesity and Type 2 (non-insulin-dependent) diabetes mellitus. *Diabetologia*, 1985; 28:881-90.

7. Bjorntorp P, Krotkiewski M. Exercise treatment in diabetes mellitus. *Acta Med Scand*, 1985; 217:3-7.

8. Schneider SH, Ruderman NB. Exercise and physical training in the treatment of diabetes mellitus. *Compr Ther*, 1986; 12:49-56.

9. Holloszy JO, Schultz J, Kusnierkiewicz J, Hagberg JM, Ehsani AA. Effects of exercise on glucose tolerance and insulin resistance. Brief review and some preliminary results. *Acta Med Scand* (Suppl), 1986; 711:55-65.

10. Schwartz RS. Exercise training in the treatment of diabetes mellitus in elderly patients. *Diabetes Care*, 1990; 13 (Suppl 2):77-85.

11. Horton ES. Exercise and diabetes mellitus. *Med Clin North Am*, 1988; 72:1301-21.

12. Gautier JF, Scheen A, Lefebvre PJ. Exercise in the management of non-insulin-dependent (Type 2) diabetes mellitus. *Int J Obesity*, 1995; 19 (Suppl 4):S58-S61.

13. Stout RW. Overview of the association between insulin and atherosclerosis. *Metab*, 1985; 34 (Suppl 1):7-12.

14. Miller JP, Pratley RE, Goldberg AP et al. Strength training increases insulin action in healthy 50- to 65-yr-old men. *J Appl Physiol*, 1994; 77:1122-7.

15. Smutok MA, Reece C, Kokkinos PF et al. Effects of exercise training modality on glucose tolerance in men with abnormal glucose regulation. *Int J Sports Med*, 1994; 15:283-9.

16. Schwartz RS, Shuman WP, Larson V et al. The effect of intensive endurance exercise training on body fat distribution in young and older men. *Metab*, 1991; 40:545-51.

17. Pavlou KN, Krey S, Stefee WP. Exercise as an adjunct to weight loss and maintenance in moderately obese subjects. *Am J Clin Nutr*, 1989; 49:1115-23.

18. Kriska AM, Blair SN, Pereira MA. The potential role of physical activity in the prevention of non-insulin-dependent diabetes mellitus: The epidemiological evidence. *Exercise Sport Sci Rev*, 1994; 22:121-43.

19. Helmrich SP, Ragland DR, Paffenbarger RS Jr. Prevention of non-insulin-dependent diabetes mellitus with physical activity. *Med Sci Sports Exercise*, 1994; 26:824-30.

20. Manson JE, Rimm EB, Stampfer MJ et al. Physical activity and incidence of non-insulin-dependent diabetes mellitus in women. *Lancet*, 1991; 338:774-8.

21. Manson JE, Nathan DM, Krolewski AS, Stampfer MJ, Willett WC, Hennekens CH. A prospective study of exercise and incidence of diabetes among US male physicians. *JAMA*, 1992; 268:63-7.

22. Kriska AM, LaPorte RE, Pettitt DJ et al. The association of physical activity with obesity, fat distribution and glucose intolerance in Pima Indians. *Diabetologia*, 1993; 36:863-9.

23. Williamson DF, Madans J, Anda RF, Kleinman JC, Kahn HS, Byers T. Recreational physical activity and 10-year weight change in a US national cohort. *Int J Obesity*, 1993; 17:279-86.

24. Kahn SE, Larson VG, Beard JC et al. Effect of exercise on insulin action, glucose tolerance, and insulin secretion in aging. *Am J Physiol*, 1990; 258:E937-43.

25. Noble JD, Farrell PA. Effect of exercise training on the onset of type I diabetes in the BB/Wor rat. *Med Sci Sports Exercise*, 1994; 26:1130-4.

26. Eriksson KF, Lindgarde F. Prevention of type 2 (non-insulin-dependent) diabetes mellitus by diet and physical exercise. The six-year Malmo feasibility study. *Diabetologia*, 1991; 34:891-8.

27. Mahler DA, Froelicher VF, Miller NH, York TD. In Kenney WL (Ed): *ACSM's guidelines for exercise testing and prescription*. Baltimore, MD: Williams & Wilkins, 1995.

Physical Activity, Physical Fitness, and Blood Pressure

James M. Hagberg
University of Pittsburgh Medical Center, Pittsburgh, Pennsylvania, USA

Recent data indicate that over 50 million people in the United States, or 20% of the American population, have hypertension.[1] Ninety percent of hypertensives have mild to moderate hypertension, which are defined by the Joint National Committee on the Detection, Evaluation, and Treatment of High Blood Pressure Report V (JNC V) as Stage 1 or 2 hypertension with blood pressures (BPs) in the range 140-179/90-109 mmHg.[1] While antihypertensive medications are clearly the first line of treatment for Stage 3 or greater hypertension, physical activity is a nonpharmacological treatment that is often featured prominently in the treatment of Stage 1 or 2 hypertension.

Forty-seven full-length English publications have reported the results of studies assessing the effects of endurance exercise training on individuals with essential hypertension.[2] These studies vary widely in terms of their design, with very few being randomized clinical trials and many not even including hypertensive control groups. The sample sizes, and the age, gender, and ethnicity of the subjects also varied widely among these studies. Exercise training intensity, frequency, duration, and length also varied markedly among these studies, as did the BP measurement techniques and other mechanistic measurements that were made.

Seventy percent of the groups that initially had systolic BP greater than 140 mmHg in these 47 studies decreased casual systolic BP significantly with exercise training.[2] The sample size-weighted average reduction in casual systolic BP was 10.5 mmHg from an initial systolic BP of 154 mmHg. Seventy-eight percent of the groups that initially had diastolic BP greater than 90 mmHg reduced casual diastolic BP significantly with exercise training. The average diastolic BP reduction was 8.6 mmHg from an initial value of 98 mmHg. Thus, the average BP reduction associated with endurance exercise training does not "normalize" BP in the large majority of hypertensive subjects. It is important to note that only one group showed a significant increase in casual BP with exercise training.[3] Thus, beneficial BP responses are eighty times more frequent than are negative responses, and beneficial responses are three times more frequent than are equivocal responses.

It is now clear that ambulatory BP measured during a person's usual daily lifestyle is a better indicator of cardiovascular disease risk and hypertensive end-organ damage than is casual BP. Reductions in ambulatory BP with exercise training are less consistent and smaller than those summarized above for casual BP.[4] However, few studies have quantified changes in ambulatory BP with exercise training in hypertensive subjects.[5-7] In addition, these studies generally had small sample sizes, which limits the statistical power of these comparisons given the inherent variability in ambulatory BP.

Endurance Exercise Training

Endurance exercise training is the type of exercise primarily addressed in this review. Such exercise is dynamic and rhythmic in nature and involves the major skeletal muscle groups of the body. General recommendations are that it must elevate heart rate for at least 20 to 30 minutes every other day. A recent joint statement by the Centers for Disease Control and the American College of Sports Medicine recommends that people accumulate 30 minutes of structured or lifestyle physical activity on most days of the week.[8] While some epidemiological data support this recommendation, at present no data are available from experimental studies to support the conclusion that lifestyle activities can beneficially affect BP in hypertensive individuals. Resistance or weight training is not recommended as the sole mode of exercise training for hypertensives because it has not consistently been shown to reduce BP in hypertensive individuals and because of the risks resulting from the marked pressor BP response to such exercise.[4] Circuit weight training does lower BP in hypertensive individuals, probably as a result of the endurance exercise component that is included in such training programs.[4]

The hemodynamic mechanisms underlying the BP reductions resulting from exercise training are unclear, as both cardiac output and peripheral vascular resistance have been reported to be reduced with equal frequency.[4] One relatively consistent finding with exercise training in hypertensives is reduced sympathetic nervous system activity, whether measured as plasma norepinephrine levels, plasma norepinephrine turnover, or peripheral muscle sympathetic nerve activity. On the other hand, changes in variables related to the renin-angiotensin-aldosterone system (decreased blood and plasma volume, increased sodium excretion) have generally only been found in Asian/Pacific Islander hypertensives with exercise training.[2]

The lack of a relationship between weight loss or changes in body composition and the BP reductions resulting from exercise training indicates that anthropomorphic changes are not a primary mechanism underlying BP reductions. However, it is not known if a substantial weight loss in obese hypertensives resulting from the increased energy expenditure associated with exercise training will reduce BP to a greater degree than exercise training or weight loss alone.

Seventy percent of the hypertensive groups in the 47 studies included in this review decreased systolic BP significantly, whether they trained at greater or less than 70% $\dot{V}O_2$max.[2] However, groups that trained at less than 70% $\dot{V}O_2$max decreased systolic BP 3.0 mmHg more than did those that trained at greater than 70% $\dot{V}O_2$max. Seventy-five percent of the groups decreased diastolic BP significantly, whether they trained at greater or less than 70% $\dot{V}O_2$max, and the diastolic

BP reductions were also the same at both training intensities. This same general trend is also evident in studies that compared the effects of different training intensities in hypertensive persons.[9-11] In addition, training at less than 70% $\dot{V}O_2max$ slows the increase in BP as spontaneously hypertensive rats mature, whereas training at intensities greater than 70% $\dot{V}O_2max$ did not.[12] Thus, training intensities of 40% to 70% $\dot{V}O_2max$ appear to reduce systolic BP more, and diastolic BP the same, as does training at greater than 70% $\dot{V}O_2max$. This is advantageous from a public-health point of view because such training intensities are associated with better adherence, lower musculoskeletal and cardiovascular risks, and are easier to implement on a community-wide basis.

Seventy percent of groups in these 47 studies reduced systolic BP significantly independent of the length of their exercise training programs.[2] Reductions in systolic BP were, however, 1 to 2 mmHg greater with training programs greater than 10 weeks in duration. Exercise training elicited significant diastolic BP reductions in 75% of the groups regardless of the length of training, but again the reductions were 2 to 2.5 mmHg greater with training programs greater than 10 weeks in duration. This trend is also generally evident in studies that assessed the time course of the BP-lowering effect of endurance exercise training in hypertensives.[10] Exercise in sedentary hypertensives also has an acute BP-lowering effect that persists for up to 8 to 12 hours after a single exercise session and results in a significant 6 mmHg reduction in average 24-hour systolic BP.[13-16] It is not known if exercise training might amplify, prolong, or, on the other hand, ameliorate this response following acute exercise.

The age range of subjects in these 47 studies was 11 to 77 years.[2] The systolic BP-lowering effect of exercise training appears to be largest in 41 to 60 year olds, and a larger percentage of groups in this age range reduced systolic BP significantly with exercise training compared to 21-to-40- and 61+-year-old groups. However, three times as many 41 to 60 year olds have been studied compared to the other two age groups. Diastolic BP reductions with exercise training, in terms of both the percentage of groups eliciting significant reductions and the average reductions, appear to be independent of age. No studies have directly compared the effect of endurance exercise training on the BP of hypertensives of different ages.

Half of these 47 studies included only men as subjects, and only 3 studies reported data separately for female hypertensives.[2] Many studies state that the BP reductions associated with exercise training did not differ between male and female hypertensives, though minimal statistical power was available to address this issue. The minimal data that are available indicate that hypertensive women may elicit greater and more consistent reductions in BP with exercise training than hypertensive men. However, no studies have directly assessed this possibility with appropriate statistical power.

Caucasians and Asians/Pacific Islanders are the primary races that have been studied with respect to the BP-lowering effect of exercise training.[2] The data from the 47 studies indicate that systolic BP is decreased more consistently (in 92% vs

46% of groups) and to a greater extent (11.9 vs 7.3 mmHg) in Asian/Pacific Islanders compared to Caucasian hypertensives. The consistency and extent of the diastolic BP-lowering response to endurance exercise training is similar in both of these ethnic groups (85% vs 70%; 6.6 vs 6.8 mmHg).

Only two studies have assessed the BP-lowering effects of endurance exercise training in African Americans.[17,18] This glaring lack of a critical mass of data in African American hypertensives is especially disconcerting since they exhibit one of the highest prevalences of hypertension of any population in the world and very high morbidity and mortality rates associated with hypertension. The first study in African Americans included 11 children with an average age of 11 years and found that 12 weeks of endurance exercise training increased their cardiovascular fitness and reduced both systolic and diastolic BP significantly.[17] A very recent study assessed the effect of exercise training on the BP of African American hypertensive men with initial BP values greater than 180/110 mmHg.[18] All subjects were first treated with antihypertensive medications to reduce diastolic BP by 10 mmHg from the initial diastolic BP or to less than 90 mmHg. Subjects were then maintained on these medications and randomized to an exercise or a control group. Sixteen weeks after randomization, the exercise training group had a significantly lower diastolic BP and a trend toward a lower systolic BP compared to the control group. After an additional 16 weeks of exercise training, subjects also required fewer antihypertensive medications to maintain this reduced BP.

Risk Factors

The primary causes of morbidity and mortality in hypertensives are stroke and coronary heart disease (CHD),[19] and while hypertension is the primary risk factor for stroke, it is only one of a multitude of risk factors for CHD. It is also important to keep in mind that many CHD risk factors, such as obesity, glucose intolerance, insulin resistance, and dyslipidemia, cluster in hypertensives, perhaps as a result of the Metabolic Syndrome proposed to be initiated by insulin resistance and hyperinsulinemia.[20] In this regard, exercise training may be especially advantageous for hypertensives because it has been shown to beneficially affect these other CHD risk factors in normotensives.

The minimal data that are available from hypertensives indicate that exercise training increases HDL-C and HDL_2-C levels and decreases the cholesterol/HDL-C ratio.[21,22] Exercise training also reduced insulin levels and improved insulin sensitivity and glucose tolerance in the few studies that have assessed these responses in hypertensives.[10,23] Endurance exercise training also beneficially affects body composition in hypertensives. Though two previous studies have provided mixed results,[24,25] the recent study in hypertensive African American men indicated that exercise training decreased left ventricular mass by more than 10% compared to the pharmacologic intervention group that lowered BP to only a slightly lesser degree.[18] However, most previous exercise training studies in hypertensives have been unidimensional in that they only assessed BP. Very few studies have assessed the potential beneficial "side effects" of exercise training on major CHD risk factors other than BP in hypertensives.

Risk estimation equations from Framingham can be used to estimate the overall effect of different interventions on the eventual development of CHD in hypertensives.[26] These equations indicate that a 55-year-old male smoker with a BP of 160/100 mmHg, cholesterol of 240 mg/dl, and HDL-cholesterol of 40 mg/dl without diabetes or ECG evidence of left ventricular hypertrophy has a 32% chance of developing CHD during the subsequent 12 years. Treatment with diuretics to lower his BP to 140/90 would also result in a 15 mg/dl average increase in total cholesterol levels,[27] so that his risk of developing CHD in 12 years is only reduced to 30%. Lowering his BP to 140/90 with beta-blockers would decrease his HDL-cholesterol levels to 35 mg/dl (27), so that his 12-year risk of developing CHD is only decreased to 31%. These estimations are similar to the results of a number of clinical trials where treatment with diuretics or beta-blockers substantially reduces strokes in hypertensives, which is a direct function of the change in BP, but has only a minimal effect on CHD.[19] Again, most previous studies investigating the effects of antihypertensive medications on hypertensives focused on BP, largely ignoring other CHD risk factors.

Beneficial Effects of Exercise Training

While JNC V first-line antihypertensive medications generally have adverse effects on CHD risk factors other than BP,[27] endurance exercise training generally has beneficial effects on these same risk factors, even though most of the evidence to date is from normotensive individuals. Endurance exercise training results in, on average, a 5 mg/dl increase in HDL-cholesterol levels.[28] Endurance exercise training also generally results in an average reduction in total cholesterol levels of 10 mg/dl, a change that may or may not be statistically significant, depending on the study sample size.[28]

Thus, even though exercise training would not lower our reference hypertensive man's BP to the same degree as would antihypertensive medications, the beneficial changes in total and HDL-cholesterol add to the benefit so that his risk of developing CHD over the next 12 years, as estimated from the Framingham equation,[26] is reduced from 32% to 25.5%. This amounts to a 20% reduction in his risk, which is substantially greater than the benefit obtained from diuretic or beta-blocker therapy. This is also still probably a conservative estimate of the benefit because some data indicate that endurance exercise training will beneficially affect other CHD risk factors, such as glucose tolerance, insulin resistance, left ventricular hypertrophy, and cardiovascular fitness. Thus, a multidimensional assessment of the benefits of exercise training for hypertensives will probably indicate that it is much more advantageous in the long-term than are first-line JNC V antihypertensive medications.

These benefits of exercise training for hypertensives estimated from Framingham risk equations already appear to be borne out in two large epidemiological studies that have shown that physically fit or physically active hypertensives had 40% to 60% lower mortality rates than did otherwise comparable unfit or sedentary hypertensives.[29,30] Even though the BP of these trained/fit individuals remained in hypertensive range, their overall major CHD risk factor profiles were probably better than those of the sedentary hypertensives, resulting in a lower rate of development of CHD. In one study, the mortality rate for fit hypertensives was actually lower than that for unfit normotensives, indicating that enhanced cardiovascular fitness could overcome the negative mortality consequences of a hypertensive BP.[29] Similar studies have demonstrated that physically active individuals generally have lower BP than sedentary persons.

The ultimate potential benefit of exercise training would be the primary prevention of hypertension. Retrospective epidemiologic studies demonstrate that physically active men are 20% to 35% less likely to develop hypertension than are their sedentary counterparts.[31] Only one hypertension primary prevention trial used a substantive physical activity component, and it was only part of an overall hygienic intervention that was applied to persons at high risk for developing hypertension.[32] Over five years the intervention group, who improved treadmill performance compared to the control group, developed hypertension at a 54% lower rate than did the control group (8.8% vs 19.2%). These results, along with the epidemiological results presented above, are consistent with the possibility that increased physical activity may be effective in the primary prevention of hypertension.

Summary

Low-to-moderate intensity endurance exercise training is a beneficial intervention in JNC V Stage 1 and 2 hypertensives. The overall benefit of exercise as an intervention for hypertensives is probably underestimated, as little is known about its effects on other major CHD risk factors. Increased fitness and physical activity levels result in lower mortality rates even in individuals that remain hypertensive. Physical activity and physical fitness also appear to diminish the rate of development of hypertension. Thus, increased physical activity should play a major role in the primary prevention of hypertension and in the treatment of the large majority of hypertensives.

References

1. Joint National Committee on Detection, Evaluation, and Treatment of High Blood Pressure Report V. *Arch Int Med*, 1993; 153:154-184.

2. Hagberg JM, Brown MD. Does exercise training play a role in the treatment of essential hypertension? *J Cardiovasc Risk*, 1995; 2:296-302.

3. Attina DA, Giuliano G, Arcangeli G, Musante R, Cupelli V. Effects of 1 yr of physical training on borderline hypertension: An evaluation by bicycle ergometer exercise testing. *J Cardiovasc Pharmacol*, 1986; 8 (Suppl 5):S145-S147.

4. American College of Sports Medicine Position Stand. Physical activity, physical fitness, and hypertension. *Med Sci Sports Exercise*, 1993; 25:i-x.

5. Seals DR, Reiling M. Effect of regular exercise on 24 hour arterial pressure in older hypertensive humans. *Hypertension*, 1991; 18:583-592.

6. Gilders RM, Voiner C, Dudley GA. Endurance training and blood pressure in normotensive and hypertensive adults. *Med Sci Sports Exercise*, 1989; 21:629-636.

7. Blumenthal JA, Siegel WC, Appelbaum M. Failure of exercise to reduce blood pressure in patients with mild hypertension. *JAMA*, 1991; 266:2098-2104.

8. Pate RR, Pratt M, Blair SN et al. Physical activity and public health: Recommendations from the Centers for Disease Control and Prevention and the American College of Sports Medicine. *JAMA*, 1995; 273:402-407.

9. Matsusaki M, Ikeda M, Tashiro E et al. Influence of workload on the antihypertensive effect of exercise. *Clin Exp Pharmacol Physiol*, 1992; 19:471-479.

10. Hagberg JM, Montain SJ, Martin WH, Ehsani AA. Effect of exercise training on 60-69 yr old persons with essential hypertension. *Am J Cardiol*, 1989; 64:348-353.

11. Roman O, Camuzzi AL, Villalon E, Klenner C. Physical training program in arterial hypertension: A long-term prospective follow-up. *Cardiology*, 1981; 67:230-243.

12. Tipton CM, Matthes RD, Marcus KD, Rowlett KA, Leininger JR. Influences of exercise intensity, age, and medication on resting blood pressure in SHR populations. *J Appl Physiol*, 1983; 55:1305-1310.

13. Pescatello LS, Fargo AE, Leach CN, Scherzer HH. Short-term effect of dynamic exercise on arterial blood pressure. *Circulation*, 1991; 83:1557-1561.

14. Hagberg JM, Montain SJ, Martin WH. Blood pressure and hemodynamic responses after exercise in older hypertensives. *J Appl Physiol*, 1987; 63:270-276.

15. Brown MD, Taylor-Tolbert N, Dengel D, McCole SD, Hagberg JM. Ambulatory systolic blood pressure is reduced following a single bout of exercise. *Med Sci Sports Exercise*, 1994; 26:S163.

16. Kaufman FL, Hughson RL, Schaman JP. Effect of exercise on recovery blood pressure in normotensive and hypertensive subjects. *Med Sci Sports Exercise*, 1987; 19:17-20.

17. Danforth J, Allen K, Fitterling J et al. Exercise as a treatment for hypertension in low-socioeconomic-status black children. *J Consult Clin Psychol*, 1990; 58:237-239.

18. Kokkinos PF, Narayan P, Colleran JA et al. Effects of regular exercise on blood pressure and left ventricular hypertrophy in African-American men with severe hypertension. *N Engl J Med*, 1995; 333:1462-1467.

19. Kaplan, N. *Clinical hypertension* (5th edition). Baltimore: Williams & Wilkins, 1990.

20. Reaven GM. Role of insulin resistance in human disease. *Diabetes*, 1988; 37:1595-1607.

21. Tanabe Y, Sasaki J, Urata H et al. Effect of mild aerobic exercise on lipid and apolipoprotein levels in patients with essential hypertension. *Jpn Heart J*, 1988; 29:199-206.

22. Sasaki J, Urata H, Tanabe Y et al. Mild exercise therapy increases serum high density lipoprotein 2 cholesterol levels in patients with essential hypertension. *Am J Med Sci*, 1989; 297:220-223.

23. Bursztyn M, Ben-Ishay D, Shochina M, Mekler J, Raz I. Disparate effects of exercise training on glucose tolerance and insulin levels and on ambulatory blood pressure in hypertensive patients. *Hypertension*, 1993; 11:1121-1125.

24. Kelemen MH, Effron MB, Valenti SA, Stewart KJ. Exercise training combined with antihypertensive drug therapy. *JAMA*, 1990; 263:2766-2771.

25. Baglivo HG, Fabregues G, Burrieza H et al. Effect of moderate physical training on left ventricular mass in mild hypertensive persons. *Hypertension*, 1990; 15 (Suppl. 1):I153-I156.

26. Anderson KM, Wilson PWF, Odell PM, Kannel WB. An updated coronary risk profile. *Circulation*, 1991; 83:356-362.

27. Weinberger MH. Antihypertensive therapy and lipids: Evidence, mechanisms, and implications. *Arch Int Med*, 1985; 145:1102-1111.

28. Wood PD, Stefanick ML. Exercise, fitness, and atherosclerosis. In: *Exercise, fitness, and health*. Eds.: C Bouchard, RJ Shephard, T Stephens, JR Sutton, BD McPherson. Champaign, IL: Human Kinetics, 1988, pp 409-423.

29. Blair SN, Kohl HW III, Paffenbarger R Jr et al. Physical fitness and all-cause mortality: A prospective study of healthy men and women. *JAMA*, 1989; 262:2395-2401.

30. Paffenbarger RS Jr, Jung DL, Leung RW, Hyde RT. Physical activity and hypertension: An epidemiological view. *Ann Med*, 1991; 23:319-327.

31. Paffenbarger RS Jr, Wing AL, Hyde RT, Jung DL. Physical activity and incidence of hypertension in college alumni. *Am J Epidemiol*, 1983; 117:245-257.

32. Stamler R, Stamler J, Gosch FC et al. Primary prevention of hypertension by nutritional-hygienic means: Final report of a randomized clinical trial. *JAMA*, 1989; 262:1801-1807.

Physical Activity, Coagulability, and Fibrinolysis

E. Randy Eichner
University of Oklahoma Health Sciences Center,
Oklahoma City, Oklahoma, USA

Burgeoning research is beginning to elucidate how blood rheology and hemostatic function relate to risk of cardiovascular disease (CVD), especially heart attack and stroke. From this broad and emerging field, this review keys on how physical activity relates to hematocrit, fibrinogen, platelet function, and fibrinolysis. Epidemiological studies are considered first.

Hematocrit and CVD

Research from the Framingham Heart Study and elsewhere suggests that hematocrit per se is a CVD risk factor. Hematocrit was shown to be a risk factor for coronary heart disease (CHD) in men in Puerto Rico and in men in the British Regional Heart Study. Also, epidemiologic studies from Japan and from the British Regional Heart Study implicate hematocrit as a risk factor in stroke, especially thrombotic stroke.[1]

Fibrinogen and CVD

Prospective epidemiological studies agree that fibrinogen level is an independent risk factor for stroke or acute myocardial infarction (AMI). In Gothenburg, when a random sample of 792 middle-aged men was followed for nearly 14 years, fibrinogen level was tied to occurrence of stroke and AMI, a direct relationship that persisted for stroke even when blood pressure, cholesterol, and smoking were considered.[2] In Framingham, 1 315 people free of CVD had fibrinogen levels measured. During the next 12 years, for both sexes, the risk of CVD in general and of CHD in particular increased in proportion to baseline fibrinogen level. The risk of stroke rose steadily with fibrinogen level in men but not women. It was concluded that elevated fibrinogen level is a CVD risk factor.[3]

A meta-analysis of six prospective epidemiological studies (including Gothenburg, Framingham, and Northwick Park) also concluded that fibrinogen is a major CVD risk factor. In that analysis, people in the high versus low tertile of fibrinogen level had about twice the risk of later developing heart attack or stroke.[4]

Cross-sectional studies support the fibrinogen hypothesis by linking fibrinogen level to markers of subclinical CVD in middle-aged and elderly people. Also, a two-year follow-up of nearly 3 000 angina patients finds that the level of fibrinogen (and levels of von Willebrand factor antigen and tissue plasminogen activator antigen) predict the risk of AMI or sudden death: A high fibrinogen level predicts high risk; a low level predicts low risk, even when cholesterol level is high.[5]

Platelets and CVD

Diverse evidence suggests a role for platelets in CVD. Studies by autopsy in sudden cardiac death, arteriography in AMI, and angioscopy in unstable angina show that such events begin when platelets adhere to a damaged atherosclerotic plaque and initiate clotting. Research suggests that diurnal (morning) peaks in platelet aggregability may contribute to morning peaks in incidence of angina, AMI, stroke, and sudden cardiac death.[6] A five-year follow-up of AMI survivors in Holland ties platelet reactivity to prognosis: Patients with the most "hyperreactive" platelets have the greatest risk of cardiac events or death.[7] Other prospective studies suggest that platelet aggregability (as well as platelet count and platelet size) may influence the natural history of CHD in men.[8]

Fibrinolysis and CVD

Another key hemostatic function in CVD is impaired fibrinolysis,[9] usually due to high plasma levels of plasminogen-activator inhibitor type I (PAI-1), the rapid inhibitor of endogenous tissue-type plasminogen activator (t-PA). In a three-year follow-up of young survivors of AMI, high PAI-1 activity predicted second AMI.[10] High t-PA antigen also predicts reinfarction; this paradox is explained by an increase in circulating complexes of t-PA and its inhibitor PAI-1; such complexes impair fibrinolysis, not enhance it.[11]

Other research agrees that impaired fibrinolysis predicts or augments CVD. Northwick Park reports a strong, independent relation between impaired fibrinolysis and higher 16-year risk of coronary events in men middle-aged at entry.[12] In a prospective study, atherosclerotic patients at high risk for thrombotic CVD events were marked by impaired fibrinolysis due to high PAI-1 levels.[13] In the follow-up of nearly 3 000 angina patients, high t-PA antigen levels predicted AMI or sudden death.[5] High t-PA antigen levels (presumably bound to and thus inactivated by PAI-1) predict the seven-year risk of death in angina patients,[11] as well as the risk of first-ever AMI or stroke (thromboembolic) in apparently healthy US male physicians.[14,15]

Finally, fibrinolysis, like platelet reactivity, has a diurnal cycle. Research on healthy volunteers suggests that, in the afternoon and evening, t-PA activity tends to predominate, making for brisk fibrinolysis; whereas in the early morning, PAI-1 activity tends to predominate, making for sluggish fibrinolysis.[16] The morning peak in coronary events may thus owe in part to diurnal cycles in both platelet function and fibrinolysis.

In summary, abnormalities in blood rheology and hemostatic function have been tied to CVD. Unclear is whether such abnormalities are "horse or cart"—whether they contribute to atherothrombosis or merely mark it. Probably, they are cart and horse. Probably, measures to improve rheology and hemostasis can help prevent CVD.[9] One such measure is physical activity. Considered next is how regular physical activity influences hematocrit, fibrinogen, platelet function, and fibrinolysis.

Physical Activity and Hematocrit

High hematocrit impairs blood rheology by increasing blood viscosity, and promotes coagulability by enhancing platelet-endothelial contact. The latter effect is in part "physical," from a churning effect of flowing red cells that drives platelets toward the vessel wall,[17] and —if turbulent blood flow causes hemolysis—in part "chemical," from the release of ADP by hemolyzed red cells.[18]

It is established that regular physical activity, especially endurance (aerobic) exercise, lowers hematocrit by increasing the plasma volume. This expansion of plasma volume occurs within days of beginning regular exercise. The low baseline hematocrit of endurance athletes (compared to the population norm) has been termed "sports anemia," but really is a dilutional pseudoanemia that likely helps prevent CVD.[19]

Although the precise "exercise prescription" to optimize this "blood-thinning" benefit is not known, there is a "dose-effect": Expansion of plasma volume in exercisers ranges from about 5% in brisk walkers or joggers up to 20% in elite marathoners. If regular exercise is stopped, this benefit is lost as fast as it was gained; within days, plasma volume "shrinks" to the sedentary baseline.[20]

Physical Activity and Fibrinogen

Fibrinogen level, like hematocrit, tends to be lower in active people versus sedentary counterparts. In middle-aged British men, a habit of strenuous exercise, compared to mild exercise, is linked with a lower fibrinogen level. Another cross-sectional study ties upper-body obesity with higher fibrinogen levels in premenopausal women. An Italian study finds higher fibrinogen in obese versus nonobese children. Finnish studies tie fibrinogen level inversely to physical activity and fitness in middle-aged men and to physical activity in postmenopausal women. The Postmenopausal Estrogen/Progestin Interventions (PEPI) study also ties baseline fibrinogen level inversely to self-reported habits of leisure-time physical activity (and/or to body mass index) in middle-aged women.[21]

Longitudinal studies—a handful of pilot studies as a group—suggest that regular physical activity can reduce fibrinogen in healthy subjects and in patients with diabetes or CVD. In an uncontrolled study with few subjects, mean fibrinogen level fell a significant 13% in older men, but not in younger men (perhaps because younger men began with lower baseline levels) who trained for six months.[22] In another study, a 6% fall in fibrinogen level in young exercisers was not significant (compared to nonexercisers), but the chance of a type II error was high.[23] Most of the other training studies here are limited by sketchy design, lack of controls, or few subjects.

All considered, it is likely that regular physical activity does reduce baseline fibrinogen level—perhaps just by diluting fibrinogen in an expanded plasma volume (the same way physical activity reduces hematocrit). But more research is needed to be certain whether (and how) regular physical activity reduces fibrinogen.

Physical Activity and Platelets

How physical activity affects basal platelet function is still unclear. Cross-sectional studies of platelet aggregability in athletes versus nonathletes are few and inconclusive. One longitudinal study of exercise training and platelet function lacks nontraining controls.[24]

Only two longitudinal studies in this area include proper controls. In one study, 12 weeks of endurance training (brisk walking to jogging) reduced platelet aggregability in middle-aged, overweight Finnish men.[25] In the other, 8 weeks of training (cycling) reduced platelet aggregability and adhesiveness in young Taiwanese men; this "benefit" disappeared after 12 weeks of detraining.[26] More research is needed to learn whether—and by what mechanisms, including changes in lipid profile[27]—regular exercise can reliably reduce platelet hyperreactivity.

Physical Activity and Fibrinolysis

Finally, physical activity clearly enhances fibrinolysis. Indeed, we have known for decades that exercise (or adrenaline) spurs fibrinolysis and that basal fibrinolysis tends to be brisk in active people but sluggish in obese or inactive people, mainly because the latter have elevated levels of the fibrinolytic inhibitor, PAI-1.[28]

Recent cross-sectional research finds the following: Obese children have high levels of PAI-1; fibrinolysis is impaired in sedentary diabetics; inactive men and women have higher PAI-1 levels than do physically active people; and PAI-1 levels correlate with fatness, especially upper-body obesity.[29,30] In fact, emerging studies seem to agree that elevated PAI-1 levels are part of the abdominal-obesity, insulin-resistance syndrome ("Syndrome X") that raises the risk of CVD.[31]

Longitudinal studies on physical training and fibrinolysis are few and poorly controlled, but as a group suggest that endurance training can enhance baseline fibrinolysis in diabetics and in healthy men and women.[32,33] It is clear that a vigorous exercise bout acutely increases fibrinolysis.[34]

During exercise, adrenaline and sheer stress from accelerated blood flow spur the vascular endothelium to release t-PA. Endothelial cells can also release PAI-1, but generally not in response to moderate exercise. Rather, endothelial cells tend to release PAI-1 in response to injury, thrombin, or inflammatory cytokines. So, regular physical activity would be expected to increase t-PA activity more than PAI-1 activity, and thus enhance baseline fibrinolysis.

Indeed, based on the few longitudinal studies, physical training seems to reduce baseline PAI-1 level.[33] This beneficial fall in PAI-1 seems to relate partly to a fall in blood triglycerides and/or to reversal of insulin resistance.[31] Some evidence suggests that dietary changes[35] or weight loss can also reduce PAI-1. More research is needed here, too.

Conclusion

All considered, it seems fair to conclude that the public can improve blood rheology and hemostatic function and thus reduce the risk of CVD by a lifestyle of prudent diet, weight control, and physical activity.

References

1. Wannamethee G, Shaper AG. Haematocrit: Relationships with blood lipids, blood pressure and other cardiovascular risk factors. *Thromb Haemostasis*, 1994; 72:58-64.

2. Wilhelmsen L, Svardsudd K, Korsan-Bengsten K et al. Fibrinogen as a risk factor for stroke and myocardial infarction. *N Engl J Med*, 1984; 311:501-05.

3. Kannel WM, Wolf PA, Castelli WP, D'Agostino RB. Fibrinogen and risk of cardiovascular disease. The Framingham Study. *JAMA*, 1987; 258:1183-86.

4. Ernst E, Resch KL. Fibrinogen as a cardiovascular risk factor: A meta-analysis and review of the literature. *Ann Intern Med*, 1993; 118:956-63.

5. Thompson SG, Kienast J, Pyke SDM et al. Hemostatic factors and the risk of myocardial infarction or sudden death in patients with angina pectoris. *N Engl J Med*, 1995; 332:635-41.

6. Eichner ER. Circadian rhythms: The latest word on health and performance. *Phys Sportsmed*, 1994; 22:82-93.

7. Trip MD, Cats VM, van Capelle FJL, Vreeken J. Platelet hyperreactivity and prognosis in survivors of myocardial infarction. *N Engl J Med*, 1990; 322:1549-54.

8. Thaulow E, Erikssen J, Sandvik L et al. Blood platelet count and function are related to total and cardiovascular death in apparently healthy men. *Circulation*, 1991; 84:613-17.

9. Hamsten A. Hemostatic function and coronary artery disease. *N Engl J Med*, 1995; 322:677-78.

10. Hamsten A, de Faire U, Walldium G et al. Plasminogen activator inhibitor in plasma: Risk factor for recurrent myocardial infarction. *Lancet*, 1987; 2:3-9.

11. Jansson JH, Olofsson BO, Nilsson TK. Predictive value of tissue plasminogen activator mass concentration on long-term mortality in patients with coronary artery disease: 7-year follow-up. *Circulation*, 1993; 88:2030-34.

12. Meade TW, Ruddock V, Stirlin Y et al. Fibrinolytic activity, clotting factors, and long-term incidence of ischaemic heart disease in Northwick Park Heart Study. *Lancet*, 1993; 342:1076-79.

13. Cortellaro M, Cofrancesco E, Boschetti C et al. Increased fibrin turnover and high PAI-1 activity as predictors of ischemic events in atherosclerotic patients. A case-control study. *Arterioscler Thromb*, 1993; 13:1412-17.

14. Ridker PM, Vaughan DE, Stampfer MJ et al. Endogenous tissue plasminogen activator and risk of myocardial infarction. *Lancet*, 1993; 341:1165-68.

15. Ridker PM, Hennekens CH, Stampfer MJ et al. Prospective study of endogenous tissue plasminogen activator and risk of stroke. *Lancet*, 1994; 343:940-43.

16. Andreotti F, Davies GJ, Hackett DR et al. Major circadian fluctuations in fibrinolytic factors and possible relevance to time of onset of myocardial infarction, sudden cardiac death and stroke. *Am J Cardiol*, 1988; 62:635-37.

17. Cadroy Y, Hanson SR. Effects of red blood cell concentration on hemostasis and thrombus formation in a primate model. *Blood*, 1990; 75:2185-93.

18. Turitto VT, Weiss HJ. Red blood cells: Their dual role in thrombus formation. *Science*, 1980; 207:541-43.

19. Eichner ER. Sports anemia, iron supplements, and blood doping. *Med Sci Sports Exercise*, 1992; 24:S315-18.

20. Selby GB, Eichner ER. Hematocrit and performance: Effect of endurance training on blood volume. *Semin Hematol*, 1994; 31:122-27.

21. Stefanick ML, Legault C, Tracy RP et al. Distribution and correlates of plasma fibrinogen in middle-aged women. *Arterioscler Thromb Vasc Biol*, 1995; 15:2085-93.

22. Stratton JR, Chandler WL, Schwartz RS et al. Effects of physical conditioning on fibrinolytic variables and fibrinogen in young and old healthy adults. *Circulation*, 1991; 83:1692-97.

23. El-Sayed MS, Davies B. A physical conditioning program does not alter fibrinogen concentration in young healthy subjects. *Med Sci Sports Exercise*, 1995; 27:485-89.

24. Davis RB, Boyd DG, McKinney ME, Jones CC. Effects of exercise and exercise conditioning on blood platelet function. *Med Sci Sports Exercise*, 1990; 22:49-53.

25. Rauramma R, Salonen JT, Seppanen K et al. Inhibition of platelet aggregability by moderate-intensity physical exercise: A randomized clinical trial in overweight men. *Circulation*, 1986; 74:939-44.

26. Wang J, Hen CJ, Chen H. Effects of exercise training and deconditioning on platelet function in men. *Arterioscler Thromb Vasc Biol*, 1995; 15:1668-74.

27. Lacoste L, Lam JYT, Hung J et al. Hyperlipidemia and coronary disease. Correction of the increased thrombogenic potential with cholesterol reduction. *Circulation*, 1995; 92:3172-77.

28. Chandler WL, Veith RC, Fellingham GW et al. Fibrinolytic response during exercise and epinephrine infusion in the same subjects. *J Am Coll Cardiol*, 1992; 19:1412-20.

29. Szymanski LM, Pate RR. Fibrinolytic responses to moderate intensity exercise. Comparison of physically active and inactive men. *Arterioscler Thromb*, 1994; 14:1746-50.

30. Szymanski LM, Pate RR, Durstine JL. Effects of maximal exercise and venous occlusion on fibrinolytic activity in physically active and inactive men. *J Appl Physiol*, 1994; 77:2305-10.

31. Vague P, Raccah D, Scelles V. Hypofibrinolysis and the insulin resistance syndrome. *Int J Obesity*, 1995; 19:S11-13.

32. Williams RS, Logue EE, Lewis JL et al. Physical conditioning augments the fibrinolytic response to venous occlusion in healthy adults. *N Engl J Med*, 1980; 302:987-91.

33. Gris JC, Schved JF, Feugeas O et al. Impact of smoking, physical training and weight reduction on FVII, PAI-1, and hemostatic markers in sedentary men. *Thromb Haemostasis*, 1990; 64:516-20.

34. Szymanski LM, Pate RR. Effects of exercise intensity, duration, and time of day on fibrinolytic activity in physically active men. *Med Sci Sports Exercise*, 1994; 26:1102-08.

35. Mehrabian M, Peter JB, Barnard RJ, Lusis AJ. Dietary regulation of fibrinolytic factors. *Atherosclerosis*, 1990; 84:25-32.

Effects of Physical Activity on Cardiovascular Disease Mortality Independent of Risk Factors

Steven N. Blair
Cooper Institute for Aerobics Research, Dallas, Texas, USA

Physical inactivity and low physical fitness increase risk for cardiovascular disease (CVD), whereas regular activity also has beneficial effects on other CVD risk factors. Both of these issues are examined in detail in other reports in this volume. The purposes of this chapter are to evaluate the independent effects of physical activity on CVD mortality and to characterize the relation between physical fitness or physical activity and CVD and all-cause mortality within and across strata of other factors, such as smoking habit, lipoprotein profile, blood pressure, glucose tolerance, family history of CVD, and body composition. Earlier reports on physical activity or physical fitness and CVD and all-cause mortality will be reviewed briefly, and recent analyses of the relation of physical fitness to mortality in various risk groups in the Aerobics Center Longitudinal Study will be presented.

Studies on both physical activity and cardiorespiratory fitness are included in this report. Most of the recent population-based studies evaluating the role of sedentary living habits in CVD used self-report of leisure-time physical activity as the exposure. These studies contribute much to understanding the important role of physical activity in the prevention of CVD, but have limitations due to the relatively imprecise assessment of activity patterns by their questionnaire methods. Cardiorespiratory fitness, defined here as aerobic power, can be measured objectively by exercise tests on ergometers, although there are obvious limitations in using these data as a marker for activity pattern. The inverse gradient of mortality risk across categories of physical fitness has a steeper slope than does the gradient across categories of physical activity; the relative risk (RR) of CVD mortality is approximately 2.0 when the least- and most-active groups are compared, and as high as 7.0 or more when the least-fit individuals are compared with the most-fit.[1]

Physical Inactivity or Low Cardiorespiratory Fitness as an Independent Risk Factor for Mortality

Virtually all recent mortality studies on cardiorespiratory activity or physical fitness include consideration of potentially confounding variables, such as blood pressure, blood glucose, lipid levels, family history, obesity, health status, and age.[2-4] The possible influence of these variables on the relation between activity or fitness and mortality typically was adjusted for in multivariable statistical models, with the results usually indicating an attenuation of the association, but still with significantly higher risk of dying in the sedentary or unfit groups.

Low physical fitness is one of the strongest independent predictors of all-cause mortality in the Aerobics Center Longitudinal Study. My research group recently reported mortality data from a follow-up of 25 341 men and 7 080 women.[5] There were 601 deaths during 211 996 man-years and 89 deaths during 52 982 woman-years of follow-up after a baseline clinical examination that included a maximal exercise test on a treadmill. All-cause relative risks, adjusted for age, examination year, and nine other mortality predictors, are shown in Figures 1 and 2.

The strongest precursors of mortality in men are low cardiorespiratory fitness, cigarette smoking, an abnormal electrocardiogram (ECG), and the presence of chronic disease at baseline. Elevated systolic blood pressure and serum cholesterol also were significant predictors, and elevated fasting blood glucose was of borderline significance. In women, of all the characteristics considered only low cardiorespiratory fitness and cigarette smoking were significant, and similar strength, mortality predictors. Adjustment for multiple precursors in this study attenuated the relative risk of low fitness. The age and exam year adjusted risk of low fitness was 2.03 in men and 2.23 in women. As shown in Figures 1 and 2, these risks dropped to 1.52 in men and 2.10 in women after additional adjustment for all other precursors included in the figures. The percent decline for risk of low fitness in the fully adjusted model was similar to the attenuation of risk seen in the other predictors in the fully adjusted model. The primary conclusions from this study are that low cardiorespiratory fitness is an independent predictor of all-cause mortality, is of similar strength to cigarette smoking, and may be a stronger predictor than elevated blood pressure or cholesterol.

Further evidence of the independent association of activity or fitness to mortality risk is available from recent studies on change in activity or fitness. In these reports, initially sedentary or unfit men who improved their status on these variables had a substantial reduction in mortality rates when compared with men who did not improve their activity or fitness.[2,4] Initially sedentary college alumni who increased their physical activity to 2,000 kcal/week in moderately vigorous sports had a 41% reduction risk of coronary heart disease (CHD) death when compared with men who remained sedentary.[4] Cooper Clinic men who initially were in the least-fit one-fifth of the population, but who had become at least moderately fit by the time of a subsequent examination, had an all-cause death rate about 60% lower than did unfit men who remained unfit.[2] These risk reductions with improvements in activity or fitness are comparable to the reduction in risk associated with stopping smoking, 44% and 50% for the two studies, respectively. These analyses included adjustment for age, family history of CHD, health status, and other risk factors. In summary, low activity or fitness appears to be an independent risk factor for CVD, and has a comparable effect on risk at least as great as do other established precursors of mortality.

Activity, Fitness, and Mortality Risk in Risk Subgroups

The studies briefly reviewed above confirm the independent role of activity or fitness as precursors for mortality as demonstrated by multivariable analysis tech-

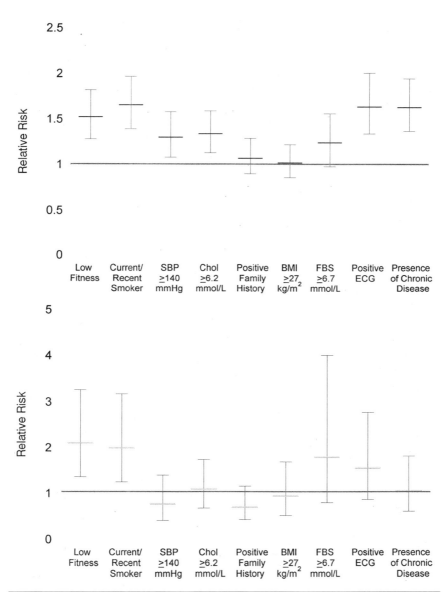

Figures 1 and 2.   Relative risks are adjusted for age, examination year, and each of the other characteristics in the figures. Low fitness is the least-fit one-fifth in each age group; current/recent smoker refers to those who smoked within the past two years; a positive family history indicates at least one parent dead of CHD; a positive ECG refers to an abnormal ECG (either at rest or during the exercise test); and presence of chronic disease refers to physician-diagnosed disease present at baseline (stroke, hypertension, CHD, diabetes, or cancer). Cut-points for other mortality predictors are indicated in the figure label. The relative risks are for the comparison of the high-risk category as specified with all others. The error bars indicate the 95% confidence intervals.[5]

niques. A more illustrative demonstration of these associations is seen in stratified analyses. Table 1 displays death rates across physical activity or cardiorespiratory fitness categories within strata of other mortality predictors for all-cause CVD or CHD. The intent of this presentation is to examine how the relation between activity or fitness and disease might differ for various profiles. Other standard precursors of mortality, such as obesity, cigarette smoking, high blood pressure, elevated cholesterol, and positive family history of CVD, are included. There is consistency across the different analyses and studies and for men and women. The general pattern of results indicates an inverse gradient of risk across categories of activity or fitness within various strata of individual mortality precursors.

Similar results are available from other publications for glucose intolerance and diabetes,[6] hypertension,[7] family history of hypertension,[8] and body stature.[8] The data presented here are from three large cohort studies on activity or fitness and disease where stratified analyses are published. Most other recent papers on this topic used multivariate adjustment for potential confounders rather than presenting stratified or cross-tabulation analyses, so it is not possible to determine if the results shown in the table are broadly representative. However, several reports on physical activity and incidence of non-insulin-dependent diabetes mellitus also show an inverse gradient of risk with higher levels of activity, especially in individuals at high risk.[9-11]

My colleagues and I recently conducted analyses in the Aerobics Center Longitudinal Study specifically to evaluate the relation of cardiorespiratory fitness to all-cause mortality in low and high risk strata of other precursors of mortality.[5] There were similar inverse gradients for all-cause death rates across low, moderate, and high categories of cardiorespiratory fitness in smokers and nonsmokers and for men and women in low and high risk strata for systolic blood pressure or cholesterol. Figure 3 shows comparable analyses in men for low and high risk strata for parental history of CHD, body mass index, fasting blood glucose, and baseline health status. The death rates are adjusted for age, examination year, and other mortality predictors. There were too few deaths in many of the cells to perform the same analyses for women. The results in Figure 3 show lower death rates in moderate- and high-fit men when compared with low-fit men in both low and high risk strata of the other characteristics. The linear trends are significant for all analyses, indicating that cardiorespiratory fitness appears to delay death in men regardless of their parental history of CHD, body mass index, fasting blood glucose value, or status of health at baseline. The consistency of the results shown here, and those published earlier,[5] make it unlikely that the inverse association between fitness and mortality is due to confounding by conventional mortality predictors.

Additional evidence for the strength of low cardiorespiratory fitness as a precursor of mortality is shown in Figure 4. These data indicate that the inverse gradient of death rates across fitness categories shown earlier persists when combinations of mortality predictors are used to assign men and women to risk strata. The other three major mortality predictors—elevated blood pressure or cholesterol, or cigarette smoking—were used in these analyses. Whether men had none of these

Table 1.   Cardiovascular Disease or All-Cause Death Rates Across Physical-Activity or Physical-Fitness Categories Within Various Risk Factor Subgroups

Study risk factor	Activity or fitness category[a]			
	1 (low)	2	3	4 (high)
British Civil Servants (9,376 men, fatal and nonfatal CHD)[3]				
Family history				
Parent(s) alive	5.7[b]	5.1	4.2	2.0
Parents(s) died CVD	8.8	6.5	6.8	3.6
Cigarette smoking				
Never	5.7	4.5	3.2	2.2
Ex-smoker	4.6	4.7	3.9	1.8
Current	8.7	7.1	4.8	2.8
Body mass index (kg/m^2)				
< 24	5.5	4.3	3.5	1.9
24-26.9	6.2	5.7	6.0	2.4
≥ 27	7.3	7.1	4.8	1.3
Harvard Alumni Study (16,936 men, all-cause mortality)[12]				
Family history, parents died before age 65				
Neither	90[c]	63	46	
One	102	79	69	
Both	93	80	71	
Blood-pressure status				
Hypertensive as an adult	173	117	79	
College SBP < 130 mmHg	79	59	50	
College SBP ≥ 130 mmHg	77	69	60	
Cigarette smoking				
None	79	54	44	
< 20/day	104	71	41	
≥ 20/day	136	113	91	

(continued)

characteristics (front row of the top panel of Figure 4) or had any two or all three of these characteristics (back row of top panel), death rates were progressively lower for moderate and high fitness categories when compared with the low fit. In fact, high-fit men with any two or all three of these characteristics had a lower death

Table 1. *(continued)*

Study risk factor	Activity or fitness category[a]			
	1 (low)	2	3	4 (high)
Aerobics Center Longitudinal Study (ACLS)				
(3,120 women, all-cause mortality)[13]				
Family history of CHD death				
No	50[d]	9	5	
Yes	37	19	8	
Cigarette smoking				
Never	25	13	5	
Ex-smoker	50	11	10	
Current	57	23	22	
Systolic blood pressure (mmHg)				
< 120	32	16	8	
120-140	38	19	6	
> 140	347	19	0	
Cholesterol level (mmol/L)				
< 5.20	19	11	7	
5.20-6.75	40	24	5	
>6.75	83	5	25	
ACLS				
(10,224 men, all-cause mortality)[13]				
Family history of CHD death				
No	57[c]	16	18	
Yes	66	30	21	
Cigarette smoking				
Never	26	16	16	
Ex-smoker	44	13	19	
Current	80	47	41	
Systolic blood pressure (mmHg)				
< 120	60	19	20	
120-140	76	28	20	
> 140	54	29	24	
Cholesterol level (mmol/L)				
< 5.20	68	17	14	
5.20-6.75	53	29	28	
>6.75	95	54	27	

Study risk factor	Activity or fitness category[a]			
	1 (low)	2	3	4 (high)
ACLS				
(25389 men, all-cause mortality)[14]				
Body mass index (kg/m²)				
< 27	52[c]	29	20	
27-30	49	30	20	
>30	62	18		

[a]Number of categories range from 2 to 4 across the various studies. British Civil Servants and Harvard Alumni study categories are of physical activity. ACLS categories are of physical fitness based on a maximal exercise test on a treadmill. Categories are not comparable across studies. For example, category 3 (top category) in the Harvard Alumni Study may indicate as much physical activity as category 4 (top category) in the British Civil Servants Study. The activity and fitness categories should be viewed as an index rather than a specific amount. [b]Rate per 1,000 man-years. [c]Age-adjusted rate per 10,000 man-years. [d]Age-adjusted rate per 10,000 woman-years. [e]Unpublished data. [f]Number of other risk factors. Risk factors and cut-points were any cigarette smoking, systolic blood pressure ≥ 140 mmHg, total cholesterol ≥ 6.2 mmol/L.

rate than did low-fit men with none of the mortality predictors. Although a smaller number of deaths required combining moderate and high fitness categories in women, a similar pattern of results is seen as shown for men. Fit women in all risk strata had lower death rates than did low-fit women, and fit women with any two or all three mortality precursors had lower death rates than did low-fit women with none of these characteristics.

Multivariable adjustment also attentuates the relative risks for other characteristics, such as cigarette smoking, elevated blood or cholesterol, family history of premature disease, and presence of chronic disease. However, after multivariable adjustment, low cardiorespiratory fitness is one of the strongest predictors of mortality.

Summary

The association of physical activity or cardiorespiratory fitness to all-cause and CVD mortality is not likely to be due to confounding by other well-established mortality predictors. Multivariable adjustment for an extensive list of potential confounders frequently reduces the strength of the activity-disease relation, but does not eliminate it. Stratified analyses show similar inverse gradients of disease risk across categories of activity or fitness in men and women at low, moderate, and high risk for CVD, based on their other risk characteristics. An active and fit way of life appears to attenuate the force of these other predictors on mortality.

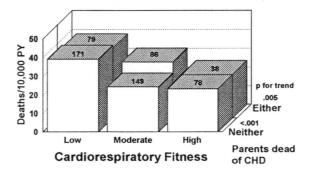

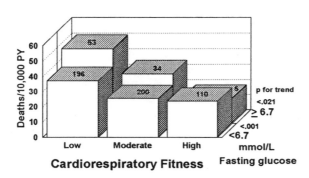

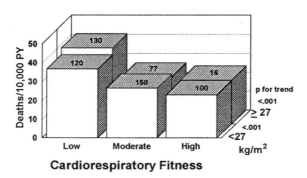

(continued)

Figure 3. Categories of cardiorespiratory fitness and all-cause mortality by strata of family history of CHD, body mass index (kg/m²), fasting blood glucose, and health status (positive resting or exercise ECG, CHD, stroke, hypertension, diabetes, or cancer) in 25,341 men in the Aerobics Center Longitudinal Study. Height of the bars shows the all-cause death rates adjusted for age, year of baseline examination, systolic blood pressure, total serum cholesterol, cigarette smoking habit, and each of the other characteristics in the figure. Numbers atop the bars represent the number of deaths. The p values are for a test of trend across cardiorespiratory fitness categories (low fitness = least-fit 20%, moderate fitness = next 40%, and high fitness = most-fit 40%).

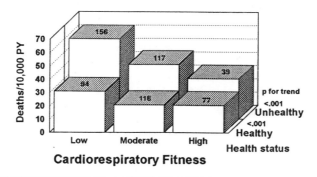

Figure 3.   *(continued)*

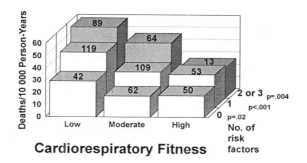

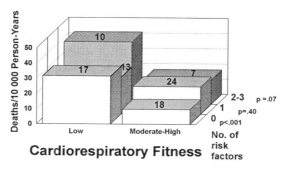

Figure 4.   Cardiorespiratory fitness and all-cause mortality by the number of multiple mortality predictors in 25 341 men (top panel) and 7 080 women (bottom panel) in the Aerobics Center Longitudinal Study. Height of the bars shows all-cause death rates adjusted for age, year of baseline examination, chronic illness (CHD, stroke, hypertension, diabetes, or cancer), abnormal resting or exercise ECG, parental history of CHD death, fasting blood glucose, and body mass index. Numbers atop the bars indicate the number of deaths. Cardiorespiratory fitness categories for men are low fitness = least-fit 20%, moderate fitness = next 40%, and high fitness = most-fit 40%; for women the moderate and high fitness categories are combined. The three categories of multiple mortality predictors are none, any one, and any two or all three among current or recent smoking, total cholesterol >6.2 mmol/L, and systolic blood pressure >140 mmHg.[5]

References

1. Blair SN. Physical activity, fitness, and coronary heart disease. In Bouchard C, Shephard RJ, Stephens T (Eds): *Physical activity, fitness, and health: International proceedings and consensus statement.* Champaign, IL,: Human Kinetics, 1994; 579-590.

2. Blair SN, Kohl HW III, Barlow CE, Paffenbarger RS Jr, Gibbons LW, Macera CA. Changes in physical fitness and all-cause mortality: A prospective study of healthy and unhealthy men. *JAMA*, 1995; 273:1093-1098.

3. Morris JN, Clayton DG, Everitt MG, Semmence AM, Burgess EH. Exercise in leisure time: Coronary attack and death rates. *Br Heart J*, 1990; 63:325-334.

4. Paffenbarger RS Jr, Hyde RT, Wing AL, Lee I, Jung DL, Kampert JB. The association of changes in physical-activity level and other lifestyle characteristics with mortality among men. *N Engl J Med*, 1993; 328:538-545.

5. Blair SN, Kampert JB, Kohl HW III, Barlow CE, Macera CA, Paffenbarger RS Jr, Gibbons LW. Influences of cardiorespiratory fitness and other precursors on cardiovascular disease and all-cause mortality in men and women. *JAMA*, 1996; 276:205-210.

6. Kohl HW, Gordon NF, Villegas JA, Blair SN. Cardiorespiratory fitness, glycemic status, and mortality risk in men. *Diabetes Care*, 1992; 15:184-192.

7. Blair SN, Kohl HW, Barlow CE. Physical fitness and all-cause mortality in hypertensive men. *Ann Med*, 1991; 23:307-312.

8. Paffenbarger RS Jr, Wing AL, Hyde RT. Physical activity as an index of heart attack risk in college alumni. *Am J Epidemiol*, 1978; 108:161-175.

9. Helmrich SP, Ragland DR, Leung RW, Paffenbarger RS Jr. Physical activity and reduced occurrence of non-insulin-dependent diabetes mellitus. *N Engl J Med*, 1991; 325:147-152.

10. Manson JE, Nathan DM, Krolewski AS, Stampfer MJ, Willett WC, Hennekens CH. A prospective study of exercise and incidence of diabetes among US male physicians. *JAMA*, 1992; 268:63-67.

11. Manson JE, Rimm EB, Stampfer MJ, Colditz GA, Willett WC, Krolewski AS et al. Physical activity and incidence of non-insulin-dependent diabetes mellitus in women. *Lancet*, 1991; 338:774-778.

12. Paffenbarger RS Jr, Hyde RT, Wing AL, Hsieh CC. Physical activity, all-cause mortality, and longevity of college alumni. *N Engl J Med*, 1986; 314:605-613.

13. Blair SN, Kohl HW, III, Paffenbarger RS Jr, Clark DG, Cooper KH, Gibbons LW. Physical fitness and all-cause mortality: A prospective study of healthy men and women. *JAMA*, 1989; 262:2395-2401.

14. Barlow CE, Kohl HW III, Gibbons LW, Blair SN. Physical fitness, mortality and obesity. *Int J Obesity*, 1995; 19(Suppl 4):S41-S44.

The Cardiac Risks of Vigorous Physical Activity

Paul D. Thompson and Geoffrey E. Moore
University of Pittsburgh Heart Institute, Pittsburgh, Pennsylvania, USA

Causes of Sudden Death During Physical Exertion

Atherosclerotic coronary artery disease is the major cause of exercise-related sudden death during exercise in adults.[1] Cardiomyopathies,[2,3] cerebrovascular events, and aortic dissection[1] also occasionally cause exercise-related deaths in this age group. Among previously asymptomatic subjects dying from coronary disease during exertion, there is usually evidence of atherosclerotic plaque rupture and acute coronary artery thrombosis.[4-6] Among previously asymptomatic survivors of an exercise-related myocardial infarction (MI), coronary angiography often demonstrates coronary thrombosis or an eccentric atherosclerotic plaque consistent with prior plaque rupture.[6,7] In contrast, patients with diagnosed coronary disease who die during exertion often lack evidence of an acute coronary event,[8] suggesting that ventricular fibrillation arising from scarred myocardium is the proximate cause of death.

Whereas acquired heart disease is the primary cause of exertion-related deaths in adults, congenital cardiac abnormalities are the primary cause of exercise-related cardiac deaths in young people.[9-11] Definite or probable hypertrophic cardiomyopathy (HCM) causes the majority of these deaths. Coronary artery anomalies, myocarditis, aortic stenosis, and dilated cardiomyopathy cause most of the remaining deaths.[10]

Several reports suggest that there is an excess of sudden deaths during exertion due to rhabdomyolysis in individuals with sickle cell trait.[11,12] One report examined deaths during basic training in 2 million US military recruits between 1977 and 1981.[12] All of the sudden deaths unexplained by prior disease were related to physical exertion and were caused by cardiac events, heat illness, or exertional rhabdomyolysis. The relative risk of sudden, unexplained death among African Americans with sickle cell trait was 27 times higher than in African Americans without sickle cell trait and 40 times higher than in other races. Extreme exertion in physically untrained subjects, such as military recruits, could induce hypoxia, lactic acidosis, red cell sickling, and ultimately rhabdomyolysis.[13]

The Risk of Exercise

Since the incidence of occult heart disease varies among populations, the risk of exercise also varies with the population studied. Most studies of exercise-related cardiac death are based on few events so that minor variance in the numerator can greatly alter the estimate. Few studies have examined well-defined, unselected populations, and results from selected populations are not applicable to the general population.

Nevertheless, an estimated 0.75 per 100,000 men and 0.13 per 100,000 women die during high school and college athletics per year.[11] This yields an absolute death rate of one per 133,000 men and per 769,000 women. These estimates include all sports-related nontraumatic deaths and are not restricted to cardiac events. The absolute death rate in African Americans with sickle cell trait during 8 to 11 weeks of basic training was one death for every 3,105 recruits or 32 per 100,000 individuals.[12] This yields an annual rate of one death for every 478 to 660 recruits, which is a remarkably high rate.

The annual incidence of exercise-related cardiac arrests among previously healthy adults in Seattle has been estimated as 5.4 deaths per 100,000 individuals or one for every 18,000 active men.[14] A similar incidence of one death per 15,000 previously healthy joggers has been estimated in Rhode Island,[15] but this study assumed that Rhode Island men with known heart disease did not jog. Only 9[14] and 10[15] deaths were reported in these studies, so confidence limits are wide. In Rhode Island, for example, the 95% confidence limits suggest that one death during jogging will occur per year for every 4,000 to 26,000 asymptomatic men.[15]

Both of the studies conclude that exercise transiently increases the risk of sudden cardiac death.[14,15] The relative risk of sudden death was sevenfold higher during jogging than during other activities in Rhode Island.[15] The incidence of cardiac arrest in Seattle was 56 times higher during vigorous exercise for men who rarely exercised and 5 times higher for men who regularly exercised.[14] This apparently protective effect of regular exercise may be misleading, however, because it is based on the risk per person-hours of exercise. Men exercising more hours, therefore, could have lower death rates per hour of exercise, but similar absolute death rates during exercise.

The risk of myocardial infarction is also increased two to six times during vigorous exercise than during other activities,[16,17] although no studies to our knowledge provide an absolute incidence of MI during exercise in healthy individuals. The absolute incidence of MI during exertion has been estimated as one per year per 2,142 to 2,571 exercising men,[18] with 95% confidence limits of one per 571 to 3,714 men. This risk is consistent with reports that 4% to 20% of acute MIs are associated with moderate or heavy physical exertion.[16,17]

Preventing Exercise-Related Acute Cardiac Events

The prevention of exercise-related sudden deaths is difficult. Routine cardiovascular testing using echocardiography has been advocated to detect hypertrophic cardiomyopathy, the leading cause of exercise-related sudden deaths in young subjects. Five studies[19-23] examined 5,458 high school and collegiate athletes, using screening echocardiography. No cases of hypertrophic cardiomyopathy were detected. Approximately 11 cases would be expected, given the population prevalence of hypertrophic cardiomyopathy of approximately 0.2%.[24]

Similar problems plague routine exercise testing to screen exercising adults. The American College of Sports Medicine recommends that high-risk individuals undergo exercise stress testing prior to vigorous exercise.[25] The high-risk classification includes men over 40 and women over 50 years of age, individuals with more than one coronary disease risk factor, and those with known coronary disease.[25] The American Heart Association, however, considers exercise testing prior to exercise programs as controversial.[26]

Exercise testing in asymptomatic adults is a poor predictor of the major cardiac complications during exercise, acute myocardial infarction, and sudden cardiac death. A true positive exercise test requires a hemodynamically significant coronary obstruction, whereas acute coronary events often involve plaque rupture and thrombosis at the site of previously nonobstructive atherosclerotic plaque.[27]

Studies evaluating the utility of exercise testing in ostensibly healthy populations support this hypothesis. McHenry et al. reported a study of 916 Indiana State Troopers who underwent maximal exercise tests, had repeat testing at intervals of one to five years, and were followed for a mean of 12.7 years.[28] Only 61 men (6.6%) ever demonstrated a positive ECG response to exercise. Of these, 21 (32%) developed clinical signs of coronary disease—including angina pectoris in 18, an acute MI in 1, and sudden death in 1. An additional asymptomatic man underwent coronary bypass surgery. Among the 833 men with normal ECG responses, only 44 (5%) subsequently developed clinical coronary disease: 25 developed an infarct, 7 died suddenly, and 12 developed angina. These data suggest that a positive exercise test identifies individuals with hemodynamically significant coronary lesions, but that these lesions are often tolerated until the appearance of angina.

Screening only individuals at high risk produces similar results. Exercise testing was used to screen for heart disease in 3,617 men participating in the Lipid Research Clinics Primary Prevention Trial.[29] All men had prerandomization low density lipoprotein cholesterol values above 4.91 (190) mmol/L (mg/dl). Exercise tests to 90% of age-predicted maximal heart rate were performed at baseline and annually thereafter. Sixty-two men developed an exercise-related event: 54 acute myocardial infarctions and eight sudden deaths. Only 11 of the 62 events occurred in men with a positive exercise test. The predictive value of a positive exercise test for an acute exercise event was only 4%, in part because such events are rare. The authors concluded that routine exercise testing is not effective in preventing acute cardiac events even in high-risk populations.

Recommendations

Despite the problems with routine testing, we do recommend that all young athletes undergo a brief cardiovascular exam by a practitioner who is aware of those conditions causing exercise-related cardiac events.[30] Many of the conditions associated with sudden death in athletes can be detected by simple inspection and cardiac auscultation. The examination should look for the connective tissue stigmata of Marfan's Syndrome. Cardiac auscultation should be done with subjects sitting or standing to reduce ventricular volume and thereby maximize the chance of eliciting the murmur of hypertrophic cardiomyopathy. The Valsalva maneuver also reduces ventricular volume and augments the murmur of hypertrophic cardiomyopathy. Athletes with possible abnormalities should undergo further evaluation. Guidelines exist for determining eligibility for athletic participation.[31]

Practitioners should inform exercising adults of the nature of prodromal cardiac symptoms, especially the fact that cardiac discomfort is often not perceived as "pain" but as discomfort, tightness, or heartburn. New symptoms of exercise intolerance, such as exertional syncope, unusual dyspnea, and chest discomfort, should be carefully evaluated in athletes of all ages. Many victims of exercise-related events complained of symptoms which they or their physicians ignored.[5]

Suggested Future Research

Compared to the number of studies on the cardiovascular benefits of physical activity, there are relatively few studies on the risks of exercise. Nevertheless, these risks remain a major concern for practitioners who often fear legal liability for failing to detect cardiac abnormalities. Additional research emphasis should be placed on the risk side of the exercise risk/benefit equation.

Population-based surveillance studies are needed to define more explicitly the cardiovascular risks of exercise and to identify population subgroups who bear an increased exercise risk. For example, diabetics appear to have an increased risk of exercise-related MI,[17] possibly because their more diffusely atherosclerotic coronary arteries are less compliant and more susceptible to plaque rupture. There may also be subpopulations where the risks outweigh the benefits of exercise. Better studies are also needed to identify the dose-response relationship between exertion and cardiovascular disease risk, since it is reasonable that lower levels of activity will be associated with fewer cardiac complications.

References

1. Ragosta M, Crabtree J, Sturner WQ, Thompson PD. Death during recreational exercise in the state of Rhode Island. *Med Sci Sports Exercise*, 1984;16:339-342.

2. Siegel RJ, French WJ, Roberts WC. Spontaneous exercise testing: Running as an early unmasker of underlying cardiac amyloidosis. *Arch Int Med*, 1982;142:345.

3. Waller BF. Exercise-related sudden death in young (age <30 years) and old (age >30 years) conditioned subjects. In Wenger NK (Ed.): *Exercise and the heart*. Philadelphia: F.A. Davis, 1985, 9-73.

4. Black A, Black MM, Gensini G. Exertion and acute coronary artery injury. *Angiology*, 1975;26:759-783.

5. Thompson PD, Stern MP, Williams P et al. Death during jogging or running: A study of 18 cases. *JAMA*, 1979;242:1265-1267.

6. Ciampricotti R, Gamal MIH, Bonnier JJ, Relik THFM. Myocardial infartion and sudden death after sport: Acute coronary angiographic findings. *Catheterization and Cardiovascular Diagnosis*, 1989;17:193-197.

7. Richardson PD, Davies MJ, Born GVR. Influence of plaque configuration and stress distribution on fissuring of coronary atherosclerotic plaques. *Lancet*, 1989;2:941-944.

8. Cobb LA, Weaver WD. Exercise: A risk for sudden death in patients with coronary heart disease. *J Am Coll Cardiol*, 1986;7:215-219.

9. Maron BJ, Roberts WC, McAllister HA, Rosing DR, Epstein SE. Sudden death in young athletes. *Circulation*, 1980;62:218-229.

10. Burke AP, Farb A, Virmani R, Goodin J, Smialek JE. Sports-related and non-sports-related sudden cardiac death in young adults. *Am Heart J*, 1991;121:568-575.

11. Van Camp SP, Bloor CM, Mueller FO, Cantu RC, Olson HG. Nontraumatic sports death in high school and college athletes. *Med Sci Sports Exercise*, 1995;27:641-647.

12. Kark JA, Posey DM, Schumacher HR, Ruehle CJ. Sickle-cell trait as a risk factor for sudden death in physical training. *N Engl J Med*, 1987;317:781-787.

13. Eichner ER. Sickle cell trait, heroic exercise, and fatal collapse. *Phys and Sports Med*, 1993;21:51-64.

14. Siscovick DS, Weiss NS, Fletcher RH, Lasky T. The incidence of primary cardiac arrest during vigorous exercise. *N Engl J Med*, 1984;311:874-877.

15. Thompson PD, Funk EJ, Carleton RA, Sturner WQ. Incidence of death during jogging in Rhode Island from 1975 through 1980. *JAMA*, 1982;247:2535-2538.

16. Willich SN, Lewis M, Lowell H et al. Physical exertion as a trigger of acute myocardial infarction. *N Engl J Med*, 1993;329:1684-1690.

17. Mittleman MA, Maclure M, Tofler GH et al. Triggering of acute myocardial infarction by heavy exertion: Protection against triggering by regular exercise. *N Engl J Med*, 1993;329:1677-1683.

18. Thompson PD. The relative risk of myocardial infarction during exercise. In Fletcher GF (Ed.): *Cardiovascular response to exercise*. Mount Kisco, NY: Futura, 1994, 291-300.

19. Maron BJ, Bodison SA, Wesley YE, Tucker E, Green KJ. Results of screening a large group of intercollegiate athletes for cardiovascular disease. *J Am Coll Cardiol*, 1987;10:1214-1221.

20. Lewis JF, Maron BJ, Diggs JA et al. Preparticipation echocardiographic screening for cardiovascular disease in a large, predominantly black population of collegiate athletes. *Am J Cardiol*, 1989;64:1029-1033.

21. Murray PM, Cantwell JD, Heath DL, Shoop J. The role of limited echocardiography in screening athletes. *Am J Cardiol*, 1995;76:849-850.

22. Feinstein RA, Colvin E, Kim OM. Echocardiographic screening as part of a preparticipation examination. *Clin J Sports Med*, 1993;3:149-152.

23. Weidenbener EJ, Krauss MD, Waller BF, Taliercio CP. Incorporation of screening echocardiography in the preparticipation exam. *Clin J Sports Med*, 1995;5:86-89.

24. Maron BJ, Gardin JM, Gidding SS, Kurosaki TT, Bild DE. Prevalence of hypertrophic cardiomyopathy in a general population of young adults: Echocardiographic analysis of 4 111 subjects in the CARDIA study. *Circulation*, 1995;92:785-789.

25. Mahler DA, Froerlicher VF, Miller NH, York TD. *ACSM's guidelines for exercise testing and prescription*. 5th edition. Philadelphia, PA: A. Waverly, 1995, 5.

26. Schlant RC, Blomqvist CG, Brandenburg RO et al. Guidelines for exercise testing: A report of the Joint American College of Cardiology/American Heart Association Task Force on assessment of cardiovascular procedures (subcommittee on exercise testing). *Circulation*, 1986;74:653A-667A.

27. Little WC, Constantinescu M, Applegate RJ et al. Can coronary angiography predict the site of a subsequent myocardial infarction in patients with mild-to-moderate coronary artery diseae? *Circulation*, 1988;78:1157-1166.

28. McHenry PL, O'Donnell J, Morris SN, Jordan JJ. The abnormal exercise electrocardiogram in apparently healthy men: A predictor of angina pectoris as an initial coronary event during long-term follow-up. *Circulation*, 1984;70:547-551.

29. Siscovick DS, Ekelund LG, Johnson JL, Truong Y, Adler A. Sensitivity of exercise electrocardiography for acute cardiac events during moderate and strenuous physical activity: The Lipid Research Clinics Coronary Primary Prevention Trial. *Arch Int Med*, 1991;151:325-330.

30. Fahrenbach MC, Thompson PD. The preparticipation sports examination: Cardiovascular considerations for screening. *Cardiology Clinics*, 1992;10:319-328.

31. Maron BJ, Mitchell JH. 26th Bethesda Conference: Recommendations for determining eligibility for competition in athletes with cardiovascular abnormalities. *J Am Coll Cardiol*, 1994;24:845-899.

Part V

SECONDARY PREVENTION OF CARDIOVASCULAR DISEASE AND CARDIAC REHABILITATION

Cardiac Rehabilitation as Secondary Prevention: A Synopsis of the Clinical Practice Guideline for Cardiac Rehabilitation

L. Kent Smith
Arizona Heart Institute and Foundation for the Guideline Expert Panel, Phoenix, Arizona, USA

Cardiovascular disease is the leading cause of morbidity and mortality in the United States, accounting for over 50% of all deaths. Coronary heart disease (CHD), with its clinical manifestations of stable angina pectoris, unstable angina, acute myocardial infarction, and sudden cardiac death, affects 13.5 million Americans. The almost 1 million annual survivors of myocardial infarction and the 7 million patients with stable angina pectoris are candidates for cardiac rehabilitation, as are the more than 300,000 patients who undergo coronary artery bypass graft (CABG) surgery and the 360,000 patients who undergo percutaneous transluminal coronary angioplasty (PTCA) and other transcatheter procedures each year. An estimated 4.7 million patients with heart failure may also be eligible. Although beneficial outcomes from cardiac rehabilitation services can be expected in most of these patients, only about 20% of such patients currently participate in cardiac rehabilitation programs.[1]

Definition

The US Public Health Service definition of cardiac rehabilitation, used by the guideline, states that "cardiac rehabilitation services are comprehensive, long-term programs involving medical evaluation, prescribed exercise, cardiac risk factor modification, education, and counseling. These programs are designed to limit the physiologic and psychological effects of cardiac illness, reduce the risk for sudden death or reinfarction, control cardiac symptoms, stabilize or reverse the atherosclerotic process, and enhance the psychosocial and vocational status of selected patients." This guideline provides recommendations for cardiac rehabilitation services for patients with CHD and with heart failure, including those following cardiac transplantation.

Purpose of Guideline

This guideline is designed for use by health practitioners who provide care to patients with cardiovascular disease. These include physicians (primary care, cardiologists, and cardiovascular surgeons), nurses, exercise physiologists, dietitians, behavioral medicine specialists, psychologists, and physical and occupational thera-pists. The information can guide clinical decision making regarding referral and follow-up of patients for cardiac rehabilitation services, as well as administrative decisions regarding the availability of and access to cardiac rehabilitation services.

This guideline details the outcomes that result from cardiac rehabilitation ser-vices. The interventions examined involve two parallel applications: (1) exercise training and (2) education, counseling, and behavioral interventions. The guide-line emphasizes the added effectiveness of multifactorial cardiac rehabilitation services integrated in a comprehensive approach.

Outcomes of Cardiac Rehabilitation Services

Exercise tolerance.   Cardiac rehabilitation exercise training consistently improves objective measures of exercise tolerance, without significant cardiovascular com-plications or other adverse outcomes. Appropriately prescribed and conducted ex-ercise training is recommended as an integral component of cardiac rehabilitation services, particularly for patients with decreased exercise tolerance. Continued exercise training is required to sustain improved exercise tolerance.[2]

Strength training.   Strength training improves skeletal muscle strength and en-durance in clinically stable coronary patients. Training measures designed to in-crease skeletal muscle strength can safely be included in the exercise-based reha-bilitation of clinically stable coronary patients, when appropriate instruction and surveillance are provided.[3]

Exercise habits.   Cardiac rehabilitation exercise training promotes increased par-ticipation in exercise by patients after myocardial infarction and coronary artery bypass surgery. This effect does not persist long-term after completion of exercise rehabilitation. Long-term exercise training is recommended to provide the benefit of enhanced exercise tolerance and exercise habits.[4]

Symptoms.   Exercise rehabilitation decreases angina pectoris in patients with CHD and decreases symptoms of heart failure in patients with left ventricular sys-tolic dysfunction.[5] Exercise training is recommended as an integral component of the symptomatic management of these patients. Symptoms of angina pectoris are also reduced by cardiac rehabilitation education, counseling, and behavioral inter-ventions alone or as a component of multifactorial cardiac rehabilitation.

Smoking.   A combined approach of cardiac rehabilitation education, counseling, and behavioral interventions results in smoking cessation and relapse prevention.[6] Smoking cessation and relapse prevention programs should be offered to patients who are smokers to reduce their risk of subsequent coronary events. Smoking cessation is achieved by specific smoking cessation strategies.

Lipids.   Intensive nutrition education, counseling, and behavioral interventions improve dietary fat and cholesterol intake. Education, counseling, and behavioral interventions about nutrition—with and without pharmacologic lipid-lowering therapy—result in significant improvement in blood lipid levels and are recommended as a component of cardiac rehabilitation. Optimal lipid management requires specifically directed dietary and, as medically indicated, pharmacologic management, in addition to cardiac rehabilitation exercise training.[7]

Body weight.   Multifactorial cardiac rehabilitation that combines dietary education, counseling, and behavioral interventions designed to reduce body weight can help patients lose weight. Education or cardiac rehabilitation exercise training as sole interventions are unlikely to achieve and maintain weight loss. The optimal management for overweight patients to promote maintenance of weight loss requires multifactorial rehabilitation, including nutrition education and counseling and behavioral modification, in addition to exercise training.[8]

Blood pressure.   Expert opinion supports a multifactorial education, counseling, behavioral, and pharmacologic approach as the recommended strategy for the control of hypertension. This approach is documented to be effective in nonrehabilitation populations. Neither education, counseling, and behavioral interventions nor cardiac rehabilitation exercise training as sole interventions have been shown to control elevated blood pressure levels.

Psychological well-being.   Education, counseling and/or psychosocial interventions, either alone or as a component of multifactorial cardiac rehabilitation, result in improved psychological well-being and are recommended to complement the psychosocial benefits of exercise training.[9]

Social adjustment and functioning.   Cardiac rehabilitation exercise training improves social adjustment and functioning and is recommended to improve social outcomes.

Return to work.   Cardiac rehabilitation exercise training exerts less of an influence on rates of return to work than many nonexercise variables, including employer attitudes, prior employment status, economic incentives, and the like. Exercise training as a sole intervention is not recommended to facilitate return to work. Nor have education, counseling, and behavioral interventions resulted in improvement in rates of return to work. Many patients return to work without formal interventions. However, in selected patients, formal cardiac rehabilitation vocational counseling may improve rates of return to work.

Morbidity and safety issues.   The safety of exercise rehabilitation is well established; rates of myocardial infarction and cardiovascular complications during exercise training are very low.[10] Cardiac rehabilitation exercise training does not change rates of nonfatal reinfarction.[11] Education, counseling, and behavioral interventions, as components of multifactorial cardiac rehabilitation, may decrease progression of coronary atherosclerosis and lower recurrent coronary event rates.

Mortality and Safety Issues: Based on meta-analyses, total and cardiovascular mortality are reduced in patients following myocardial infarction who participate in cardiac rehabilitation exercise training, especially as a component of multifactorial rehabilitation. Education, counseling, and behavioral interventions reduce cardiac and overall mortality rates and are recommended in the multifactorial rehabilitation of patients with CHD.[12]

Pathophysiologic measures, coronary atherosclerosis.   Cardiac rehabilitation exercise training as a sole intervention does not result in regression or limitation of progression of angiographically documented coronary atherosclerosis. Exercise training, combined with intensive dietary intervention, with and without lipid-lowering drugs, results in regression or limitation of progression of angiographically documented coronary atherosclerosis and is recommended.[2]

Hemodynamic measurements.   Cardiac rehabilitation exercise training has no apparent effect on development of coronary collateral circulation and produces no consistent changes in cardiac hemodynamic measurements at cardiac catheterization. Exercise training in patients with heart failure and a decreased ventricular ejection fraction produces favorable hemodynamic changes in the skeletal musculature and is recommended to improve skeletal muscle functioning.

Myocardial perfusion and/or evidence of myocardial ischemia.   Cardiac rehabilitation exercise training decreases myocardial ischemia as measured by exercise ECG, ambulatory ECG recording, and radionuclide perfusion imaging and is recommended to improve these measures of myocardial ischemia.[13]

Myocardial contractility, ventricular wall motion abnormalities, and/or ventricular ejection fraction.   Cardiac rehabilitation exercise training has little effect on ventricular ejection fraction and regional wall motion abnormalities and is not recommended to improve measures of ventricular systolic function. The effect of exercise training on left ventricular function in patients after anterior Q wave myocardial infarction with left ventricular dysfunction is inconsistent.

Occurrence of cardiac arrhythmias.   Cardiac rehabilitation exercise training has inconsistent effects on ventricular arrhythmias.

Effects of Cardiac Rehabilitation Services on Special Populations

Patients with heart failure and cardiac transplantation.   Cardiac rehabilitation exercise training in patients with heart failure and moderate-to-severe left ventricular systolic dysfunction improves functional capacity and symptoms, without changes in left ventricular function,[14] and is recommended to attain functional and symptomatic improvement. Such training in patients following cardiac transplantation improves measures of exercise tolerance and is recommended for this purpose.

Elderly patients.   Elderly coronary patients have exercise trainability comparable to younger patients participating in similar cardiac rehabilitation exercise training.[15] Elderly female and male patients show comparable improvement. Referral to, and participation in, exercise rehabilitation is less frequent at elderly age, especially for elderly females. No complications or adverse outcomes of exercise training at elderly age were described in any study. Elderly patients of both genders should be strongly encouraged to participate in exercise-based cardiac rehabilitation.

Alternate Approaches to the Delivery of Cardiac Rehabilitation Services

Alternate approaches to the delivery of cardiac rehabilitation services, other than traditional supervised group interventions, can be implemented effectively and safely for carefully selected clinically stable patients.[7] Transtelephonic and other means of monitoring and surveillance of patients can extend cardiac rehabilitation services beyond the setting of supervised, structured, group-based rehabilitation. These alternate approaches have the potential to provide cardiac rehabilitation services to low- and moderate-risk patients who comprise the majority of patients with stable CHD, most of whom do not currently participate in structured supervised cardiac rehabilitation.

Cost Outcomes

The Clinical Practice Guideline addressed the issue of cost effectiveness of cardiac rehabilitation programs. As with other outcomes covered in the guideline, this issue was based upon scientific evidence in the medical literature. There were a limited number of studies of cardiac rehabilitation services, including randomized controlled trials and nonrandomized controlled trials, that addressed the cost-effectiveness issue. Although variation was noted, the average cost of a 12-week cardiac rehabilitation program was approximately $1,000 per patient. Regarding the issue of cost effectiveness or actual savings of medical care costs, several points were addressed and conclusions made.

It is difficult to estimate the savings that widespread use of cardiac rehabilitation will reap. This is an area that needs greater study. However, from the limited trials that have been conducted, there are indications that the potential for cost savings is great.

In a randomized trial of an eight-week comprehensive cardiac rehabilitation program, the incremental cost (subtracting the cost of usual care) of services was $480 per patient.[16] The results of a second trial estimated that cardiac rehabilitation saved $739 per patient in reduced hospital admissions after 21 months.[17]

Comparing the estimated $480 per patient cost with the conservative savings estimate of $739 in reduced hospital admissions, the net saving would be $259 per patient. If an additional 50% of the 2.4 million Americans annually have recognition of heart disease, receive effective cardiac rehabilitation, the American health system would save more than $310 million in hospital costs alone over about a two-year period.

Guideline Availability

The Clinical Practice Guideline Cardiac Rehabilitation, AHCPR Publication No. 96-0672, as well as the *Quick Reference Guide for Clinicians, Cardiac Rehabilita-*

tion as Secondary Prevention, AHCPR Publication No. 96-0673, are available from the AHCPR Publications Clearinghouse; call toll free 800-358-9295 or write to P.O. Box 8547, Silver Spring, Maryland 20907.

Acknowledgments

The Expert Panel was co-chaired by Nanette K Wenger, MD and Erika S Froelicher, RN, PhD. Panel members were Philip A Ades, MD; Kathy Berra, BSN; James A Blumenthal, PhD; Catherine ME Certo, ScD, PT; Anne M Dattilo, PhD, RD; Dwight Davis, MD; Robert F DeBusk, MD; Joseph P Drozda Jr, MD; Barbara J Fletcher, RN, MN; Barry A Franklin, PhD; Helen Gaston; Philip Greenland, MD; Patrick E McBride, MD, MPH; Christopher GA McGregor, MB, FRCS; Neil B Oldridge, PhD; Joseph C Piscatella; Felix J Rogers, DO. L Kent Smith, MD, MPH was the project director.

References

1. Leon AS, Certo C, Comoss P, Franklin BA, Froelicher V, Haskell WL, Hellerstein HK, Marley WP, Pollock ML, Ries A et al. Scientific evidence of the value of cardiac rehabilitation services with emphasis on patients following myocardial infarction—Section 1: Exercise conditioning component [position paper]. *J Cardiopueln Rehabil*, 1990;10:79-87.

2. Haskell VL, Alderman EL, Fair JM, Maron DJ, Mackey SF, Superko HR, Williams PT, Johnstone IM, Champagne ME, Krauss RM et al. Effects of intensive multiple risk factor reduction on coronary atherosclerosis and clinical cardiac events in men and women with coronary artery disease: The Stanford Coronary Risk Intervention Project (SCRIP). *Circulation*, 1994;89:975-90.

3. McCartney N, McKelvie RS, Hasiam DR, Jones NL. Usefulness of weightlifting training in improving strength and maximal power output in coronary artery disease. *Am J Cardiol*, 1991;67:939-45.

4. Todd IC, Ballatyne D. Effect of exercise training on the total ischaemic burden: An assessment by 24 hour ambulatory electrocardiographic monitoring. *Br Heart J*, 1992;68:560-6.

5. Meyer TR, Casadei B, Coats AJ, Davey PP, Adamopoulos S, Radaelli A, Conway J. Angiotensin-converting enzyme inhibition and physical training in heart failure. *J Intern Med*, 1991;230:407-13.

6. Taylor CB, Houston-Miller N, Killen JD, DeBusk RF. Smoking cessation after acute myocardial infarction: Effects of a nurse-managed intervention. *Ann Intern Med*, 1990;113:118-23.

7. DeBusk RF, Houston-Miller N, Superko HR, Dennis CA, Thomas RJ, Lew HT, Berger WE III, Heller RS, Rompf J, Gee D et al. A case-management system

for coronary risk factor modification after acute myocardial infarction. *Ann Intern Med*, 1994;120:721-9.

8. Karvetti RL, Hamalainen H. Long-term effect of nutrition education on myocardial infarction patients: A 10-year follow-up study. *Nutr Metab Cardiovasc Dis*, 1993;3:185-92.

9. Oldridge NB, Guyatt G, Jones N, Crowe J, Singer J, Feeny D, McKelvie R, Runions J, Streiner D, Torrance G. Effects on quality of life with comprehensive rehabilitation after acute myocardial infarction. *Am J Cardiol*, 1991;67:1084-9.

10. Van Camp SP, Peterson RA. Cardiovascular complications of outpatient cardiac rehabilitation programs. *JAMA*, 1986;256:1160-3.

11. O'Connor GT, Buring JE, Yusuf S, Goldhaber SZ, Olmstead EM, Paffenbarger RS Jr, Hennekens CH. An overview of randomized trials of rehabilitation with exercise after myocardial infarction. *Circulation*, 1989;80:234-44.

12. Oldridge NB, Guyatt GH, Fischer ME, Rimm AA. Cardiac rehabilitation after myocardial infarction: Combined experience of randomized clinical trials. *JAMA*, 1988;260:945-50.

13. Sebrechts CP, Klein JL, Ahnve S, Froelicher VIF, Ashburn WL. Myocardial perfusion changes following 1 year of exercise training assessed by thallium-201 circumferential count profiles. *Am Heart J*, 1986;112:1217-26.

14. Meyer TR, Casadei B, Coats AJ, Davey PP, Adamopoulos S, Radaelli A, Conway J. Angiotensin-converting enzyme inhibition and physical training in heart failure. *J Intern Med*, 1991;230:407-13.

15. Ades PA, Waldmann ML, Gillespie C. A controlled trial of exercise training in older coronary patients. *J Gerontol*, 1995;50A:M7-11.

16. Oldridge N, Furlong W, Feeny D, Torrance G, Guyatt G, Crowe J, Jones N. Economic evaluation of cardiac rehabilitation soon after acute myocardial infarction. *Am J Cardiol*, 1993;72:154-61.

17. Ades PA, Huang D, Weaver SO. Cardiac rehabilitation participation predicts lower rehospitalization costs. *Am Heart J*, 1992;123:916-21.

Update on Secondary Prevention of Cardiovascular Disease and Exercise-Based Cardiac Rehabilitation

Barry A. Franklin
William Beaumont Hospital, Royal Oak, Michigan, USA
Wayne State University School of Medicine, Detroit, Michigan, USA

Cardiovascular disease is the leading cause of mortality in the US, accounting for almost 50% of all deaths. More than 1.5 million Americans sustain myocardial infarction (MI) each year; of these, almost 500,000, or one-third, will die. The 1 million survivors of MI and 7 million patients with stable angina pectoris are candidates for exercise-based cardiac rehabilitation, as are the nearly 700,000 patients who undergo coronary revascularization procedures annually.[1] An estimated 4.7 million patients with heart failure may also be eligible for cardiac rehabilitation. However, only 15% to 20% of all patients with heart disease who are candidates for cardiac rehabilitation actually participate in formal programs.

What Is Cardiac Rehabilitation?

The objectives of contemporary cardiac rehabilitation are to increase functional capacity, decrease symptoms, stop cigarette smoking, modify lipids and lipoproteins, reduce blood pressure, and improve psychosocial well-being. Interventions designed to retard the progression or induce regression of the underlying atherosclerotic process and to restore and maintain optimal physical, psychological, emotional, social, and vocational functioning are paramount. As is indicated in Figure 1, comprehensive or multidisciplinary programs should include the following major components:

- Exercise training
- Risk-factor modification
- Medical surveillance/emergency support
- Psychosocial/vocational counseling

Candidates for Cardiac Rehabilitation

Exercise-based cardiac rehabilitation has become the "standard of care" within the medical community, by which a broad spectrum of patients are restored to their optimal physical, medical, and psychosocial status after an acute cardiac event. Included are the traditional patients of past years: MI, coronary artery bypass graft

CONTEMPORARY CARDIAC REHABILITATION

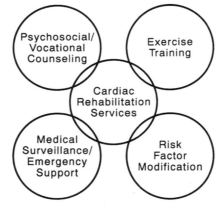

Figure 1.   Key components of a contemporary rehabilitation program for patients with heart disease.

surgery (CABGS), and percutaneous transluminal coronary angioplasty (PTCA) patients. The following are also treated with exercise-based cardiac rehabilitation:

- Coronary patients with or without residual myocardial ischemia
- Compensated heart failure, cardiomyopathies, and threatening ventricular arrhythmias
- A variety of categories of patients with nonischemic heart disease
- Patients with concomitant pulmonary disease
- Patients who have undergone pacemaker or cardioverter-defibrillator implantation, heart valve repair or replacement, and cardiac transplantation
- Elderly patients
- Medically complex patients taking multiple medications

Recently, concerns have been raised regarding the potential deleterious effects of exercise training for patients with silent myocardial ischemia or those recovering from large anterior wall MI. Some clinicians have suggested that asymptomatic patients who demonstrate significant ST-segment depression should refrain from vigorous exercise training, citing biopsy studies of ischemic myocardium showing increased fibrosis.[2] Silent myocardial ischemia may also increase the risk of cardiac arrest during vigorous physical exertion.[3] A nonrandomized, controlled study of patients with anterior MI and diminished ejection fraction showed a significantly greater deterioration in global and regional left ventricular function in exercising patients compared with nonexercising patients.[4] However, other investigations of painless exercise-induced ST-segment depression have allayed concerns regarding risk, demonstrating better survival, milder disease, and higher exercise training intensities in such patients compared with those with angina.[5,6] In addition, randomized, controlled trials[7,8] in patients with anterior Q-wave MI and decreased ejection fraction showed no significant difference in left ventricular dysfunction between exercise and control patients.

Modifying the Patient's Risk Status

Although the degree of left ventricular dysfunction (i.e., ejection fraction) and residual myocardial ischemia largely determine the risk of future cardiac events, risk status can be influenced by numerous interventions and lifestyle habits (Figure 2). Multicenter trials have confirmed that mortality from acute MI can be decreased by approximately 25% with early thrombolytic therapy, immediate PTCA, or both.[9] Patients at moderate risk may likely experience a reduction in mortality from successful PTCA or CABGS. Aggressive risk factor modification aimed at smoking cessation and cholesterol reduction, and efficacious drugs, including beta-blockers, aspirin, angiotensin-converting enzyme inhibitors, and lipid-lowering agents, have produced regression or limitation of progression of angiographically-documented coronary atherosclerosis and significant reductions in subsequent cardiac events.[10] Moreover, randomized trials of secondary prevention have demonstrated increased survival with regular dynamic exercise. In contrast, time (disease progression), poor patient management or compliance, and psychological dysfunction, manifested as Type-A behavior pattern, hostility, depression, vital exhaustion, or social isolation, can lead to increased risk and an adverse prognosis.

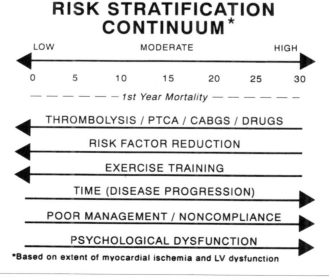

Figure 2.   Variables that may potentially influence the patient's risk status (PTCA = percutaneous transluminal coronary angioplasty; CABGS = coronary artery bypass graft surgery).

Outcomes of Exercise-Based Cardiac Rehabilitation

Benefits of Exercise Training

Common rationale for exercise training of patients with cardiovascular disease include increases in exercise tolerance, particularly for patients with reduced functional capacity, improved skeletal muscle strength and endurance, and relief of symptoms of myocardial ischemia.[11] Favorable risk factor modification, improved psychosocial well-being, and increased survival are also expected outcomes, especially when exercise is combined with education and behavior modification in a multifactorial program.

Exercise tolerance.   A "spontaneous" increase in aerobic fitness or peak oxygen consumption ($\dot{V}O_2$ peak) generally occurs within 3 to 11 weeks after clinically uncomplicated MI, CABGS, or PTCA, even in patients who undergo no formal exercise training.[11] Nevertheless, improvement in aerobic capacity can be further augmented by gymnasium or home-based physical conditioning programs.[12] Increases in $\dot{V}O_2$ peak among cardiac patients range from 11% to 66% after three to six months of exercise training, with the greatest improvements among the most unfit.[13] The most consistent benefit appears to occur with exercise training at least three times per week for 12 or more weeks duration, 20 to 40 minutes/session, at an intensity approximating 70% to 85% of maximal heart rate.[1] However, exercise training intensities in the 50% to 70% heart-rate range, corresponding to 40% to 60% of $\dot{V}O_2$ peak, have been shown to effect comparable improvement in functional capacity in deconditioned patients (Figure 3). Improved $\dot{V}O_2$ peak is particularly beneficial, since most patients with clinically manifest heart disease have a subnormal aerobic capacity (50%-70% age, gender-predicted). Because a given submaximal task or work rate requires a relatively constant aerobic requirement, cardiac patients find that after an exercise training program, they are working at a lower percentage of their $\dot{V}O_2$ peak, with greater reserve (Figure 4).

Upper-body training.   Upper-body aerobic exercise and mild-to-moderate resistance training can safely and effectively improve muscular strength and endurance in clinically stable coronary patients.[14] Moreover, recent studies suggest that the arms respond to aerobic exercise training in a similar quantitative and qualitative manner as do the legs.[15] Adjunctive upper-body and resistance exercise programs also facilitate increased transfer of training benefits to occupational and recreational activities and provide greater diversity to the conditioning regimen, which may increase patient interest and adherence.

Symptoms.   Exercise-based cardiac rehabilitation decreases angina pectoris in patients with coronary disease and improves symptoms of heart failure in patients with left ventricular systolic dysfunction.[1] Some of the greatest increases in exercise tolerance occur in patients with angina on exertion. Reductions in myocardial oxygen demand via decreases in the submaximal rate-pressure product are largely responsible (Figure 5). Nevertheless, several studies have now documented a reduction in exercise-induced ischemia, manifested by decreased ST segment de-

THEORETICAL THRESHOLD INTENSITIES FOR TRAINING CARDIAC PATIENTS

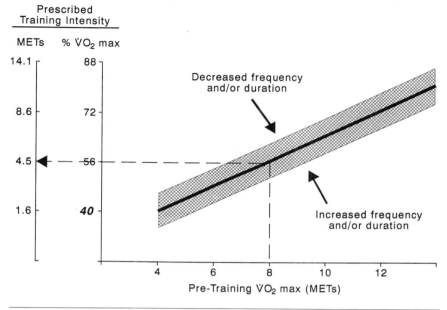

Figure 3.   The threshold intensity for training increases in direct proportion to $\dot{V}O_2$ peak before training; however, it can be modulated by altering the exercise duration or frequency, or both. For example, patients with an initial aerobic capacity of 8 METs would exercise at approximately 56% of their $\dot{V}O_2$ peak, or 4.5 METs, to further increase their functional capacities.

pression or thallium perfusion abnormalities at matched rate-pressure products after exercise training.[13]

Coronary risk factors.   Aerobic exercise training can result in modest decreases in body weight, fat stores, and blood pressure (in hypertensives).[16] A meta-analysis of statistically aggregated data from 15 longitudinal studies of the effect of moderate exercise training in 490 male post-MI patients has demonstrated beneficial alterations in lipids and lipoproteins.[17] However, exercise alone should not be expected to alter global coronary risk status. Rehabilitation regimens reporting the most favorable impact on coronary risk factors are multifactorial; that is, they provide exercise training, dietary education and counseling, and, in some studies, pharmacologic therapy, psychological support, and behavior training.[1] There is little or no evidence of smoking cessation resulting from exercise training as an isolated intervention. Nevertheless, between 17% and 26% of patients can be expected to stop smoking after participating in a formal smoking cessation program.

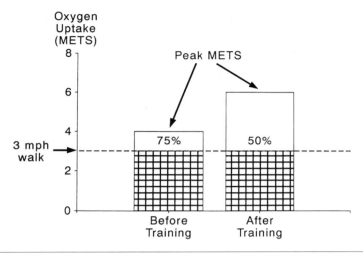

Figure 4.   Effect of exercise training on peak oxygen uptake (METs) and relative oxygen cost (activity METs/peak METs) of walking at three miles per hour (mph) on a level grade. Following a physical-conditioning program, peak oxygen uptake increased from 4 to 6 METs, decreasing the relative oxygen cost of a three-mph walk from 75% to 50%.

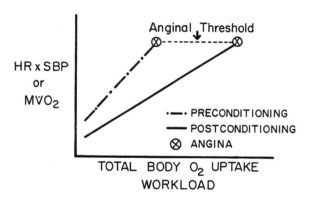

Figure 5.   The effect of physical conditioning on the rate-pressure product (HR <x> SBP) and myocardial oxygen consumption ($M\dot{V}O_2$) at submaximal and peak exercise. Peak body oxygen uptake and workload are augmented by exercise training. Myocardial oxygen requirements are reduced at a given workload or oxygen uptake, but angina occurs at the same rate-pressure product.

Psychological well-being.   Exercise-based cardiac rehabilitation, either alone or as a component of multifactorial intervention, often results in improvement in measures of psychological status and functioning, such as enhanced well-being and self-efficacy.[11] On the other hand, exercise training per se does not consistently improve measures of anxiety and depression.[1] Group therapy or stress management may be more effective interventions in this regard.

Morbidity/mortality.   Three meta-analyses of randomized, controlled clinical trials in post-MI patients have now shown that exercise-based cardiac rehabilitation provides a 20% to 25% reduction in total and cardiovascular-related mortality, especially as component of multifactorial rehabilitation (i.e., 26% mortality vs 15% in exercise-only trials), with no difference in the rate of nonfatal recurrent events.[18-20] These results, however, cannot necessarily be extrapolated to patients following CABGS and/or PTCA.[16] In addition, contemporary thrombolytic and revascularization procedures, and newer pharmacologic agents, which markedly decrease early postinfarction mortality, may diminish the impact of adjunctive exercise-based cardiac rehabilitation programs on survival.

Limitations of Exercise Training

Exercise training as a sole intervention does not necessarily halt the progression of coronary artery disease or, for that matter, prevent restenosis or reinfarction. However, intensive multifactorial intervention (including exercise) can result in regression or limitation of progression of angiographically documented coronary atherosclerosis.[1] Conventional exercise training does little to improve left ventricular ejection fraction, regional wall motion abnormalities, resting hemodynamics, and collateral circulation.[11] Studies describing changes in ventricular arrhythmias following exercise rehabilitation have also produced inconsistent results.[1]

Safety of Exercise-Based Cardiac Rehabilitation

According to 1980 to 1984 survey data, the incidence of cardiovascular complications was one cardiac arrest per 111,996 patient-hours, one MI per 292,990 patient-hours, and one fatality in 783,972 patient-hours of exercise-based cardiac rehabilitation.[21] However, this low mortality rate applies only to medically supervised programs equipped with a defibrillator and appropriate emergency drugs. Up to 90% of all patients with cardiac arrests occurring under such conditions were successfully resuscitated.

Special Populations

Women.   The effects of exercise rehabilitation in women with coronary artery disease have been less well studied than in men.[13] Only 3% of the 4,500 patients evaluated in a meta-analysis of randomized trials of cardiac rehabilitation after MI were women.[19] Nevertheless, recent studies suggest comparable exercise trainability in age-matched men and women in cardiac rehabilitation programs.[22,23]

Elderly.   Older coronary patients show improvements similar to those seen in younger patients participating in exercise-based rehabilitation programs.[1] Elderly female and male patients also demonstrate comparable exercise trainability. However, referral to and participation in exercise rehabilitation is less frequent in older adults, especially women.

Heart failure.   Exercise training in patients with heart failure and moderate-to-severe left ventricular dysfunction results in improved functional capacity and reduced symptoms. Peripheral (skeletal muscle) adaptations are largely responsible for the increase in exercise tolerance.[13]

Cardiac transplantation.   Rehabilitation in patients after cardiac transplantation increases effort tolerance, raises the anaerobic threshold, and improves the ventilatory response to exercise.[13]

Deficiencies in Our Current Knowledge

The expansion of population of patients eligible for and receiving exercise-based cardiac rehabilitation, the changing spectrum of medical and surgical interventions for cardiac illness, and new approaches to the delivery of cardiac rehabilitation have highlighted a number of critical gaps in our current knowledge base. Areas for future research include the following:

- Outcomes of cardiac rehabilitation in post-MI patients treated with contemporary therapies
- Cost-effectiveness outcomes resulting from new approaches to deliver cardiac rehabilitation services
- Safety and effectiveness outcomes of exercise rehabilitation with and without supervision and/or electrocardiographic monitoring in the surveillance and treatment of selected patient subsets

Conclusion

The treatment of heart disease has evolved from simple lifestyle modification in the mid to late 1960s, to an array of costly medical and surgical interventions which, oftentimes, fail to address the underlying causes: high-fat and cholesterol diets, cigarette smoking, hypertension, lack of exercise, and psychological dysfunction. As the year 2000 approaches, we have come full circle (Figure 6) in that new studies have shown that aggressive risk factor modification can result in regression or limitation of progression of angiographically-documented coronary atherosclerosis and significant reductions in subsequent cardiac events.[10]

We must conclude, as did Herman K. Hellerstein, MD in 1972,[24] that: ". . . a planned program featuring exercise training among other measures (e.g., control of coronary risk factors) may tangibly reduce the risk of reinfarction and greater myocardial damage." Like all statements of wisdom, this thesis is both time-tested and well-founded, so clearly evident and acceptable today that we feel we should have known it all along.

Evolutionary Treatment
of Heart Disease

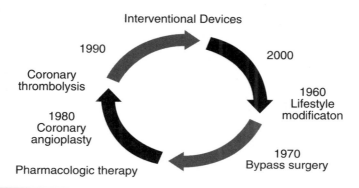

Figure 6.   Lifestyle modification is strongly emphasized in the treatment of heart disease.

References

1. Wenger NK, Froelicher ES, Smith LK et al. *Clinical practice guideline: Cardiac rehabilitation.* Rockville, MD: US Department of Health Services, Agency for Health Care Policy and Research and National Heart, Lung, and Blood Institute, 1995.

2. Hess OM, Schneider J, Nonogi H et al. Myocardial structure in patients with exercise-induced ischemia. *Circulation,* 1988;77:967-77.

3. Hoberg E, Schuler G, Kunze B et al. Silent myocardial ischemia as a potential link between lack of premonitoring symptoms and increased risk of cardiac arrest during physical stress. *Am J Cardiol,* 1990;65:583-9.

4. Jugdutt BI, Michorowski BL, Kappagoda CT. Exercise training after anterior Q wave myocardial infarction: Importance of regional left ventricular function and topography. *J Am Coll Cardiol,* 1988;12:362-72.

5. Mark DB, Hlatky MA, Califf RM et al. Painless exercise ST deviation on the treadmill: Long-term prognosis. *J Am Coll Cardiol,* 1989;14:885-92.

6. Schuler G, Shlierf G, Wirth A et al. Low-fat diet and regular, supervised physical exercise in patients with symptomatic coronary artery disease: Reduction of stress-induced myocardial ischemia. *Circulation,* 1988;77:172-81.

7. Giannuzzi P, Temporelli PL, Tavazzi L et al. EAMI—Exercise training in anterior myocardial infarction: An ongoing multicenter randomized study; Preliminary results on left ventricular function and remodeling. *Chest,* 1992;101 (Suppl 5):315S-21S.

8. Giannuzzi P, Tavazzi L, Temporelli PL et al. Long-term physical training and left ventricular remodeling after anterior myocardial infarction: Results of the Exercise in Anterior Myocardial Infarction (EAMI) trial. *J Am Coll Cardiol*, 1993;22:1821-9.

9. Grines CL, Browne KF, Marco J et al. A comparison of immediate angioplasty with thrombolytic therapy for acute myocardial infarction. *N Engl J Med*, 1993;328:673-9.

10. Haskell WL, Alderman EL, Fair JM et al. Effects of intensive multiple risk factor reduction on coronary atherosclerosis and clinical cardiac events in men and women with coronary artery disease: The Stanford Coronary Risk Intervention Project (SCRIP). *Circulation*, 1994;89:975-90.

11. Franklin BA, Gordon S, Timmis GC. Amount of exercise necessary for the patient with coronary artery disease. *Am J Cardiol*, 1992;69:1426-31.

12. DeBusk RF, Houston N, Haskell W, Fry G, Parker M. Exercise training soon after myocardial infarction. *Am J Cardiol*, 1979;44:1223-9.

13. Balady GJ, Fletcher BJ, Froelicher ES et al. Cardiac rehabilitation programs. A statement for healthcare professionals from the American Heart Association. *Circulation*, 1994;90:1602-10.

14. Franklin BA, Bonzheim K, Gordon S et al. Resistance training in cardiac rehabilitation. *J Cardiopul Rehabil*, 1991;11:99-107.

15. Franklin BA, Vander L, Wrisley D et al. Trainability of arms versus legs in men with previous myocardial infarction. *Chest*, 1994;105:262-4.

16. American College of Sports Medicine Position Stand: Exercise for patients with coronary artery disease. *Med Sci Sports Exercise*, 1994;26:i-v

17. Tran ZV, Brammell HL. Effects of exercise training on serum lipid and lipoprotein levels in post-MI patients. A meta-analysis. *J Cardiopul Rehabil*, 1989;9:250-5.

18. Oldridge NB, Guyatt GH, Fisher ME et al. Cardiac rehabilitation after myocardial infarction: Combined experience of randomized clinical trials. *JAMA*, 1988;260:945-50.

19. O'Connor GT, Buring JE, Yusuf S et al. An overview of randomized trials of rehabilitation with exercise after myocardial infarction. *Circulation*, 1989;80:234-44.

20. Lau J, Antman EM, Jimenez-Silva J et al. Cumulative meta-analysis of therapeutic trials for myocardial infarction. *N Engl J Med*, 1992;327:248-54.

21. Van Camp SP, Peterson RA. Cardiovascular complications of outpatient cardiac rehabilitation programs. *JAMA*, 1986;256:1160-3.

22. Ades PA, Waldman ML, Polk DM, Coflesky JT. Referral patterns and exercise response in the rehabilitation of female coronary patients aged ≥ 62 years. *Am J Cardiol*, 1992;69:1422-5.

23. Cannistra LB, Balady GJ, O'Malley CJ, Weiner DA, Ryan TJ. Comparison of the clinical profile and outcome of women and men in cardiac rehabilitation. *Am J Cardiol*, 1992;69:1274-9.

24. Hellerstein HK. Rehabilitation of the postinfarction patient. *Hospital Practice*, July 1972; 45-53.

Behavioral and Psychosocial Issues of Cardiac Rehabilitation

James A. Blumenthal, Elizabeth D. Gullette, Melissa Napolitano, and Renata Szczepanski
Duke University Medical Center, Durham, North Carolina, USA

In addition to the physical health benefits of exercise outlined in other chapters of the Proceedings, the present chapter presents an overview of the psychological benefits of physical fitness and exercise training. For the purposes of this review, psychological benefits are considered in four domains: (1) mood, (2) personality, (3) psychophysiologic reactivity, and (4) cognitive function. Although space limitations preclude a comprehensive survey of this voluminous literature, key studies are cited, along with major review papers for interested readers.

Mood

In addition to the many potential cardiovascular and other health benefits associated with exercise, there is increasing evidence that exercise may provide a number of psychological benefits. Numerous empirical studies have documented the benefits of acute and chronic exercise in improving mood, including anxiety, depression, tension, and fatigue. For example, in a study of the acute effects of exercise, Roth[1] randomly assigned 80 college students, including both active and inactive individuals, to an aerobic exercise or a waiting-list control group. Self-report measures of mood before and after a 20-minute exercise session revealed that tension and anxiety were significantly reduced by the exercise, regardless of students' activity status. Similar acute studies of other groups, including women and older adults, also have found improved psychological well-being following a single bout of exercise.

In an attempt to determine the effects of habitual exercise on psychological well-being, a number of cross-sectional studies have examined anxiety and depression levels among subjects who differ in physical fitness. In general, such studies have found that sedentary subjects obtain significantly higher scores on measures of negative mood states than did active subjects. In a representative study of 22 healthy, middle-aged men, Lobstein, Mosbacher, and Ismail[2] found depression to be the most powerful discriminator between physically active and sedentary men.

Risk of depression has also been shown to be altered by exercise. Camacho et al.[3] observed that those individuals who increased their activity levels from 1965 to 1974 were at no greater risk for depression than were those who had been active all along, suggesting that the high risk of depression among inactive adults may be modified if the activity level is increased. In contrast, by 1983, those individuals who had been active but then became inactive were 1.5 times more likely to become depressed than were those who had maintained their high levels of activity.

Longitudinal studies, like cross-sectional studies, have provided support for the mood-enhancing effects of physical exercise. For example, Blumenthal et al.[4] compared changes in psychological functioning in a group of 32 men and women who engaged in 10 weeks of aerobic exercise with a matched group of subjects who did not engage in any exercise during the same time interval. Although there were no group differences prior to treatment, the exercise group obtained lower scores on measures of anxiety, tension, and depression, and reported less fatigue and increased vigor after the 10-week program.

The use of exercise for the treatment of clinical depression has received particular attention. The most comprehensive review of the literature on exercise and depression is a recent meta-analysis by North, McCullagh, and Tran.[5] Their review of 80 studies concluded that exercise decreased symptoms of depression significantly more than did control conditions, regardless of age, sex, health, or source of subject recruitment. Research specifically focusing on cardiac patients, however, has been more equivocal, with the majority of studies failing to find significant reductions in depressive symptoms associated with exercise, although those individuals who were depressed prior to treatment have exhibited the largest reductions in depression scores.[6]

Although the precise mechanisms by which exercise improves mood are not known, several biologic factors may be relevant. Findings from several cross-sectional studies have suggested that the antidepressant effect of chronic exercise may be mediated by increased central norepinephrine neurotransmission. Exercise also may improve mood via changes in the hypothalamo-pituitary-adrenocortical axis (HPA) via a lessened cortisol response to submaximal exercise after exercise training, or by increased levels of beta-endorphins.

Psychological mechanisms may also be responsible for the effects of exercise on mood, alone or in combination with the physiological adaptations mentioned above. Increased self-efficacy, increased positive thoughts, distraction from negative thoughts, enhanced self-concept, and other factors all have been suggested, although there are no definitive conclusions about what psychological processes may be responsible for exercise-related changes in mood. It is likely that rather than any single mechanism, a combination of physiological, psychological, and social adaptations associated with exercise contributes to improvements in mood.

Personality

Personality refers to a pattern of enduring dispositional characteristics or traits, as contrasted to mood, which is defined as a transient and situationally dependent emotional state. Research on the effects of exercise on personality has resulted in mixed findings. Some studies have found no evidence for global changes in personality as a result of exercise, while others show moderate effects. For example, in a cross-sectional study, Plante and Karpowitz[7] found that males who were classified as intense aerobic exercisers, moderate aerobic exercisers, or nonexercisers did not differ on any of the personality dimensions assessed. Other studies have reported that athletes are more self-assured and nonaggressive than are nonathletes and more extroverted and less neurotic than are the population norms.[8]

Interventional studies have reported conflicting results. Emery and Gatz[9] studied older adults who were randomized to either an aerobic exercise, social activity and exercise, or waiting-list group. After a 12-week intervention, no change on personality measures was found. However, Jasnoski, Holmes, and Banks[10] found that after a 10-week intervention, positive changes in personality (as measured by the Sixteen Factor Personality Questionnaire) were associated with changes in aerobic, but not with anaerobic, fitness.

One aspect of personality functioning that does appear to change consistently is self-concept. Self-concept refers to a person's conscious awareness of the self, including physical traits and abilities. It has been proposed that exercise can alter self-concept through changes in body image, through a sense of mastery and competence over one's environment and health, or through the social interaction often co-occurring with exercise.

In an early review of the effects of physical fitness training on mental health, Folkins and Sime[11] concluded that fitness training improves self-concept in such diverse populations as adult male rehabilitation patients, adult females, college students, adolescent males and females, and obese teenage males. Cross-sectional studies also have shown that physically active subjects score higher on measures of self-esteem than do sedentary subjects.

Recently, research on self-concept and exercise has been extended to the elderly. Perri and Templer[12] studied 9 men and 14 women with a mean age of 65 who were assigned either to a 14-week aerobic exercise condition or to a nonrandom control group. They found the exercise group improved on all measures, including self-concept. Although Blumenthal, Emery, Madden et al.[13] reported that there were no significant changes on measures of reported self-esteem among 101 healthy adults aged 60 to 83 as a result of exercise compared with yoga and waiting-list controls, exercisers reported significant improvements in perceptions of self-worth, suggesting that perceptions may change more than do "objective" scores on psychometric tests.

The Type A Behavior Pattern (TABP) is another personality dimension that has been widely studied. TABP refers to a constellation of overt behaviors and psychological traits, including explosive, loud, and rapid speech; excessive competitiveness; hostility; a sense of time urgency; and impatience.

Four out of 5 interventional studies have demonstrated exercise-related changes in measures of TABP. In the first study, Blumenthal, Williams, Williams, and Wallace[14] found that a 10-week, supervised exercise program was associated with a significant reduction in Type A scores on the Jenkins Activity Survey, especially among Type A individuals. One limitation of the study, however, was the lack of a nonexercise control group. A subsequent study by Blumenthal et al.[15] randomly assigned Type A men either to an aerobic exercise condition or to a strength and flexibility training group for 12 weeks. Both groups exhibited decreases in overt behavioral manifestations of TABP, including volume and speed of speech and potential for hostility. Because similar changes were associated with aerobic exercise and anaerobic exercise, it was suggested that improvements in aerobic fitness were not responsible for behavioral changes. Roskies et al.[16] examined the effects of three treatments (aerobic exercise, cognitive-behavioral stress management, and weight training) in 107 healthy Type A men. Results indicate that the stress management group, but not the exercise group, significantly reduced TABP. Taken together, results suggest that manifestations of TABP can be altered with exercise, although the mechanisms by which exercise alters behavior are not clear.

Psychophysiologic Reactivity

Exaggerated cardiovascular and neuroendocrine responses to stress have been associated with increased risk for subsequent development of hypertension and coronary heart disease. It has been proposed that heightened physiological responses may mediate the relationship between stress and cardiovascular disease.[17] Hence, researchers have examined the extent to which chronic and acute exercise may decrease cardiovascular and neurohumoral responses to stress.

In 1987, a meta-analytic review of 34 studies examined the relationship between aerobic exercise and reactivity to psychosocial stressors.[18] From this review, it was concluded that more-fit subjects, compared with less-fit subjects, show reduced psychophysiological reactivity to mental stressors. However, of the 34 studies reviewed, only 3 were randomized, controlled studies published in peer-reviewed journals. Since their review, there have been a number of randomized trials of exercise training and psychophysiological reactivity, which have been reviewed elsewhere.[19]

Table 1 shows that of 9 published intervention trials, 4 studies showed attenuated cardiovascular responses for subjects who participated in aerobic exercise compared with nonaerobic controls; 1 study reported mixed results; 3 studies showed no significant differences among groups; and 1 study showed that aerobic fitness was associated with greater, not less, cardiovascular reactivity. These inconsistencies are not surprising because the studies utilized different control conditions, different stressors, varying exercise-training protocols, and different methods of assessing physical fitness. Generally, aerobic exercise seems to be more effective than is nonaerobic exercise in reducing cardiovascular stress responses, and *levels* of cardiovascular and neurohumoral *responses* appear to be affected more consistently by exercise than change scores (i.e., *reactivity* or change from resting or baseline levels).[20]

Studies of *acute* exercise generally have found reduced cardiovascular responses to mental stress. The effects of exercise on psychophysiological stress *recovery* have also been examined. Four studies showed that exercise was associated with faster recovery from stressful laboratory tasks, although results were not consis-

Table 1. Randomized, Controlled Trials of Exercise and Reactivity

Authors	Sample	Control condition	Exercise training	Significant effects
Roskies, et al. (*Health Psychol* 1986, 5, 45-49)	107 males Mean age = 37	No control	3x weekly for 10 weeks	No changes
Sinyor, et al. (*Physio Behav*, 1987, 42, 293-296)	6 males Mean age = 22.5	Strength training	3x weekly for 12 weeks	No changes
Blumenthal, et al. (*Psychosom Med*, 1988, 50, 418-433)	36 Type A men Mean age = 44.4	Strength training	3x weekly for 12 weeks	Lower HR, BP
Sherwood, et al. (*Psychosom Med*, 1989, 51, 123-156)	27 Type A men Mean age = 41.4	Strength training	3x weekly for 12 weeks	Lower DBP
Blumenthal, et al. (*Am J Cardiol*, 1990, 65, 93-98)	37 Type A men Mean age = 42	Strength training	3x weekly for 12 weeks	Lower HR, BP
Blumenthal, et al. (*Health Psychol*, 1991, 10, 384-391)	50 women Mean age = 50	Strength training	3x weekly for 12 weeks	Mixed pattern
Stein & Boutcher (*Int. J Psychophysiol*, 1992, 13, 215-223)	40 men Mean age = 45.6	No exercise	3x weekly for 8 weeks	Lower HR
Albright et al. (*Psychosom Res*, 1993, 36, 25-36)	83 men and women Mean age = 47.5	No exercise	5x weekly for 6 months	No changes
De Geus, et al. (*Psychosom Med*, 1993, 55, 347-363)	62 subjects	No exercise	1.5 to 2.5 hours weekly for 4 or 8 months	More-fit subjects had higher HR, BP

tent across all studies. Taken together, results generally show that enhanced physical fitness is associated with decreased cardiovascular and neuroendocrine responses during stress. Potential mechanisms include decreases in sympathetic nervous system activation, increased parasympathetic functioning, and changes in receptor structure and function. Further research in this area needs to be conducted in order to examine mechanisms for the apparent reduction in stress responses and to examine the effects of exercise on physiologic responses during daily life.

Cognitive Function

Interest in the use of exercise to improve cognitive performance also has received much attention.[21] Cognitive declines have been shown to accompany normal aging and are associated with various medical conditions, such as chronic obstructive pulmonary disease and hypertension. Consequently, research on the effects of exercise on cognitive functioning has focused upon the elderly and different clinical populations.

Early support for an association between chronic exercise and cognitive functioning was obtained primarily from cross-sectional research, which suggested that individuals who are aerobically fit perform better on cognitive performance tasks than do less-fit individuals.[22] Because such studies do not allow for the delineation of causal relationships and are subject to selection bias, more recent studies have employed interventional designs. These studies have varied widely in their methodologies, however, which has resulted in inconsistent findings.

There have been eight randomized, controlled trials of exercise and cognitive function (Table 2). In one of the earliest controlled exercise interventions, Dustman and colleagues[23] randomly assigned 43 adults for four months of aerobic exercise or strength/flexibility training; a third group of sedentary individuals formed a nonrandom, nonexercise control group. Although both exercise groups improved their cognitive performance, the aerobic exercise group demonstrated greater improvements than did the other groups. In a subsequent study, Blumenthal and colleagues[13] randomly assigned a group of 101 older adults to aerobic exercise, yoga, or waiting-list control groups. At the four-month posttreatment assessment, no significant group differences were observed in neuropsychological functioning.

A semicrossover design was employed, such that aerobic exercise participants continued aerobic exercise training while subjects in the other groups engaged in aerobic exercise for 4 months. Again, there were no group differences in neuropsychological functioning. A subset of 50 participants subsequently engaged in 6 additional months of aerobic exercise, so that some individuals engaged in exercise for as long as 14 months. Despite increasing levels of physical fitness and improvements on some indices of psychological adjustment, exercise participants failed to demonstrate significant changes in neuropsychological functioning. Interestingly, even in the absence of objectively assessed cognitive changes, individuals who completed the exercise interventions reported perceiving improvement in their cognitive performance.[24] It is possible that the neuropsychological

Table 2. Randomized, Controlled Exercise Interventions

Authors	Sample	Design	Results
Blumenthal, et al. (*J Gerontol*, 1989, 44, M147-157)	Healthy men (n = 50) and women (n = 51) Mean age = 67	Randomized to aerobic exercise, yoga, or wait list. Duration = 4 months	No effects[a]
Dustman, et al. (2) (*Neurobiol Aging*, 1984, 5, 33-42)	Healthy men (n = 27) and women (n = 16) Mean age = 60	Randomized to aerobic exercise or strength/flexibility, but inclusion of a nonrandom, nonexercise control group	Improved on reaction time and psychomotor performance[b]
Emery & Gatz (*Gerontology*, 1990, 30, 184-18)	Healthy men (n = 8) and women (n = 40) Mean age = 72	Randomized to aerobic exercise, social activity, or control. Duration = 3 months	No effects[c]
Hawkins, et al. (*Psychol Aging*, 1992, 7, 643-653)	Healthy men (n = 10) and women (n = 26) Mean age = 68	Randomized to aquatic exercise or control. Duration = 10 weeks	Improved information processing[d]
Madden, et al. (*Psychol Aging*, 1989, 4, 307-320)	Healthy men (n = 40) and women (n = 39) Mean age = 67	Randomized to aerobic exercise, yoga, or control. Duration = 4 months	No effects[e]
Molloy, et al. (*Age & Aging*, 1988, 17, 303-310)	Institutionalized women (n = 45) Mean age = 83	Randomized to aerobic exercise or control group. Duration = 3 months	No effects[f]

Authors	Sample	Design	Results
Panton, et al. (*J Gerontol*, 1990, 45, M26-31)	Sedentary men (n = 23) and women (n = 26) Mean age = 72	Randomized to walk/jog, strength training, or nonexercise. Duration = 6 months	No effects[g]
Pierce, et al. (*Health Psych*, 1993, 12, 286-291)	Hypertensive men (n = 62) and women (n = 38) Mean age = 45	Randomized to aerobic exercise, strength training/flexibility, or waiting list. Duration = 4 months	No effects[h]

Cognitive Assessment Instruments

[a]Finger Tapping, Grip Strength, Randt Story Memory, Digit Span, Benton Visual Retention, Selective Reminding, Digit Symbol, Trail Making, 2&7 Test, Verbal Fluency, Non-Verbal Fluency, Stroop Word-Color

[b]Critical Flicker Function, Culture Fair IQ, Digit Span, Digit Symbol, Dots Estimation Reaction Time, Stroop Word-Color

[c]Digit Symbol, Digit Span, 2 tests of writing speed

[d]Time sharing and attention flexibility tasks

[e]Simple reaction time tasks, Primary task reaction time and Secondary task reaction time (using letter search and word comparison tasks)

[f]Color Slide Test (a test of memory, language, and visual perception), Recognition tests, Digit Symbol, Digit Span, Logical Memory, Word Fluency

[g]Total reaction time, speed of movement tasks

[h]Wechsler Memory Scales, Digit Span, Digit Symbol, Trail Making, Stroop Word-Color, Paired Associates Learning, Sternberg Memory Search Task

procedures that are typically used to assess cognitive performance are not sensitive to the cognitive changes that result from increased physical activity. Perceptions may be equally important and may be more sensitive to cognitive changes associated with exercise.

In addition to examining the effects of chronic exercise on cognitive function, a number of studies have examined the acute effects of exercise.[25] Forty-five-minute bouts of moderate exercise in older adults with memory complaints have been found to contribute to short-term improvements during postexercise cognitive testing. In contrast, shorter-term exercise, such as having a duration of six minutes, does not appear to contribute to postexercise cognitive improvements, and acute exercise of greater intensity has been associated with declines in cognitive functioning.

At the present time, the specific mechanisms through which exercise and fitness impact cognitive functioning remain unclear. Alterations in central nervous system (CNS) functioning have been related to age- and pathology-related declines, and thus may explain improvements in cognitive functioning associated with physical fitness or exercise. Enhanced transport and consumption of oxygen in the brain resulting from exercise may enhance the metabolism of neurotransmitters critical to optimal neuropsychological functioning, such as acetylcholine, dopamine, serotonin, and norepinephrine. Exercise also could contribute to direct alterations of neurotransmitter levels, increased blood flow to the brain, or reductions in sympathetic tone. Future research will need to determine what kind of exercise over what duration improves which specific cognitive functions in which individuals.

Exercise Compliance

Despite the well-documented benefits of physical activity, the problem of nonadherence to exercise is significant, with more than 50% of all persons who begin an exercise program dropping out within six months. This is a particularly important issue for cardiac rehabilitation patients for whom long-term adherence to an exercise program may improve outcome, including increased functional capacity, reduced risk factors, improved psychosocial well-being, and increased survival. A major challenge in increasing compliance is to understand the factors that affect exercise behavior in order to devise an exercise program that is appropriate to the specific needs, preferences, and health status of a given individual.

Research has identified a number of determinants of exercise behavior, including demographic variables, health-risk behaviors, exercise factors, and psychological traits. Demographic variables associated with lower levels of physical activity include gender, age, race, and socioeconomic status. For example, women, older adults, African Americans, and blue collar workers tend to be more sedentary. Similarly, smokers and individuals who are overweight are generally less physically active. With regard to exercise factors, exercise intensity and program location have both been found to be important predictors of exercise adherence. In a community sample of 1,411 adults, Sallis et al.[26] found moderate activity to be associated with better adherence relative to vigorous activity over a period of one year. Interestingly, King et al.[27] found similar improvements in fitness in a 12-month randomized, controlled trial of group versus home-based exercise of varying intensities.

Among cardiac rehabilitation patients, research also has demonstrated a relationship between compliance and both demographic and health factors. For example, Oldridge et al.[28] examined predictors of exercise dropout in a study of 678 postmyocardial-infarction (post-MI) patients and found blue-collar occupational status, younger age, smoking, higher resting systolic blood pressure, angina, and the presence of cough or sputum to be significantly associated with program dropout. In a study of 35 consecutive post-MI patients referred to a cardiac rehabilitation program, Blumenthal et al.[29] found that those individuals who dropped out of the program, compared to those who remained in the program, had lower resting left ventricular ejection fraction and were more depressed, hypochondriacal, anxious, and socially introverted. Interestingly, individuals with these characteristics have been shown to benefit the most from exercise, underscoring the importance of developing compliance strategies aimed at patients identified as being at high risk for dropout.

Drawing on this research into predictors of compliance, several behavioral models have been applied to exercise interventions. According to the theory of planned behavior, intention to exercise is influenced by personal attitudes, social norms, and perceived behavioral control. This theory has contributed to a better understanding of the process by which individuals decide to initiate an exercise program. Social-cognitive theory emphasizes the importance of goals and perceived behavioral control, including related concepts of outcome expectancies and self-efficacy. From this perspective, high self-efficacy, dissatisfaction with past behavior, and challenging goals are the ideal cognitive components for motivation.

Recently, the transtheoretical model of behavior change has been applied to several health-related behaviors, including smoking, weight loss, and exercise. According to this model, patients progress through five stages of change: precontemplation, contemplation, preparation, action, and maintenance. A 16-Item Decisional Balance Scale has been developed to identify patients' perceptions of the pros and cons of exercising, and a Processes of Change Questionnaire, consisting of 10 subscales, assesses use of various cognitive or behavioral processes for engaging in exercise behavior. Marcus et al.[30] have reported that the valence of exercise increases linearly through each stage and that precontemplators (i.e., individuals who have not thought about exercising) use each process less than do individuals in any other stage. This pattern suggests that an effective approach to helping individuals move from one stage to the next would be to encourage them to expand their repertoire of both cognitive and behavioral strategies.

In summary, a number of contributors to exercise compliance have been identified, including attention to individuals' attitudes toward exercise; cognitions regarding self-efficacy, past success, and future goals; and readiness to change. Understanding these contributors can provide potentially useful information in developing strategies for enhancing motivation and adherence to exercise. Future research should focus on developing and evaluating strategies to initiate and maintain exercise behavior in clinical and healthy populations, including women, the elderly, and children.

References

1. Roth DL. Acute emotional and psychophysiological effects of aerobic exercise. *Psychophys*, 1989; 26:593-602.

2. Lobstein DD, Mosbacher BJ, Ismail AH. Depression as a powerful discriminator between physically active and sedentary middle-aged men. *J Pychosom Res*, 1983; 27:69-76.

3. Camacho TC, Roberts RE, Lazarus NB, Kaplan G, Cohen RD. Physical activity and depression: Evidence from the Alameda County Study. *Am J Epidemiol*, 1991; 134:220-231.

4. Blumenthal JA, Williams S, Needels TL, Wallace AG. Psychological changes accompany aerobic exercise in healthy middle-aged adults. *Psychosom Med*, 1982; 44:529-535.

5. North TC, McCullagh P, Tran ZV. Effect of exercise on depression. *Exercise Sport Sci Rev*, 1990; 18:379-415.

6. Blumenthal JA, Emery CF, Rejeski WJ. The effects of exercise training on psychosocial functioning after myocardial infarction. *J Cardiopul Rehab*, 1988; 8:183-193.

7. Plante TG, Karpowitz, D. The influence of aerobic exercise on physiological stress responsivity. *Psychophys*, 1987; 24:670-677.

8. Kirkcaldy BD. Personality profiles at various levels of athletic participation. *Personality and Individual Differences*, 1982; 3:321-326.

9. Emery CF, Gatz M. Psychological and cognitive effects of an exercise program for community-residing older adults. *The Gerontologist*, 1990; 30:184-188.

10. Jasnoski NM, Holmes DS, Banks DL. Changes in personality associated with changes in aerobic and anaerobic fitness in women and men. *Psychosom Res*, 1988; 32:273-276.

11. Folkins CH, Sime WE. Physical fitness and mental health. *Am Psychol*, 1981; 36:373-389.

12. Perri S, Templer D. The effects of an aerobic exercise program on psychological variables in older adults. *Ag Hum Devel*, 1985; 20:167-172.

13. Blumenthal JA, Emery CF, Madden DJ, George LK, Coleman R et al. Cardiovascular and behavioral effects of aerobic exercise training in healthy older men and women. *J Gerontol*, 1989; 44:M147-M157.

14. Blumenthal JA, Williams RS, Williams RB, Wallace AG. Effects of exercise on the Type A (coronary prone) pattern. *Psychosom Med*, 1980; 42:289-296.

15. Blumenthal JA, Emery CF, Walsh MA, Cox DR, Kuhn CM, Williams RB, Williams RS. Exercise training in healthy Type A middle-aged men: Effects on behavioral and cardiovascular responses. *Psychosom Med*, 1988; 50:418-433.

16. Roskies E, Seraganian P, Oseasohn R, Hanley JA, Collu R, Martin N, Smilga C. The Montreal Type A intervention project: Major findings. *Health Psychol*, 1986; 5:45-69.

17. Krantz DK, Manuck SB. Acute physiologic reactivity and risk of coronary heart disease: A review and methodologic critique. *Psych Bull*, 1984; 96:435-464.

18. Crews DJ, Landers DM. A meta-analytic review of aerobic fitness and reactivity to psychosocial stressors. *Med Sci Sports Exercise*, 1987; 19:S114-S120.

19. Filligim RB, Blumenthal JA. Does aerobic exercise reduce stress responses? In Turner R, Sherwood A, Light K (Eds): *Individual differences in cardiovascular responses to stress*. New York: Plenum, 1992.

20. Blumenthal JA, Fredrikson M, Kuhn CM, Ulmer RL, Walsh-Riddle M, Applebaum M. Aerobic exercise reduces levels of cardiovascular and sympathoadrenal responses to mental stress in subjects without prior evidence of myocardial infarction. *Am Cardiol*, 1990; 65:93-98.

21. Emery CF, Blumenthal JA. Effects of physical exercise on psychological and cognitive functioning of older adults. *Ann Behav Med*, 1991; 13:99-107.

22. Spirduso WW. Reaction and movement time as a function of age and physical activity level. *Gerontology*, 1980; 30:435-440.

23. Dustman RE, Ruhling RO, Russell EM et al. Aerobic exercise training and improved neuropsychological function of older adults. *Neurobiol Aging*, 1984; 5:35-42.

24. Blumenthal JA, Emery CF, Madden DJ, Schniebolk S et al. Long-term effects of exercise on psychological functioning in older men and women. *J Gerontol: Psych Sci*, 1991; 46:P352-P361.

25. Tomporowski PD, Ellis NR. Effects of exercise on cognitive processes: A review. *Psych Bull*, 1986; 99:338-346.

26. Sallis JF, Haskell WL, Fo SP, Vranizan KM, Taylor CB, Solomon DS. Predictors of adoption and maintenance of physical activity in a community sample. *Prevent Med*, 1986; 15:331-341.

27. King AC, Haskell WL, Taylor CB, Kraemer HC, DeBusk RF. Group- vs home-based exercise training in healthy older men and women. A community-based clinical trial. *JAMA*, 1991; 266:1535-1542.

28. Oldridge NB, Donner AP, Buck CW, Jones NL, Andrew GM, Parker JO, Cunningham DA, Kavanaugh T, Rechnitzer PA, Sutton JR. Predictors of dropout from cardiac exercise rehabilitation. Ontario Exercise-Heart Collaborative Study. *Am J Cardiol*, 1983; 51:70-74.

29. Blumenthal JA, Williams RS, Wallace AG, Williams RB Jr, Needles TL. Physiological and psychological variables predict compliance to prescribed exercise

therapy in patients recovering from myocardial infarction. *Psychosom Med*, 1982; 44:519-527.

30. Marcus BH, Banspach SW, Lefebvre RC, Rossi JS, Carleton RA, Abrams DB. Using the stages of change model to increase the adoption of physical activity among community participants. *Am J Health Promotion*, 1992; 6:424-429.

Does The Mode of Delivery of Cardiac Rehabilitation Influence Outcome?

Nancy Houston Miller

Stanford University School of Medicine, Stanford, California, USA

Cardiac rehabilitation services are designed to enhance the recovery of the more than 6 million Americans who suffer coronary heart disease. Cardiac rehabilitation programs should provide multifactorial services, including exercise training, education and counseling about risk reduction and lifestyle changes, and interventions to improve psychosocial functioning. Rehabilitative services usually begin in the hospital for patients recovering from acute events, such as myocardial infarction (MI), coronary artery bypass graft (CABG) surgery, or percutaneous transluminal coronary angioplasty (PTCA). Exercise training under supervision by medical staff with ECG monitoring, if indicated, as well as education and counseling on risk factors and psychological aspects of recovery, commence one to three weeks after hospital discharge. Outpatient rehabilitation extends from four to six weeks at a minimum to six months or more. Maintenance beyond six months may or may not continue with formal supervision or monitoring.

Rehabilitation in the outpatient setting is presently offered to patients in two formats: group programs, located primarily in hospitals or community settings, or home rehabilitation programs. The traditional format for rehabilitation in the past has been a group-based approach. Group-based programs currently reach 11% to 38% of all patients with coronary heart disease.[1-3] A recent survey[3] of 163 rehabilitation programs across the country indicated that only a minority of MI, PTCA, and CABG survivors enroll in cardiac rehabilitation programs (10.8%, 10.3%, and 23.4%, respectively). Enrollment rates were found to be particularly low for women recovering from MI and CABG surgery compared to men (6.9% vs 13.3% and 20.2% vs 22.6%, respectively). Enrollment was slightly higher for women recovering from PTCA than for men (11.1% vs 10.0%, respectively). Enrollment rates for nonwhites were lower than those of whites (5.1%, 16.9%, and 5.2% of all MI, PTCA, and CABG patients, respectively). Finally, enrollment tended to be highest in the west and the midwest regions of the United States. Various patient, physician, and program-related factors have been shown to affect enrollment.[4-6] These include the degree of social support, severity of disease, strength of the physician's recommendation, and the physician's perception of the benefits of cardiac rehabilitation, as well as program costs and desirability of program schedules, facilities, and location. One study suggested that only about one-half of patients referred to cardiac rehabilitation programs actually enroll in them.[7]

The traditional setting for group rehabilitation programs has been the hospital. Most patients attend such programs for 10 to 12 weeks following an acute coronary event. The brevity of participation is generally due to a lack of reimbursement for longer term services. Other settings include universities or community-based organizations, such as the YMCA. These settings serve only about 15% of all patients receiving cardiac rehabilitation services.[3] While rehabilitation has traditionally been carried out in a supervised group, an alternate site for such services is the home.[8-10] Patients at low to moderate risk, who comprise the majority of those with coronary heart disease, have safely undertaken home-based exercise training with and without transtelephonic monitoring. It is unclear how many patients are actually participating in such programs.

The goals of cardiac rehabilitation include an improvement in the patient's prognosis, functional capacity, quality of life, and psychosocial status. Such improvement in these outcomes is also due to intensive risk-factor modification that should be included as part of cardiac rehabilitation services. The central question is, Does the mode of delivery of these services affect the outcome?

Two meta-analyses of 21 controlled trials of cardiac rehabilitation established an approximate 25% reduction in mortality at a three-year follow-up in patients participating in rehabilitation compared to controls.[11,12] The meta-analyses, which involved more than 4 000 patients with coronary heart disease, were largely based on trials conducted in the 1980s. Exercise training was the sole intervention in seven of these trials. In the remaining trials, which incorporated risk-factor modification and psychosocial advice, the mortality was lower than in those that provided exercise alone. Most of these studies involved male patients less than 65 years of age and excluded high-risk patients. These studies did not show a reduction in reinfarction favoring rehabilitation.

Do These Studies Relate to Contemporary Care in the 1990s?

Thrombolytic and adjunctive medical therapies provided within hours of an acute myocardial infarction, augmented by coronary revascularization for patients exhibiting post-MI ischemia, have decreased early acute coronary mortality to such an extent that exercise training, which begins weeks after the acute event, is unlikely to improve prognosis even further. Prophylactic therapy with aspirin and beta-blockers, and more recently the use of ACE inhibitors, commonly given after acute MI, also reduce long-term mortality. It is noteworthy in the 1990s that these therapies are more likely to influence prognosis than will the 10 to 12 weeks of exercise training most often provided under existing reimbursement guidelines for rehabilitative services. Exercise training then must be seen primarily as a method to enhance the functional capacity of patients, to optimize risk reduction, and to provide psychosocial support.

Does the Mode of Delivery of Rehabilitation Affect the Functional Capacity of Patients?

The 114 scientific reports in the Agency for Health Care Policy and Research (AHCPR) guidelines[13] on cardiac rehabilitation address the effect of cardiac rehabilitation on measures of exercise tolerance. Thirteen of 14 randomized, controlled trials performed in the United States showed statistically significant improvements in exercising versus control patient groups.[13] No significant cardiovascular complications were noted. Two-thirds of the trials, conducted in the United States and elsewhere, provided training for six months or less. Half of these studies were home-based, and half were group-based. The magnitude of improvement in functional capacity of patients appears to be comparable irrespective of the mode of delivery. Studies show that post-MI and post-CABG patients reach functional capacities equivalent to 8.0 to 9.0 METs at six months, whether assigned to group or home-based programs.[14-16] Moreover, low-to-moderate intensity activity appears to be as effective as is high-intensity exercise in increasing the functional capacity of patients in cardiac rehabilitation.[17,18]

Goble et al.[18] randomly allocated 308 men to eight weeks of group and home-based activities of high and low intensities. High-intensity exercise was carried out for 30 minutes at 70% to 85% of maximum heart rate. Patients attended a group rehabilitation program three times per week. Those assigned to low-intensity exercise worked at a heart rate of 20 beats above their resting rate in a group program for 30 minutes twice per week. Patients in both groups were asked to walk at a comfortable pace 30 minutes per day outside of the group program. While the peak exercise capacity at eight weeks was slightly higher in the high-intensity group, (11 vs 10 METs) this small difference disappeared by 12 months.

Does the Mode of Delivery of Rehabilitation Affect the Safety of Exercise Training?

Studies of the safety of exercise training in group rehabilitation programs in the 1970s and 1980s indicate that the risk of an untoward event is extremely low.[19,20] Continuous ECG monitoring in group rehabilitation has not been shown to improve the safety of exercise training.[20] Fewer patients have undergone home-based exercise training than group-based training. However, for patients with low to moderate risk, who comprise the majority of post-MI patients, and those following coronary revascularization, home-based training appears to be as safe as is group-based training. The safety of home-based exercise training is enhanced by thrombolysis and/or mechanical revascularization, which are designed to alleviate myocardial ischemia, and by afterload-reducing drugs, which are designed to mitigate left ventricular dysfunction. These two pathologic mechanisms are responsible not only for spontaneous but for exercise-induced cardiac events.

Risk stratification early in the course of recovery from an acute event enables identification of appropriate candidates for exercise training. For example, 70% of all survivors of an MI aged 70 or less are at low risk for subsequent coronary events.[21] For these patients, medically directed home-based rehabilitation and group-based exercise rehabilitation in a community setting have shown comparable efficacy and safety.[14] Home-based exercise training can be supervised by health-care professionals through periodic telephone contact, using behavioral strategies, such as activity logs and simple heart rate monitors, to promote adherence.[14,16]

Patients with heart failure who may be referred for cardiac rehabilitation services are generally at high risk for sudden cardiac death. Exercise training does not reduce this risk, whereas afterload-reducing drugs do. Group rehabilitation programs may employ continuous ECG monitoring for these sicker patients with heart failure or for those with ongoing ischemia. While programs with ECG monitoring have reported lower complication rates than those without such monitoring,[20] it is difficult to establish the contribution of such monitoring to safety separate from patient selection. Accordingly, continuous ECG monitoring is recommended only for selected high-risk patients.[22] Ongoing surveillance and prompt response to changes in patients' clinical status promotes the safety of exercise training in any delivery system.

Does the Mode of Delivery Affect the Modification of Coronary Risk Factors?

While exercise training has traditionally been the primary focus of cardiac rehabilitation, modification of cardiovascular risk factors appears to exert a stronger effect on prognosis among patients with established heart disease. Aggressive management of hyperlipidemia with diet and drug therapy in patients with ischemic heart disease has been shown to decrease not only cardiovascular mortality but total mortality as well, and to reduce the rate of subsequent MI and hospitalization for unstable angina and the need for mechanical revascularization.[23] There is little evidence to suggest that exercise training alone has a significant effect on smoking cessation, lipid modification (including a reduction in plasma LDL cholesterol or triglycerides), body weight or blood pressure, or an increase in HDL cholesterol.[13]

Specific interventions targeting education and counseling for coronary risk-factor modification have produced the most consistent results.[24] For example, interventions for smoking and hyperlipidemia, which exhibit a major impact on prognosis, have shown their greatest impact in home-based rehabilitation settings.[23,25] Patients receiving multifactorial home-based interventions have demonstrated significantly lower total and plasma LDL cholesterol levels and higher smoking cessation rates than have patients receiving usual care.[9,10] The largest trial[10] employed nurses as case managers to deliver interventions for exercise training, smoking cessation, and diet-drug management of hyperlipidemia. Telephone and mail were the primary methods used for maintaining contact with post-MI patients in the year following infarction. This study provided a convenient model of rehabilitation that is potentially more accessible to patients with coronary heart disease who may not be served by group programs. Case management by nurses also helps to ensure that patients requiring lipid-lowering agents receive them at a sufficiently high dose and for long enough periods to achieve the clinical benefits previously described.

Does the Mode of Delivery of Cardiac Rehabilitation Affect the Psychological Well-Being of Patients?

Exercise training, provided alone or as a component of multifactorial cardiac rehabilitation, often results in an improvement in psychological status. Exercise alone has not been consistently shown to improve measures of anxiety and depression.[26,27] Improvement appears to be greatest in patients with high levels of distress.[28] Much of the early work on the benefits of education and counseling to improve psychological status was conducted in groups specifically designed to reduce Type A behavior, reduce anxiety, and improve psychosocial adaptation. More recent studies have shown not only an improvement in psychological outcomes but in prognosis among depressed and socially isolated post-MI patients receiving interventions provided by telephone contacts and occasional home visits.[28] Additional research is necessary to determine the effects of exercise on psychosocial functioning of the elderly, women, and those who receive rehabilitation in a home setting.

Patients with coronary heart disease may benefit greatly from cardiac rehabilitative services. In a changing health-care environment, more cost-effective models for the delivery of such services are needed. While group programs offer a wide array of services for patients with coronary heart disease, the availability of, and enrollment in, such programs has been limited for a variety of reasons. Home-based programs offer the potential to expand rehabilitative services to a much larger number of patients. For example, the management program of multiple risk-factor interventions (MULTIFIT),[10] enrolled 65% of all consecutive post-MI patients, of whom 78% participated in home-based exercise training. Cost is an important determinant of whether such programs will be disseminated, since insurance coverage varies widely from state to state and patients may be very reluctant to pay out of pocket. Managed care programs interested in optimal risk factor management and exercise training may view this approach favorably due to its greater convenience and lower cost.

In summary: (1) The traditional group-based format has limited patients' participation in cardiac rehabilitation; women and minorities are particularly underrepresented. (2) Exercise training increases functional capacity in all patients regardless of the setting, but in the era of thrombolytic therapy, the efficacy of exercise training for enhancing prognosis is limited. (3) Reimbursement for cardiac rehabilitation limited to exercise training is threatened in today's changing health-care environment. Reimbursement for smoking cessation, treatment of hyperlipidemia, and management of other risk factors generally has been limited. (4) Newer models, such as home-based cardiac rehabilitation, not only increase functional capacity but foster smoking cessation and lipid management, which demonstrably enhance prognosis. This model, if broadly disseminated, may substantially increase the number of patients with ischemic heart disease who receive rehabilitative services.

References

1. Leon AS, Certo C, Comoss P, Franklin BA, Froelicher V, Haskell WL, Hellerstein HK, Marley WP, Pollock ML, Ries A et al. Scientific evidence of the value of cardiac rehabilitation services with emphasis on patients following myocardial infarction—Section I: Exercise, conditioning component (position paper). *J Cardiopul Rehab*, 1990;10:79-87.

2. Mark DB, Naylor CD, Hlatky MA, Califf RM, Topol EJ, Granger CB, Knight JD, Nelson CL, Lee KL, Clapp-Channing NE et al. Use of medical resources and quality of life after acute myocardial infarction in Canada and the United States. *N Engl J Med*, 1994;331:1130-5.

3. Thomas RJ, Houston Miller N, Lamendola C, Berra K, Hedback B, Durstine L, Haskell W. National survey on gender differences in cardiac rehabilitation: Patient characteristics and enrollment patterns (submitted article).

4. Oldridge NB, Ragowski B, Gottlieb M. Use of outpatient cardiac rehabilitation services: Factors associated with attendance. *J Cardiopul Rehab*, 1992;12:25-31.

5. Ades PA, Waldmann ML, McCann WJ, Weaver SO. Predictors of cardiac rehabilitation participation in older coronary patients. *Arch Int Med*, 1992;152:1033-5.

6. Ades PA, Waldman ML, Polk DM, Coflesky JT. Referral patterns and exercise response in the rehabilitation of female coronary patients aged greater than or equal to 62 years. *Am J Cardiol*, 1992;69:1422-5.

7. Sevensky K, Brubaker PH, Miller HS et al. Characteristics of patients referred to cardiac rehabilitation and factors related to entry. *J Cardiopul Rehab*, 1994;14:340 (abstract).

8. Miller NH, Haskell WL, Berra K, DeBusk RF. Home versus group exercise training for increasing functional capacity after myocardial infarction. *Circulation*, 1984;70:645-9.

9. Haskell WL, Alderman EL, Fair JM, Maron DJ, Mackey SF, Superko HR, Williams PT, Johnstone IM, Champagne ME, Krauss RM et al. Effects of intensive multiple risk factor reduction on coronary atherosclerosis and clinical cardiac events in men and women with coronary artery disease: The Stanford Coronary Risk Intervention Project (SCRIP). *Circulation*, 1994;89:975-90.

10. DeBusk RF, Houston Miller N, Superko HR, Dennis CA, Thomas RJ, Lew HT, Berger WE , Heller RS, Rompf J, Gee D et al. A case-management system for coronary risk factor modification after acute myocardial infarction. *Ann Intern Med*, 1994;120:721-9.

11. O'Connor GT, Buring JE, Yusuf S, Goldhaber SZ, Olmstead EM, Paffenbarger RS Jr, Hennekens CH. An overview of randomized trials of rehabilitation with exercise after myocardial infarction. *Circulation*, 1989;80:234-44.

12. Oldridge NB, Guyatt GH, Fischer ME, Rimm AA. Cardiac rehabilitation after myocardial infarction: Combined experience of randomized clinical trials. *JAMA*, 1988;260:945-50.

13. Wenger NK, Froelicher ES, Smith LK et al. *Cardiac rehabilitation: Clinical practice guideline No. 17.* AHCPR publication no. 96-0672, 1995;1-202.

14. DeBusk RF, Haskell WL, Miller NH, Berra K, Taylor CB, Berger WE, Lew H. Medically directed at-home rehabilitation soon after uncomplicated acute myocardial infarction: A new model for patient care. *Am J Cardiol*, 1985; 55:251-7.

15. Heath GW, Maloney PM, Fure CW. Group exercise versus home exercise in coronary artery bypass graft patients: Effects on physical activity habits. *J Cardiopul Rehab*, 1987;7:190-5.

16. Stevens R, Hanson P. Comparison of supervised and unsupervised exercise training after coronary bypass surgery. *Am J Cardiol*, 1984;53:1524-8.

17. Blumenthal JA, Rejeski WJ, Walsh-Riddle M, Emery CF, Miller H, Roark S, Ribisl PM, Morris PB, Brubaker P, Williams RS. Comparison of high- and low-intensity exercise training early after acute myocardial infarction. *Am J Cardiol*, 1988;61:26-30.

18. Goble AJ, Hare DL, Macdonald PS, Oliver RG, Reid MA, Worcester MC. Effect of early programmes of high and low intensity exercise on physical performance after transmural acute myocardial infarction. *Br Heart J*, 1991; 65:126-31.

19. Haskell WL. Cardiovascular complications during exercise training of cardiac patients. *Circulation*, 1978;57:920-4.

20. Van Camp SP, Peterson RA. Cardiovascular complications of outpatient cardiac rehabilitation programs. *JAMA*, 1986;256:1160-3.

21. DeBusk RF, Blomqvist CG, Kouchoukos NT, Luepker RV, Miller HS, Moss AJ, Pollock ML, Reeves TJ, Selvester RH, Stason WB et al. Identification and treatment of low-risk patients after acute myocardial infarction and coronary-artery bypass graft surgery. *N Engl J Med*, 1986;314:161-6.

22. Parmley, WW. Position report on cardiac rehabilitation: Recommendations of the American College of Cardiology on cardiovascular rehabilitation. *J Am Coll Cardiol*, 1986;7:451-3.

23. Pedersen TR, Kjekshus J, Berg K, Haghfelt T, Faergeman O, Thorgeirsson G, Pyorala R, Miettinen T, Wilhelmsen L, Olsson AG, Wedel H. Randomized trials of cholesterol lowering in 4 444 patients with coronary heart disease: The Scandinavian Simvastation Survival Study (4S). *Lancet*, 1994;344:1383-89.

24. Godin G. The effectiveness of interventions in modifying behavioral risk factors of individuals with coronary heart disease. *J Cardiopul Rehab*, 1989;9:923-36.

25. Cavender JB, Rogers WF, Fisher LD, Gersh BJ, Coggin CJ, Myers WO, Cass Investigators. Effects of smoking on survival and morbidity in patients randomized to medical or surgical therapy in the Coronary Artery Surgery Study (CASS): 10-year follow-up. *J Am Coll Cardiol*, 1992;20:287-94.

26. Erdman RA, Duivenvoorden HJ, Verhage F, Kazemier M, Hugenholtz PG. Predictability of beneficial effects in cardiac rehabilitation: A randomized clinical trial of psychosocial variables. *J Cardiopul Rehab*, 1986;6:206-13.

27. Worcester MC, Hare DL, Oliver RG, Reid MA, Goble AJ. Early programmes of high and low intensity exercise and quality of life after acute myocardial infarction. *Br Med J*, 1993;307:1244-7.

28. Frasure-Smith N, Prince R. The ischemic heart disease life stress monitoring program: Impact on mortality. *Psychosom Med*, 1985;47:431-45.

Health-Related Quality of Life and Economic Evaluation of Cardiac Rehabilitation

Neil B. Oldridge, PhD
University of Wisconsin, Milwaukee, Wisconsin, USA

According to the US Department of Health and Human Services (1995) mortality in the United States from heart disease has decreased by 53%, from 307 per 100,000 in 1950 to 144 per 100,000 in 1993. A possible explanation for this decrease is the increased availability of more sophisticated and effective, though expensive, health-care technologies that have provided improved preventive, diagnostic, and treatment options (of course, these technologies are not always accessible). Controlling the introduction and utilization of these technologies is a major health-care policy issue in this "era of accountability and assessment."[1] As part of the strategy to achieve appropriate control and utilization, effectiveness research (also known as outcomes research) "encompasses . . . efforts aimed at identifying broadly effective care, and efforts to develop and refine methods to support the identification of effective care."[2] The assumption underlying effectiveness research is that a better understanding of patient experience will help health-care consumers, clinicians, payers, and policy makers make rational choices about more effective and efficient health care.[2,3]

As part of this research thrust, increasing attention is being given, first, to documenting the outcomes of interventions, such as cardiac rehabilitation, by using various measures of patient-perceived health-related quality of life (HRQL) and satisfaction and, second, to economic evaluations, such as cost-effectiveness and cost-utility analyses. Documentation and evaluation both are important in light of the increasing number of people demanding access to the growing number of sophisticated, effective, and expensive health-care technologies, each of which competes for limited health-care resources.

The following four points are a response to the charges put to the Consensus Development Conference on Physical Activity and Cardiovascular Health:

1. There are only limited available data on HRQL and cost-effectiveness from randomized clinical trials or from controlled, nonrandomized studies of cardiac rehabilitation.
2. The limited data suggest that some aspects of HRQL demonstrate a significant acceleration in the improvement of patients who participated in cardiac rehabilitation as compared with patients who did not participate in rehabilitation. However, the differences in HRQL between rehabilitation and usual care for patients are minimal and not clinically significant on follow-up at 12 months or later.

3. Patients who participate in cardiac rehabilitation gain more "quality-adjusted life years" than those not participating in the intervention. Although the "productive years gained" has not been measured in cardiac rehabilitation studies, more patients who participate in cardiac rehabilitation may return to work, and may return to work sooner, than patients who don't participate in the intervention.

4. The limited economic-evaluation data demonstrate cardiac rehabilitation to be an efficient use of health-care resources, which can be justified economically. There are no comparative economic-evaluation data on managed care, fee-for-service delivery, or other forms of delivery of cardiac rehabilitation services.

Cardiac Rehabilitation

Cardiac rehabilitation services, as described in the recently published *Agency for Health Care Policy and Research (AHCPR) Clinical Practice Guidelines for Cardiac Rehabilitation*,[4] are "comprehensive long-term programs involving medical evaluation, prescribed exercise, cardiac risk factor modification, education, and counseling . . . designed to limit the physiologic and psychologic effects of cardiac illness, reduce the risk for sudden death or reinfarction, control cardiac symptoms, stabilize or reverse the atherosclerotic process, and enhance the psychosocial and vocational status of selected patients." Documented benefits of cardiac rehabilitation services, largely based on evidence from patients with myocardial infarction (MI), include improvements in exercise tolerance, symptoms, blood lipid levels, and psychological well-being and reductions in stress, smoking, and mortality.[4]

However, there is only limited evidence for patients, clinicians, payers, policy makers, or researchers about HRQL or the cost-effectiveness of cardiac rehabilitation. Of the 334 references cited in the AHCPR Guidelines,[4] only 3 of the 14 randomized clinical trials[5-7] and 2 of the 14 controlled, nonrandomized trials[8,9] utilized instruments designed to measure HRQL. In the same database,[4] economic evaluations were the focus of only three studies of cardiac rehabilitation,[10-12] in addition to one that focused on an occupational work evaluation[13] and one that focused on health-care utilization associated with rehabilitation.[14] In addition, a retrospective economic evaluation of cardiac rehabilitation following PTCA was omitted from the Guidelines.[15]

Health-Related Quality of Life

Health-related quality of life represents the effect of an illness and its treatment as perceived by the patient and is modified by impairments, functional stress, perceptions and social opportunities that are in turn influenced by disease, injury, treatment, or policy.[16,17] Patient-perceived HRQL assessment and evaluation is carried out using generic health status, utility, or specific instruments, preferably in some combination.[16,18] Health-status instruments measure a spectrum of health and quality-of-life concepts, broadly applicable across types and severity of disease, interventions, and different sociodemographic and cultural subgroups. Utility measures, on the other hand, reflect the preference of individual patients for a given health status or outcome. Specific instruments include items that patients themselves deem important and are designed to be optimally responsive or sensitive to important, but often small, changes in HRQL.[16,18] Specific HRQL instruments have been developed for patients with heart failure,[19] angina,[20] and MI.[6]

Three randomized controlled trials of multifactorial cardiac rehabilitation were specifically designed to assess HRQL, one utilizing a generic instrument,[5] one a specific instrument,[7] and one utilizing both generic and specific instruments.[6] In the trial utilizing only a generic HRQL instrument, the Sickness Impact Profile was used to assess the effects of a three-month cardiac rehabilitation intervention after acute MI, with no demonstrable benefit to the health status of the patient.[5] In the trial utilizing both generic and specific HRQL instruments, a total of 201 patients were randomized, 99 to rehabilitation and 102 to usual care within eight weeks of an acute MI; of these patients, 177 were male, the average age was 52.8 years, and randomization was successful.[6] The condition-specific questionnaire, Quality of Life After Myocardial Infarction (QLMI), which was specifically developed for the trial, consists of two dimensions: Emotions and Physical Limitations which are combined to provide an Overall QLMI score. It has been shown to be reliable, valid, and responsive.[6,21] As shown in Table 1, there was a significantly greater improvement in the rehabilitation patients at eight weeks in the Overall QLMI and the Emotions dimension of the condition-specific QLMI, in state anxiety, and in exercise tolerance when compared with the usual-care patients, with no difference in either the generic Time Trade-Off or Quality of Well-Being measures. All condition-specific and generic measures of HRQL and exercise tolerance improved significantly over the 12-month follow-up period in both groups. However, the 95% confidence intervals about the differences between groups at the 12-month follow-up effectively excluded sustained, clinically important benefits of rehabilitation in HRQL.[6] In the trial utilizing only a condition-specific instrument, the efficacy of a mail-out intervention after MI was examined, using the condition-specific QLMI to assess HRQL 6 months after the acute event.[7] HRQL was greater for each dimension in intervention patients than in control patients and, as in the previous trial, [6] the improvement was significant in the Emotions dimension.[7] In the two controlled, nonrandomized studies of cardiac rehabilitation on HRQL cited in the Guidelines,[4] one used the Sickness Impact Profile, finding a significant time effect and no main effect for HRQL,[8] while the other, which used both the Sickness Impact Profile and the Quality of Life Index, found no effect on HRQL.[9]

Economic Evaluation

With only finite and limited financial resources to invest in health care, a central issue for health-care policy makers is how to make rational decisions to get the

Table 1.   Percent Change From Baseline to 8 weeks and to 12 Months in Generic Utility and Condition-Specific Health-Related Quality of Life With 8 Weeks of Rehabilitation and Follow-Up at 12 months

	Baseline	8 weeks	12 months
Condition-specific HRQL			
QLMI † Overall			
Treatment	5.2	+13%*	+18%**¶
Usual care	5.2	+10%	+19%**
QLMI † Emotions			
Treatment	5.3	+12%	+15%**¶
Usual care	5.3	+8%	+16%**
QLMI † Limitations			
Treatment	4.9	+20%	+24%**
Usual care	5.0	+16%	+22%**
Generic utility HRQL			
TTO †††			
Treatment	0.719	+10%	+19%***
Usual care	0.766	+7%	+14%***
QWB ††			
Treatment	0.617	+17%	+26%***
Usual care	0.632	+12%	+24%***

† Quality of Life After Myocardial Infarction;   †† Quality of Well-being;
††† Time Trade-Off   Treatment effects: * p < 0.05;
Time effects:** p < 0.001;   ¶ Treatment by time effects: p = 0.003

most value for health-care expenditures. Economic evaluation assists in making these difficult decisions about health-care services, and it has been defined as "the comparative analysis of alternative courses of action in terms of both their costs and consequences."[22] Two principal questions need to be considered when reviewing health-care economic evaluations: Are both costs (inputs) and consequences (outputs) of the health-care service examined? Is there a comparison between two or more options of services?

The costs considered in an economic evaluation of illness or health-care services include the direct monetary costs incurred and may also include indirect costs, for example, lost productivity. The classification of an economic evaluation is based on how the consequences are measured.[22] In *cost-effectiveness analysis* consequences are measured either in natural units, such as deaths averted or life-years gained, or in change in some outcome, such as blood pressure or cholesterol. Consequences of health-care services also have utility, the value or worth to an individual as measured by his or her preference for a specific health status or a change in health status. *Cost-utility analysis,* a form of cost-effectiveness analysis, measures consequences in utility or preference units, such as quality-adjusted life years and healthy-year equivalents. While economic evaluations represent only one aspect of a choice between alternative health-care services, they can help to improve the quality and consistency of decision-making by consumers, providers, payers, and policy makers. Finally, economic evaluations are most useful when preceded by the assessment of the service's efficacy (can it work?), effectiveness (does it work?), and availability (does it reach all those who need it?). In the context of cardiac rehabilitation, the answers to the first two questions are probably yes, but the answer is probably no to the latter question.

Although it is difficult to conclude that universal access and coverage for rehabilitation after a coronary event is warranted on the basis of cost-effectiveness,[23] the available limited data are encouraging and suggest that cardiac rehabilitation is probably an efficient use of health-care resources, which can be economically justified. Studies from Sweden, with nonrandomized but controlled designs, have demonstrated cost-effectiveness with reduced rehospitalization and emergency visits[14] and days of rehospitalization,[10,14] and a significantly higher rate of return to work for the rehabilitation patients when compared with patients in the control group.[10] A retrospective analysis of patients in the United States who were either referred or not referred to cardiac rehabilitation, and followed up for 21 months, showed a lower incidence of rehospitalizations and lower charges per rehospitalization in rehabilitation patients, resulting in a significant saving estimated at $739 per patient (a conservative figure, as physician charges were not included).[11] Another retrospective study in the United States examined the cost-effectiveness of exercise plus education compared with education only.[15] Although total expenses were considerably lower in the exercising group at 6 months ($905) and 12 months ($2,600), the differences were not significant at either time.[15] In the only randomized trial of cardiac rehabilitation with an economic evaluation as an outcome measure, carried out in Ontario, Canada, patients referred to 8 weeks of rehabilitation within 6 weeks of an acute MI[6] incurred incremental direct costs of $790.[12] As there were direct savings of $310 per patient, primarily due to significantly fewer rehabilitation visits over a 12-month period in rehabilitation patients than in control patients, the estimated net, direct cost was $480 per patient. With patients in rehabilitation gaining 0.052 more quality-adjusted life years during the duration of the study than the control-group patients, the cost-utility ratio for cardiac rehabilitation was $9,200 per quality-adjusted life year.[12] The cost-effectiveness ratio, as estimated from previously published mortality meta-analyses,[24,25] was $21,800 per year of life saved.[12]

The data presented in Table 2 on the economic evaluation of cardiac rehabilitation can be compared in 1991 US dollars the cost-utility (per quality-adjusted life year) and cost-effectiveness (per year of life saved) of a number of selected interventions for coronary heart disease. Cardiac rehabilitation appears to have favorable cost-utility and cost-effectiveness ratios. Although not comparable, the savings of $739 per patient in reduced hospital admissions over a 21-month period of

Table 2.   Economic Evaluations (Cost-Utility per Quality-Adjusted Life-Year* and Cost-Effectiveness per Year of Life Saved**) of Various Interventions for Patients With Coronary Heart Disease in 1991 US Dollars

Cost-Utility per QALY *	
Captopril after MI † (80 years old)	$3,600
CABGS †† for 3-vessel or left main disease	$7,900
Cardiac rehabilitation after MI †	$9,200
Diastolic hypertension (>104 mm Hg)	$17,700
Diastolic hypertension (>104 mm Hg) in 40-year-old men	$35,900
Captopril after MI † (50 years old)	$60,800
Cost-Effectiveness per YOLS **	
Smoking cessation after MI †	$200-$1,200
Beta-blockers after MI † in 55-year-old men	$5,300
Lovastatin (40 mg/d) for cholesterolemia (>272 mg/dl)	$17,000
Cardiac rehabilitation after MI †	$21,800
Thrombolysis with t-PA vs streptokinase	$28,700
Lovastatin (40 mg/d) for cholesterolemia (>272 mg/dl)	$73,000

† Myocardial infarction; †† Coronary artery bypass graft surgery

time[11] and the costs of $480 per patient for an 8-week intervention,[12] have been used by the Agency for Health Care Policy and Research to generate an estimated net savings of $148 per patient per year.[26] The temptation to do this to provide evidence of potential cost savings with cardiac rehabilitation must be resisted, as the studies were generated in two locales with different health-care systems— Vermont, United States,[11] and Ontario, Canada,[12] and with different study designs, one a retrospective analysis of billing records of patients referred or not referred to cardiac rehabilitation[11] and the other a randomized controlled trial.[12] However, the limited evidence from different sources is consistent and suggests that cardiac rehabilitation is a cost-effective intervention.

Summary

The limited available data on HRQL and economic evaluations with cardiac rehabilitation are based largely on middle-aged, white, professional, male patients with MI. The available data suggest that during active participation in cardiac rehabilitation there is an accelerated improvement in some aspects of HRQL. However, most studies using either HRQL instruments or composite indices of psychological and social status and functioning demonstrate that control patients, when followed long enough, improve with the passage of time and achieve a similar level of HRQL to that seen in patients who had participated in the intervention. Exercise is considered by many to be the key component of comprehensive cardiac rehabilitation. However, the incremental value of exercise is uncertain when it is added to other cost-effective secondary prevention interventions such as smoking cessation and management of hyperlipidemia. Therefore, there is a need for considerably more research on HRQL and economic evaluation of cardiac rehabilitation in patients with MI. In addition, these kinds of data are particularly needed in patients with various presentations of coronary heart disease other than MI, in elderly patients, in female patients, in minority patients, and in patients from lower socioeconomic groups. The limited economic evaluation data do, however, suggest that cardiac rehabilitation after MI is an efficient use of health-care resources and can be economically justified, even though its worth and affordability have not been examined.

References

1. Relman AS. Assessment and accountability: The third revolution in medical care. *N Engl J Med.* 1988;319:1220-1222.

2. Office of Technology Assessment. *Identifying Health Technologies That Work: Searching for Evidence.* Washington, DC: US Government Printing Office, 1994. OTA-H-608.

3. Ellwood PM. Shattuck lecture—Outcomes management. *N Engl J Med.* 1988;318:1549-1556.

4. Wenger NK, Froelicher ES, Smith LK, Ades PA, Berra K, Blumenthal JA et al. *Cardiac Rehabilitation.* Clinical Practice Guideline #17. Rockville, MD: US Dept. of Health & Human Services, Public Health Service, Agency for Health Care Policy & Research and the National Heart, Lung, and Blood Institute, 1995. AHCPR # 96-0672.

5. Ott CR, Sivarajan ES, Newton KM, Almes MJ, Bruce RA, Bergner M et al. A controlled randomized study of early cardiac rehabilitation: The Sickness Impact Profile as an assessment. *Heart Lung.*1983;12:162-170.

6. Oldridge N, Guyatt G, Jones N, Crowe J, Singer J, Feeny D et al. Effects on quality of life with comprehensive rehabilitation after acute myocardial infarction. *Am J Cardiol.* 1991;67:1084-1089.

7. Heller RF, Knapp JC, Valenti LA, Dobson AJ. Secondary prevention after acute myocardial infarction. *Am J Cardiol.* 1993;72:759-762.

8. Munro BH, Creaner AM, Haggerty MR, Cooper FS. Effect of relaxation therapy on post-myocardial infarction patients' rehabilitation. *Nur Res.*1988;37:231-235.

9. Daumer R, Miller P. Effects of cardiac rehabilitation on psychosocial functioning and life satisfaction of coronary artery disease clients. *Rehabil Nurs.*1992;17:69-72.

10. Levin L-A, Perk J, Hedback B. Cardiac rehabilitation-cost analysis. *J Intern Med.* 1991;230:427-434.

11. Ades PA, Huang D, Weaver SO. Cardiac rehabilitation participation predicts lower rehospitalization costs. *Am Heart J.* 1992;123:916-921.

12. Oldridge N, Furlong W, Feeny D, Torrance G, Guyatt G, Crowe J et al. Economic evaluation of cardiac rehabilitation soon after acute myocardial infarction. *Am J Cardiol.* 1993;72:154-161.

13. Picard MH, Dennis C, Schwartz RG, Ahn DK, Kraemer HC, Berger WE et al. Cost-benefit analysis of early return to work after uncomplicated acute myocardial infarction. *Am J Cardiol.* 1989;63:1308-1314.

14. Bondestam E, Braikks A, Hartford M. Effects of early rehabilitation on consumption of medical care during the first year after acute myocardial infarction in patients ≥65 years of age. *Am J Cardiol.* 1995;75:767-771.

15. Edwards WW, Glickman-Weiss E, Franks BD, Iyriboz Y, Dodd SL, Quaid TP. Percutaneous transluminal coronary angioplasty rehabilitation. A cost-effectiveness analysis. *J Cardiopulmonary Rehabil.*1993;13:172-181.

16. Patrick DL, Erickson P. *Health Status and Health Policy: Quality of Life in Health Care Evaluation and Resource Allocation.* New York: Oxford University Press; 1993.

17. Schipper H, Clinch J, Olweny CLM. Quality of life studies: Definitions and conceptual issues. In: Spilker B, ed. *Quality of Life and Pharmacoeconomics in Clinical Trials* (2nd edition). Philadelphia: Lippincott-Raven Publishers; 1996:11-23.

18. Guyatt G, Feeny DH, Patrick DL. Measuring health-related quality of life. *Ann Intern Med.* 1993;118:622-629.

19. Kubo SH, Gollub S, Bourge R, Rahko S, Cobb F, Jessup M et al. Beneficial effects of pimobendan on exercise tolerance and quality of life in patients with heart failure. *Circulation.* 1992;85:942-949.

20. Spertus JA, Winder JA, Dewhurst TA, Deyo RA, Prodzinski J, McDonell M et al. Development and evaluation of the Seattle Angina Questionnaire: A new functional status measure for coronary artery disease. *J Am Coll Cardiol.* 1995;25:333-341.

21. Hillers TK, Guyatt GH, Oldridge NB, Crowe J, Willan A, Griffith L et al. Quality of life after myocardial infarction. *J Clin Epidemiol.* 1994;47:1287-1296.

22. Drummond MF, Stoddart GL, Torrance GW. *Methods for the Economic Evaluation of Health Care Programmes.* Oxford: Oxford University Press; 1988.

23. Oldridge NB. Universal access and insurance coverage: Missing pieces. *J Cardiopulmonary Rehabil.* 1995;15:9-13.

24. Oldridge NB, Guyatt GH, Fischer M, Rimm AR. Cardiac rehabilitation after myocardial infarction: Combining data from randomized clinical trials. *JAMA.* 1988;260:945-980.

25. O'Connor GT, Buring JE, Yusuf S, Goldhaber SZ, Olmstead EM, Paffenbarger RS et al. An overview of randomized trials of rehabilitation with exercise after myocardial infarction. *Circulation.*1989;80:234-244.

26. Smith LK. Guideline at work. *AACVPR News & Views.* 1996;10:5-7.

Part VI

SUCCESSFUL APPROACHES TO ADOPTING AND MAINTAINING A PHYSICALLY ACTIVE LIFESTYLE

Determinants of Physical Activity Behavior and Implications for Interventions

Bess H. Marcus and James F. Sallis

The Miriam Hospital and Brown University School of Medicine, Providence, Rhode Island, and San Diego State University, San Diego, California; USA

As physiologically oriented studies answer questions about "why" to be physically active, behaviorally oriented studies can begin to provide answers to questions about "how" to improve the health of the population of the United States through regular physical activity. This paper will focus on three key topics:

1. **Identify relevant models and theories.** Because of the complexity of physical activity behavior, it is important to have an explicit theory or model that guides the selection of variables to study. Therefore, the most influential and promising theories and models in behavioral science will be discussed.
2. **Identify determinants or factors that influence physical activity.** Observational studies of theory-derived variables can inform the researcher about which variables are most or least likely to influence physical activity in various populations. The current status of determinants research will be summarized.
3. **Apply knowledge of determinants to develop and evaluate interventions.** To be effective, interventions must alter the factors that influence physical activity. Thus, data from determinants studies, as well as theories and models, should be useful in guiding the design of interventions.

Applying theories and models can help focus on important concepts and areas of study when trying to understand complex behaviors. The theories and models presented in Table 1 are those applied most frequently in the research on determinants and interventions in physical activity.

The models vary on important dimensions, and these variations lead to differences in research methods and intervention approaches. One key dimension is the emphasis on psychological, social, or environmental influences. It can be seen in Table 1 that some models take a broad view that encompasses psychological, social, and physical environmental influences, while other models adopt a more restrictive focus. The differences between the models are important because they lead one toward measuring and eventually intervening on some variables and ignoring others.

Because of their inclusion of personal and environmental factors as well as their explicit implications for interventions, learning theories (Skinner, 1953), social-cognitive theory (Bandura, 1986), the stages of change model (Prochaska & DiClemente, 1983), and the relapse prevention model (Marlatt & Gordon, 1985) appear to be the most useful models for the field at this time.

Table 1.   Theories and Models Used in Determinants Research

Models	Features	Variables measured
Decision theory[1]	Perceived costs and benefits	Psychological
Health belief[2]	Susceptibility and cost benefit	Psychological
Planned behavior[3]	Attitudes, norms, and perceived control	Psychological
Learning theories[4]	Reinforcement	Social and environmental
Social ecology[5]	Policies, physical environment	Social and environmental
Relapse prevention[6]	Problem solving, planning for relapses	Psychological, social, and environmental
Social cognitive[7]	Self-efficacy, expectancies, modeling	Psychological, social, and environmental
Stages of change[8]	Stages and processes of change	Psychological, social, and environmental

[1]Janis & Mann, 1977
[2]Rosenstock, 1974
[3]Azjen, 1985
[4]Skinner, 1953
[5]Stokols, 1992
[6]Marlatt & Gordon, 1985
[7]Bandura, 1986
[8]Prochaska & DiClemente, 1983

Determinants of Physical Activity

The primary public health value of determinants research is to identify variables that appear to influence physical activity and which can be targeted for change in interventions. In some cases, determinants identified in descriptive research can be validated in experimental studies before being applied to larger intervention efforts.

Determinant describes a reproducible association with physical activity or exercise (Dishman & Sallis, 1994). Cross-sectional or prospective nonexperimental studies are reviewed in this section, so determinant does not imply a cause-and-effect relationship. Experimental and quasi-experimental studies are considered intervention research, and will be discussed in the chapters on intervention. Many of the determinants studies have been guided by the models described earlier. However, this summary of the literature considers all categories of potential determinants, both theoretically based and atheoretical.

Previous reviews of adult literature on physical activity determinants (Dishman & Sallis, 1994) plus recent studies total about 300. Because this chapter is focused on public-health implications, we will report on determinants of overall physical activity but not on separate effects for supervised activity. We included studies if the dependent variable was physical activity, exercise, or stage of change, but not if the dependent variable was attitude or intention. Reviews of the literature reveal consistently documented associations in many categories, which highlights the multiply determined nature of physical activity. We report on variables that can be classified into six different categories, shown in Table 2.

To identify patterns in the results of the determinants studies, we will present the percent of variables in a variety of categories that have received no, inconsistent, or consistent support as determinants. *Consistent support* does not necessarily mean high correlations; it means significant associations in multiple studies. Though the number and quality of studies contributing to the data for each category are not equivalent, the pattern of relationships may lead to improved hypotheses for future studies. Figures 1 and 2 show results for adults and youth.

Table 2   Types of Variables Used in Determinants Research

Categories	Examples
• Demographic	• Age • Gender • Ethnicity
• Psychological	• Self-efficacy • Perceived health
• Behavioral attributes & skills	• Past adult exercise • Decision making
• Sociocultural	• Social support • Physician influence
• Environmental	• Access to facilities • Season/climate
• Activity characterstics	• Intensity • Perceived effort

Determinants of Adult Physical Activity

A majority of the demographic characteristics, sociocultural factors, and activity characteristics that have been studied are consistently associated with physical activity in adults. The majority of behavioral attributes and environmental factors did not receive consistent support for associations with physical activity.

Of the numerous psychological factors studied, about one-third received no support and 40% received strong support. No single variable or category explains most adult physical activity or exercise, and there are significant variables in all categories. Figure 1 shows that many demographic, psychological, and behavioral variables have been studied, and few sociocultural, environmental, and activity characteristic variables have been studied. Further research is particularly needed in the latter categories.

Variables that are subject to modification and have consistently been associated with physical activity or found to be unrelated to physical activity among adults are summarized in Table 3. Eight variables from the psychological, behavioral, and social categories were judged to have strong support for their associations with physical activity.

A logical next step in research would be to evaluate intervention programs designed to alter these factors that may mediate physical activity. Four psychological

Table 3   Modifiable Factors

Consistently related	Consistently unrelated
Adults	
• Social support	• Health/exercise knowledge
• Past adult exercise	• Exercise in youth
• Self-efficacy	• Normative beliefs
• Expected benefits	• Perceived susceptibility to illness
• Perceived barriers	
• Intention to exercise	
• Enjoyment	
• Intensity (lower)	
Youth	
• Enjoyment	• Health/exercise knowledge
• Physical competence	• Television watching
• Self-efficacy	
• Intention to be active	
• Perceived barriers	
• Parental assistance	
• Time outdoors	

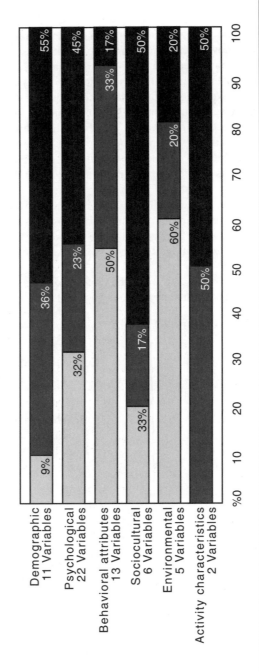

Figure 1. Determinant variables associated with overall physical activity in adults.

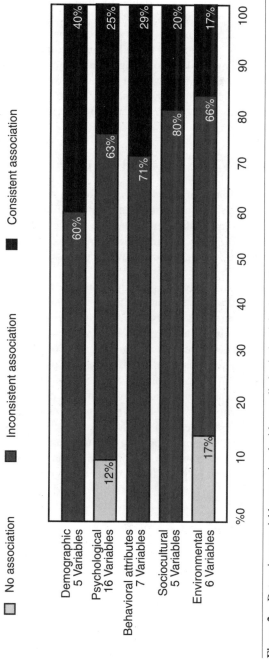

Figure 2. Determinant variables associated with overall physical activity in youth.

and behavioral variables were consistently unrelated to adult physical activity. These would appear to be poor choices as variables to attempt to change in intervention programs.

A number of nonmodifiable factors have also been found to be consistently related to physical activity participation in adults. Younger, male, educated, affluent, and childless adults are more likely to engage in higher physical activity levels.

In summary, there are determinants in all categories, so physical activity is influenced by many variables. We know something about which variables in each category are most and least important, and these findings may help us design interventions.

Determinants of Youth Physical Activity

Demographic characteristics are most likely to be consistently associated with physical activity in youth. There are many categories in Figure 2 with inconsistent associations, and this is due to the fact that many variables have been examined in only a single study. Similar to the adult literature, no one variable or category explains most youth physical activity, and all categories explain something about youth physical activity behavior.

Modifiable factors shown to be consistently related to physical activity are likely to be the most important targets for interventions. Television watching and knowledge are consistently unrelated to physical activity in youth. Interestingly, while television viewing time is not usually correlated with physical activity, an intervention that reinforced decreases in sedentary behavior (i.e., television watching) was more successful than one that reinforced increases in physical activity (Epstein, Saelens, & O'Brien, 1995). The example of television watching demonstrates that while information on determinants can provide important guidance for interventions, determinants are not the only worthwhile guide to intervention design.

In certain areas, the influences on youth physical activity are different from those on adult activity. Better understanding of determinants of youth activity can help us develop effective interventions for promoting and sustaining activity from childhood to adulthood and help us target youth at high risk for remaining or becoming sedentary.

Critique of Determinants Studies

Definitions of physical activity differ greatly across studies. In studies of adults, vigorous exercise is the most common dependent variable. A few adult studies have attempted to identify determinants of moderate intensity activities, but there are not enough studies to make statements about determinants of moderate versus vigorous physical activity. Given the recent CDC/ACSM recommendations on moderate activity (Pate et al., 1995), more attention needs to be given to the determinants of moderate-intensity activity. There are also insufficient studies to make statements about determinants of transitions to different stages of physical activity participation, such as initiation, adoption, maintenance, or relapse. Since the quality of self-report measures of physical activity varies, it is of concern that most studies rely only on self-reported physical activity. The validity of self-report measures is a particular concern in youth studies.

Few studies have specifically investigated whether some population subgroups have different determinants. In those studies, some subgroups have received more attention than have others—for example, subgroups based on gender. A consistently observed difference between these subgroups indicates that social support for exercise may be more influential for women (Sallis et al., 1992a; Duncan et al., 1993). Additionally, studies reveal that women are more likely to engage in moderate physical activity and men in vigorous activity. Women also experience a greater reduction in physical activity with age and report more demands on time that serve as a barrier to physical activity participation (Marcus et al., 1995).

There are also important gender differences in the determinants of youth physical activity behavior. Boys are more active than are girls, and this gender discrepancy increases through adolescence (Sallis, 1993). Boys also receive increased social support and parental support for physical activity (Sallis et al., 1992b).

Application of Determinants Research to Intervention Design

Results of determinants studies are not perfect guides to developing effective intervention programs for public health problems, but there are at least two important intervention-related uses of determinants research. The first use is to assist in targeting interventions to high-risk groups. Along with descriptive epidemiology studies, determinants studies identify characteristics of persons or environments with particularly low levels of physical activity. Thus, determinants research can help clarify the goals and objectives of the intervention.

The second use of determinants research is for designing specific intervention components. Knowledge of psychological correlates of physical activity should assist in developing educational and behavioral interventions. Identification of social and environmental determinants should lead to programs that enhance social and environmental support for physical activity. However, merely targeting these variables is not sufficient. Unless the intervention actually changes the mediating variables, the program is not likely to be effective.

Based on current understanding of determinants, physical activity interventions should increase their effectiveness if they are successful in changing the following mediators for adults:

- Enhance perceived benefits
- Enhance self-efficacy
- Increase intentions to exercise
- Increase enjoyment of physical activity

- Enhance social support
- Include moderate intensity activity

Physical activity interventions should be most effective when they target the following mediators in youth:

- Enhance enjoyment of physical activity
- Encourage perception of competence at physical activity
- Increase intentions to be active
- Reduce perceived barriers
- Enhance social support
- Increase time spent outdoors

The challenge is to develop and implement interventions that actually make these changes.

In summary, determinants researchers are encouraged to consider how their studies can provide hypotheses and preliminary data for intervention studies and policy changes. Intervention researchers are encouraged to make use of the results of determinants studies in the selection of goals and content for their studies and programs.

Acknowledgment

The authors acknowledge the contribution of Wendell Taylor, PhD, in reviewing literature on youth determinants.

References

Azjen I. From intentions to actions: A theory of planned behavior. In J Kuhl, J Beckman (Eds), *Action-control: From cognition to behavior.* Heidelberg: Springer, 1985; pp. 11-39.

Bandura A. *Social foundations of thought and action.* Englewood Cliffs, NJ: Prentice-Hall, 1986.

Dishman RK, Sallis JF. Determinants and interventions for physical activity and exercise. In C Bouchard, RJ Shephard, T Stephens (Eds), *Physical activity, fitness, and health: International proceedings and consensus statement.* Champaign, IL: Human Kinetics, 1994; pp. 214-238.

Duncan TE, Duncan SC, McAuley E. The role of domain and gender-specific provisions of social relations in adherence to a prescribed exercise regimen. *Journal of Sport and Exercise Psychology*, 1993;15:220-231.

Epstein LH, Saelens BE, O'Brien JG. Effects of reinforcing increases in active behavior versus decreases in sedentary behavior for obese children. *International Journal of Behavioral Medicine*, 1995:2:41-50.

Janis IL, Mann L. *Decision making: A psychological analysis of conflict, choice and commitment*. New York: Free Press, 1977.

Marcus BH, Dubbert PM, King AC, Pinto BM. Physical activity in women: Current status and future directions. In A Stanton, S Gallant (Eds), *Women's Health*. Washington, DC: American Psychological Association, 1995.

Marlatt GA, Gordon JR (Eds.). *Relapse prevention: Maintenance strategies in the treatment of addictive behaviors*. New York: Guilford, 1985.

Pate RR, Pratt M, Blair SN, Haskell WL, Macera CA, Bouchard C, Buchner D, Caspersen CJ, Ettinger W, Health GW, King AC, Kriska A, Leon AS, Marcus BH, Morris J, Paffenbarger RS Jr, Patrick K, Pollock ML, Rippe JM, Sallis J, Wilmore JH. Physical activity and public health: A recommendation from the Centers for Disease Control and Prevention and the American College of Sports Medicine. *J Am Med Assoc*, 1995;273:402-407.

Prochaska JO, DiClemente CC. Stages and processes of self-change in smoking: Towards an integrative model of change. *J Consult Clin Psychol*, 1983;51:390-395.

Rosenstock IM. Historical origins of the health belief model. *Health Education Monographs*, 1974;2:328-335.

Sallis JF. Epidemiology of physical activity and fitness in children and adolescents. *Critical Reviews in Food Science and Nutrition*, 1993;33(4/5):403-408.

Sallis JF, Hovell MF, Hofstetter CR. Predictors of adoption and maintenance of vigorous physical activity in men and women. *Prevent Med*, 1992a;21:237-251.

Sallis JF, Simons-Morton BG, Stone EJ, Corbin CB, Epsiten LH, Faucette N et al. Determinants of physical activity and interventions in youth. *Med Sci Sports Exercise*, 1992b;24(Suppl):S248-S257.

Skinner BF. *Science and human behavior*. New York: Macmillan, 1953.

Stokols D. Establishing and maintaining healthy environments. *American Psychologist*, 1992;47:6-22.

Physical Activity in Women

Patricia M. Dubbert
Jackson Veterans Affairs Medical Center and University of Mississippi School of Medicine, Jackson, Mississippi, USA

Gender differences in leisure-time physical activity in the United States are smaller than in some Western countries.[1] Unfortunately, we can take little comfort in this observation since the majority of American men are sedentary or are active on only an irregular basis. Women have much to gain from regular physical activity, and efforts to promote physical activity for women (as well as men) are a current public health priority in the United States. This chapter will briefly describe the current epidemiology of physical activity in women, examine determinants of women's physical activity, and discuss some examples of successful cognitive-behavioral interventions for increasing physical activity.

A 1991 survey by the Centers for Disease Control and Prevention revealed that 57.7% of men and 58.5% of women had sedentary lifestyles.[2] These overall similarities obscure differences within race/ethnic and age groups of men and women. Data from a 1992 survey[3] indicated that prevalence of inactivity in women increased with age from 25.6% for women 18 to 34 years to 42.1% among women > 65 years, and was greater among non-Hispanic blacks (43.6%) and Hispanics (40.2%) than non-Hispanic whites (27.6%). Women with lower levels of education and income reported the lowest levels of activity. The 1992 data indicate that less than one-third of all women in the United States meet current recommendations for either > 20 minutes of vigorous activity three days per week or the newer recommendations for > 30 minutes of moderate activity five days per week.

Existing data on gender differences in physical activity must be interpreted with caution. Comparisons of self-reported activity with fitness/physiological measures suggest that the self-report measures traditionally used (which focus on sports and higher-intensity activity) may not be as valid for women as for men.[4,5] Accurate assessments of women's activity will need to take into account housework, child and elder care activities, and walking during nonleisure activity. These activities are probably more difficult to recall accurately than are discrete periods of higher-intensity exercise or physical activity during time set aside for leisure activities.

Barriers to Increasing Physical Activity in Women

There is, as yet, relatively little empirical data to substantiate notions about the factors which facilitate or interfere with healthful physical activity in women. In part, this is because many studies of exercise determinants and barriers have not reported findings separately by gender. Interpretation of data is also complicated because it is likely that there are important differences in physical activity determinants within gender in individuals with different ethnic backgrounds, income level, and education.[1,6]

Surveys of physical activity in unsupervised community settings suggest that there is considerable variability in amount and regularity of leisure-time physical activity across time within individuals. Interruptions in regular exercise of three months or more are not unusual. Work and family demands and lack of time are frequently mentioned as causes of exercise "relapses."[7] Injury and illness also appear to have important disruptive influences on activity participation in women and men. Injury was the most frequent reason for relapses from vigorous exercise of three months or longer in one large community study,[7] and number of illness days was an important predictor of compliance in a walking program for older women.[8] However, men and women who gave up community exercise for health reasons usually returned to exercising, in contrast to those who relapsed due to lack of interest.[7]

Although concern about injuries may not be an important determinant in younger adults, fear of falling or being injured severely enough to limit functional independence may be a barrier for physical activity in older women. Cardiac-related exercise risks appear to be lower in women than in men, probably due to the later development of coronary heart disease in women.[9] Musculoskeletal injuries are fairly common in women who run or do aerobic dance, but the injury rate per hour of participation is lower in those who exercise more frequently.[10] Most current concerns about gender-specific negative effects of activity on women's health—such as training-induced amenorrhea, excessive activity associated with eating disorders, and the need for adaptations in activity during pregnancy—are relevant only for the small minority of girls and women who are already very active.[5,11]

There is considerable evidence that psychological and social factors are important determinants of exercise in women. Exercise self-efficacy (confidence in one's ability to continue activity in the face of distractions and obstacles) has been shown to be a consistent and strong predictor of exercise for both genders.[12] In a large community survey which examined responses by gender, a higher level of education and social support were significant predictors of activity for women, and younger age and environmental/neighborhood factors were significant for men.[13] Lack of interest, lack of discipline, and lack of enjoyment have been identified by women and men of varying ages as important barriers to exercise; lack of knowledge about how to exercise and lack of exercise skills are also perceived as barriers.[14] Self-consciousness in exercise settings may also be important for some women, particularly those concerned about their physical appearance.[15]

Lack of time, and work and family demands have been consistently reported by women as important barriers to exercise; however, their true impact and the mechanisms by which the demands of caring for children and elders and multiple role responsibilities affect women's physical activity are not adequately understood. Although many formal barriers to women's participation in sports have been removed during recent decades, opportunities for girls and women without special athletic abilities to participate in sports remain limited in many settings.[5,11]

Cognitive-Behavioral Intervention Strategies

Most recent studies of cognitive and behavioral interventions to increase physical activity and exercise adherence have included women participants, and, when results were examined by gender, there were typically no significant differences. However, behavioral researchers generally have not attempted to design interventions specifically to meet the unique interests or needs of women.

Behavioral theories and models—including social learning theory, the relapse prevention model, and, most recently, the transtheoretical model—have been major sources for intervention strategies used in individual counseling and small group settings for promotion of physical activity.[16] Social learning theory emphasizes cognitive mediation of the effects of environmental cues and consequences on behavior, the self-regulation of behavior through goal-setting and monitoring of progress toward these goals, and the power of modeling and observational learning.[17] The relapse prevention model attempts to explain the process of disruption of a desired behavior pattern and suggests strategies that may reduce the risk of relapse.[18] The transtheoretical model identifies the processes of change that are associated with various stages of adopting and maintaining health behaviors and suggests which strategies may be most efficacious at a specific stage of behavior change.[19]

In accord with these models, cognitive-behavioral intervention efforts are typically directed both at changing the external physical and social environment and toward changing cognitions that influence behavior choices. Typical intervention programs include an entire package of components, such as those listed in Table 1. Instructions and training need to be sufficient to ensure that women have the necessary information to plan appropriate activity and the skills to exercise in a way that is safe and enjoyable. Goals can be increased gradually to shape the individual toward more difficult (or more frequent or longer duration) activity without becoming discouraged by failure experiences. Recognizing that perfect adherence is an unrealistic goal is part of relapse prevention.

Support from others appears to be important in exercise initiation and maintenance, but may be inadequate in the natural environment for many women. Phone calls, mailed materials, or face-to-face contacts in individual or group sessions with exercise program staff have been important components of most successful intervention packages. These contacts can provide helpful feedback to women on the progress they have made and assist with problem-solving to overcome barriers. As will be seen in the following examples, some of these interventions can also be effective as independent strategies for increasing physical activity, at least on a short-term basis.

Contracting and rewards for exercise program attendance. Making an agreement for performance of specified behaviors with some type of reward contingent

Table 1.   Components of Successful Exercise Interventions

- Exercise instructions
- Graded goals appropriate for the individual
- Regular attention/support from program staff
- Exercise logs or diaries
- Identification of personal risks and benefits
- Planning strategies to minimize personal barriers
- Progress feedback
- Instruction in relapse prevention strategies

upon adhering to the agreement is a common type of behavioral intervention. A study of college women evaluated the effectiveness of these interventions, using the return of a small monetary deposit or chances for a larger lottery prize as rewards for achieving weekly attendance goals in an exercise program.[20] Other program factors, such as recording exercise data for each session and feedback to participants, were the same for the experimental groups and a control group that did not participate in contracting or in the lottery. Women in all the contracting groups and the lottery group had significantly better exercise-class attendance than did the control group.

Examining personal costs and benefits. The effects of a single motivational phone contact examining costs and benefits of exercise were examined in a study with women who had signed up for an early morning gym class.[21] Callers contacted each student, asked them to get some writing materials, and then asked them to develop a "balance sheet" of costs and benefits of relevant health behaviors, including gains and losses they expected for themselves, gains and losses to important people in their lives, and approval and disapproval from others.

One group responded in terms of their upcoming exercise class, and a second group made similar lists but in reference to quitting smoking; a third group was not asked to develop a balance sheet. Although all groups showed a decrement in attendance over time, the average weekly attendance for those who had developed the exercise balance sheet was twice as good as for those who did a smoking balance sheet and for the control-group students. This kind of intervention can be helpful both in initiating and maintaining exercise.

Self-monitoring of activity. Studies in a number of areas of behavioral intervention have demonstrated the value of self-monitoring behaviors that are targeted for change. Keeping a log or diary helps the individual compare current performance to the desired goal. The importance of frequency of monitoring exercise was evaluated in a study of home-based moderate-exercise maintenance in middle-aged adults.[22] An equal number of men and women were randomized to monitor daily and to mail in reports to the program staff monthly versus monitoring weekly and mailing in reports quarterly. After six months, there were no differences between men and women in exercise adherence, and those monitoring daily reported more frequent exercise.

Frequent contacts by program staff. Support and encouragement from others can occur in one-to-one or group contacts during exercise classes,[23] or—as in more recent studies of home- or community-based exercise—by means of individual telephone contacts.[22,24] A series of telephone contacts during the first few weeks after an individualized exercise instruction appears to be a very cost-effective type of intervention strategy. A recent study[24] with women working in a university setting compared two months of telephone prompts from student assistants on a weekly basis versus prompts only every three weeks. Women receiving weekly calls were more likely to meet their goals for walking with a partner for at least 20 minutes three days per week than were women receiving the less-frequent calls. Other results from this study suggested that giving specific performance feedback during the calls was no more effective than simply calling to inquire how the walking was going.

Mailed motivational materials. As part of a community health promotion project, written materials were developed for mailing to adults at various stages of readiness to initiate or maintain regular exercise.[25] Participants (many of them women) indicated whether they were thinking about becoming more active (contemplation stage), already trying to become more active (preparation stage), or already active (action stage) and were mailed the materials with suggestions targeted to their current behavior and motivation to change. Follow-up telephone interviews with a sample of participants revealed that many of the recipients became more active as a result of this campaign: Nearly one-third of the contemplators had advanced to the preparation stage and almost two-thirds of those who were in the preparation stage had advanced to action.

Environmental cues promoting exercise. Two studies in community settings illustrated the potential effect of simple prompts as a method of increasing the use of stairs instead of escalators by women and men.[26] One study evaluated response to a sign encouraging taking the stairs for a healthy heart in bus and train commuter stations and a shopping mall. Stair use was greater in men than in women throughout the study, but women responded as well as did men in the percent who used stairs when the sign was posted. The second study addressed longer-term effects of the sign at the train commuter station by continuing observations for a time after the sign had been removed. A similar proportion of women as men responded to the sign by taking the stairs instead of the escalator, but more men took the stairs throughout the study and women returned to taking the escalator more rapidly after the sign had been removed.

Physical activity and public health experts generally agree that interventions like those described here can produce reliable but modest improvements in adherence in comparison to control conditions.[6,27] In interpreting the results, it is important to keep in mind that most exercise adherence studies with cognitive-behavioral interventions have had small numbers of participants, been of short duration, and have lacked measures to validate participants' self-reported activity. Gender differences in response to interventions often have not been reported.

For the future, randomized, controlled trials are needed to provide clearer evidence about which of the strategies are most effective and about the participant and setting factors that may influence their effectiveness. Studies utilizing the family, other social groups, and entire communities as units of intervention may yield valuable results.[5] At the same time, effective interventions will likely involve improved matching of behavior-change strategies to individuals' physical/health, psychological/motivational, and social/economic status.

References

1. Dishman RK, Ed. *Advances in Exercise Adherence*. Champaign, IL: Human Kinetics, 1994.

2. Centers for Disease Control and Prevention. Prevalence of recommended levels of physical activity among women—Behavioral Risk Factor Surveillance System, 1992. *Morbid Mortal Weekly Rep*, 1995;44(6):105-113.

3. Centers for Disease Control and Prevention. Prevalence of sedentary lifestyle—Behavioral Risk Factor Surveillance System, US, 1991. *Morbid Mortal Weekly Rep*, 1993;42:576-579.

4. Blair SN, Kohl HW III, Paffenbarger RS Jr, Clark DG, Cooper KH, Gibbons LW. Physical fitness and all-cause mortality. *J Am Med Assoc*, 1989;262(17):2395-2401.

5. Marcus BH, Dubbert PM, King AC, Pinto BM. Physical activity in women: Current status and future directions. In Stanton AL, Gallant SJ, Eds: *Psychology of Women's Health*. Washington, DC: American Psychological Association; 1995;349-379.

6. Dishman RK, Sallis JF. Determinants and interventions for physical activity and exercise. In Bouchard C, Shephard RJ, Stephens T, Eds: *Physical activity, fitness, and health*. Champaign, IL: Human Kinetics, 1994.

7. Sallis JF, Hovell MF, Hofstetter CR, Elder JP, Faucher P, Spry VM, Barrington E, Hackley M. Lifetime history of relapse from exercise. *Addict Behav*, 1990;15:573-579.

8. Kriska AM, Bayles C, Cauley JA, LaPorte RE, Sandler RB, Pambianco G. A randomized exercise trial in older women: Increased activity over 2 years and the factors associated with compliance. *Med Sci Sports Exercise*, 1986;18(5):557-562.

9. Thompson PD, Fahrenbach MC. Risks of exercising: Cardiovascular including sudden cardiac death. In Bouchard C, Shepard RJ, Stephens T, Eds: *Physical activity, fitness, and health*. Champaign, IL: Human Kinetics, 1994;1019-1028.

10. Pate RR, Macera CA. Risks of exercising: Musculoskeletal injuries. In Bouchard C, Shephard RJ, Stephens T, Eds: *Physical activity, fitness, and health.* Champaign, IL: Human Kinetics, 1994;1008-1018.

11. Dubbert PM, Martin JE. Exercise. In Blechman EA, Brownell KD, Eds: *Handbook of behavioral medicine for women.* 1st edition. New York: Pergamon, 1988;291-304.

12. King AC, Blair SN, Bild DE, Dishman RK, Dubbert PM, Marcus BH, Oldridge NB, Paffenbarger RS Jr, Powell KE, Yeager KK. Determinants of physical activity and interventions in adults. *Med Sci Sports Exercise*, 1992;24:S221-S236.

13. Sallis JF, Hovell MF, Hofstetter CR. Predictors of adoption and maintenance of vigorous physical activity in men and women. *Prevent Med*, 1992;21:237-251.

14. Sallis JF, Hovell MF, Hofstetter CR, Faucher P, Elder JP, Blanchard J, Caspersen CJ, Powell KE, Christenson GM. A multivariate study of determinants of vigorous exercise in a community sample. *Prevent Med*, 1989;18:20-34.

15. Hart EA, Leary MR, Rejeski WJ. The measurement of social physique anxiety. *Journal of Sport & Exercise Psychology.* 1989;11:94-104.

16. Dubbert PM. Exercise in behavioral medicine. *J Consult Clin Psychol*, 1992;60(4):613-618.

17. Bandura A. *Social learning theory.* Englewood Cliffs, NJ: Prentice-Hall, 1977.

18. Marlatt GA, Gordon JR. *Relapse prevention.* New York: Guilford Press, 1985.

19. Prochaska JO, Marcus BH. The transtheoretical model: Applications to exercise. Dishman RK, Ed: *Advances in exercise adherence.* Champaign, IL: Human Kinetics, 1994:161-180.

20. Epstein LH, Wing RR, Thompson JK, Griffin W. Attendance and fitness in aerobic exercise. *Behavior Modification*, 1980;4(4):465-479.

21. Hoyt MF, Janis IL. Increasing adherence to a stressful decision via a motivational balance-sheet procedure: A field experiment. *J Pers Soc Psychol*, 1975;31:833-839.

22. King AC, Taylor CB, Haskell WL, DeBusk RF. Strategies for increasing early adherence to and long-term maintenance of home-based exercise training in healthy middle-aged men and women. *Am J Cardiol*, 1988;61:628-632.

23. Martin JE, Dubbert PM, Katell AD, Thompson JK, Raczynski JR, Lake M, Smith PO, Webster JS, Sikora T, Cohen RE. Behavioral control of exercise in sedentary adults: Studies 1 through 6. *J Consult Clin Psychol*, 1984;52:795-811.

24. Lombard DN, Lombard TN, Winett RA. Walking to meet health guidelines: The effect of prompting frequency and prompt structure. *Health Psychol*, 1995;14(2):164-170.

25. Marcus BH, Banspach SW, Lefebvre RC, Rossi JS, Carleton RA, Abrams D. Increasing the adoption of physical activity among community participants. *American Journal of Health Promotion*, 1992;6:424-429.

26. Brownell KD, Stunkard AJ, Albaum JM. Evaluation and modification of exercise patterns in the natural environment. *Am J Psychiatry*, 1980;137(12):1540-1545.

27. Dishman RK. Increasing and maintaining exercise and physical activity. *Behavior Therapy*, 1991;22:345-378.

Physical Activity in Children and Adolescents

Russell R. Pate
University of South Carolina, Columbia, South Carolina, USA

The promotion of physical activity in children and youth has long been a recognized goal of the physical education and recreation professions. Only recently, however, has this issue become a focus of the public-health community. *Healthy People 2000* includes several national health objectives that call for increased physical activity in children and youth,[1] and several prestigious organizations have taken stands noting the importance of promoting physical activity in young people.[2,3]

Much of the existing research on physical activity in children and youth has focused on the development of motor skills, measurement and enhancement of physical fitness, and psychosocial aspects of sport participation. However, the recent increase in interest in the relationship between physical activity and health has stimulated public-health researchers to investigate various additional issues related to promoting physical activity in children and youth. This paper is intended to summarize the existing body of knowledge in three relevant areas. First, it will give an overview of the physical-activity behavior of children and youth, as assessed in large-scale surveys and small group observations. Second, our knowledge of the psychosocial, environmental, and physiological determinants of physical activity in youth will be summarized. Last, the available studies on the promotion of physical activity in youth will be reviewed.

Descriptive Epidemiology of Physical Activity in Children and Youth

It is widely acknowledged that children and youth need regular physical activity for normal growth and development, maintenance of good health and fitness, and development of physical activity skills and behaviors that will carry into adulthood.[2,3] Whereas the importance of physical activity during childhood and adolescence is accepted, however, the precise amounts, intensities, and modes of physical activity youngsters need are not known with certainty. Nonetheless, public-health authorities and expert panels have established general recommendations. Table 1 lists the *Healthy People 2000* physical activity objectives that apply to children and youth;[1] in addition, this table lists the two physical activity objectives identified by an international consensus panel.[4] These recommendations establish a basis for evaluating the physical activity levels of American children and youth.

Information on the physical activity levels and patterns of children and youth is available from two major sources: population-based surveys, using self-report measures, and small group observational studies, employing more burdensome

Table 1.   Summary of Physical Activity Objectives and Recommendations for Children and Adolescents

Healthy People 2000 Physical Activity Objectives

Objectives 1.3, 15.11, 17.13 Increase to at least 30 percent the proportion of people aged 6 and older who engage regularly, preferably daily, in light to moderate physical activity for at least 30 minutes per day.

Objective 1.4 Increase to at least 20 percent the proportion of people aged 18 and older and to at least 75 percent the proportion of children and adolescents aged 6 through 17 who engage in vigorous physical activity that promotes the development and maintenance of cardiorespiratory fitness 3 or more days per week for 20 or more minutes per occasion.

Objective 1.6 Increase to at least 40 percent the proportion of overweight people aged 6 and older who regularly perform physical activities that enhance and maintain muscular strength, muscular endurance, and flexibility.

Objective 1.8 Increase to at least 50 percent the proportion of children and adolescents in 1st through 12th grade who participate daily in school physical education.

Objective 1.9 Increase to at least 50 percent the proportion of school physical education class time students spend being physically active, preferably engaged in lifetime physical activities.

International Consensus Conference 1994
1. All adolescents should be physically active daily, or nearly every day, as part of play, games, sport, work, transportation, recreation, physical education, or planned exercise in the context of family, school, and community activities.
2. Adolescents should engage in 3 or more sessions per week of activities that last 20 minutes or more at a time and that require moderate to vigorous levels of exertion.

measures, such as heart rate monitors or accelerometers.[5] In the United States a nationally representative sample of 10- to 17-year-old youths was surveyed in the mid 1980s as part of the National Children and Youth Fitness Study (NCYFS).[6] More recently the US Centers for Disease Control and Prevention implemented the Youth Risk Behavior Survey (YRBS) system, which assesses the health habits of American high school students. The YRBS questionnaire includes several items that solicit information on participation in exercise.[7] The data from both NCYFS and YRBS carry the benefit of having been drawn from large, representative samples of American youth. However, they also have the disadvantages of having been collected only with older youth and only by self-report instruments. The NCYFS physical activity instrument was designed to provide a very comprehensive and inclusive examination of physical activity habits. In contrast, the YRBS instrument provides information that reflects participation in structured exercise. Not surprisingly, the results from these two surveys provide somewhat different views of the physical activity habits of American youth. NCYFS found that, on average, American youth report engaging in some 700 to 800 minutes of physical activity per week (i.e., about 100 to 110 minutes per day). It should be noted that large standard deviations were observed at each age and that there was a modest decline in reported activity with increased age. No pronounced sexual difference was observed in the NCYFS data. The 1993 YRBS data show that 62% to 70% of boys and 38% to 51% of girls reported engaging in moderate or vigorous physical activity for 20 or more minutes at least three days per week.[7] These ranges reflect an inverse relationship with age: That is, the high end of the range is observed in 9th graders and the low end, in 12th graders.

Another approach to assessing the physical activity level of youth is to employ objective monitoring techniques. Devices such as heart rate monitors and accelerometers can be used with minimal subject reactivity to quantify accumulated participation in physical activity at selected intensity levels. Studies using such procedures, though limited by their small and possibly nonrepresentative groups, can be helpful in indirectly "validating" the findings of the population-based surveys. A previous review of several studies that used objective monitors concluded that the youth being observed engaged in moderate-intensity physical activity for 0.5 to 1.5 hours per day, yielding an average of about 1 hour per day. For vigorous physical activity the range was 0.4 to 0.7 hours per day, with the average approximating 0.5 hours per day.[4] These findings suggest that the protocols of some population surveys may provide overestimates of total physical activity time but may be reasonably accurate in providing information on participation in structured, vigorous physical activity.

Based on a review of all the available information, it seems reasonable to conclude that more than 80% of adolescents (and probably a higher percentage of children) meet the *Healthy People 2000* objective calling for 30 minutes or more of moderate-intensity physical activity on a daily basis. A smaller percentage of adolescents (38% to 70%) meet accepted guidelines for participation in vigorous exercise sessions, the percentage varying rather dramatically with age and sex. In general, participation declines with age and is lower in females than males.[4]

Determinants of Physical Activity Behavior in Children and Youth

The available body of knowledge suggests that physical activity is a complex behavior that, in children and youth as well as in adults, is associated with a diverse set of factors. As was noted earlier, age and sex are among the strongest and most consistent predictors of physical activity participation. However, no single factor is powerfully predictive of physical activity behavior. Indeed, even studies using multivariate procedures to examine a broad array of potential predictors have been able to account for only modest fractions of the total variance in physical activity levels.[8-10] Evidence indicates that physical activity is moderately associated with a sizable number of demographic, physiological, psychosocial, and environmental factors.

Among the demographic determinants other than sex and age, race or ethnicity is predictive of physical activity behavior, but more strongly in girls than boys. Among girls, African American and Hispanic girls tend to be less active than non-Hispanic, Caucasian girls.[7,10] In boys this relationship is much less pronounced. With regard to physiological factors, physical fitness and obesity status are the most frequently studied potential predictors of physical activity in youth. Youngsters who are less physically fit tend to be less physically active than their more fit counterparts, though it should be noted that the association between physical activity and physical fitness is of no more than modest magnitude ($R^2 = .25$).[11] Obese youth typically have been reported to be less physically active than nonobese youth; however, body composition within the normal, healthy range is not consistently associated with physical activity.[6,12] Also, motor-skill level and heredity are thought to be determinants of physical activity behavior, but the existing scientific literature includes little documentation of these associations.[8]

Numerous psychosocial variables have been examined as potential predictors of physical activity in children and youth. Those that have most consistently been found associated with physical activity are exercise self-efficacy, perceived competence, perceived benefits, perceived barriers, social norms for physical activity, intentions to be physically active, and attitudes toward physical activity and physical education.[8-10]

Both social and physical environmental factors appear to be significant determinants of physical activity in children and youth. Parental physical activity and parental support for physical activity appear to be important in children,[9] but peer influences become more powerful than parental influences during adolescence.[13,14] Access to attractive exercise and sport facilities, space, equipment, and programs have been shown to be associated with participation in physical activity.[8,15,16] It is known also that time spent outdoors and in participating in school sports is positively associated with overall physical activity level.[8,17] Some studies have found participation in sedentary pursuits, such as television, video games, and computer use, to be inversely related to overall physical activity level.[8,16] However, there is some inconsistency across studies in the findings, and the relationship between watching television and physical inactivity is neither as consistent nor strong as has sometimes been thought.

Interventions to Promote Physical Activity in Children and Youth

In theory, interventions to promote physical activity among youngsters could be implemented in the home, school, community, and/or health-care settings. To date, most experimental examinations of physical activity interventions targeted at children and youth have been based in schools, and some have been family-based. Very few studies have examined the promotion of physical activity in either the community or health-care settings. In general, the published studies have been focused on short-term enhancement of physical activity behavior, and little is known about the relationship between physical activity experiences in childhood and adolescence and physical activity behavior during adulthood.

In the school setting, several large-scale investigations have focused on modifying the physical education program to provide increased in-class physical activity. The Go For Health project demonstrated that teacher behaviors could be modified to increase the fraction of class time in elementary school physical education during which students engaged in moderate to vigorous physical activity.[18] Project SPARK found that in-class physical activity was greatest in classes taught by physical education specialists who were employed by the project, but also that nonspecialist, elementary classroom teachers could be trained to deliver physical education lessons that provided substantially more student physical activity than provided in classes taught by control classroom teachers.[19] The recently completed multicenter CATCH study also reported findings consistent with those of Go for Health and SPARK.[20] In addition, it has been demonstrated that interventions that succeed in increasing in-class physical activity can produce significant increases in physical fitness.[21] Collectively, the results of these studies indicate that (a) it is feasible to modify existing physical education programs to provide increased physical activity and (b) programs that provide increased physical activity can produce measurable physiological benefits in students.

The scientific evidence for the successful promotion of physical activity in other school and nonschool settings is much less extensive than that related to physical education. Studies of interventions operating through a school's health education curriculum have tended to show little impact on physical activity behavior;[8] however, one study in a high school setting did observe increased physical activity and some physiological changes that were consistent with increased physical fitness.[22]

Attempts to increase child physical activity through family-based interventions have yielded mixed success. In general, comprehensive family-health promotion programs have not succeeded in producing increased physical activity in children.[23] However, an intervention that involved training parents to reinforce the child's physical activity was successful.[24]

Interventions to promote physical activity in children and youth could be implemented in community[25] and health-care settings,[26] but to date these approaches have received little attention from researchers. It has been demonstrated that when parents are included in the counseling protocols, weight-management programs for obese youth can successfully increase physical activity.[27] Promotion of physical activity has been included as one component of community-based interventions to reduce the risk of cardiovascular disease,[28] but it has yet to be demonstrated that such efforts have a measurable impact on physical activity participation of children and youth.

Summary

Available evidence indicates that physical activity levels steadily decline during childhood and adolescence and that girls tend to be less physically active than boys. Among adolescents a sizable percentage of boys and an even larger percentage of girls fail to meet prevailing guidelines for participation in vigorous physical activity. Physical activity behavior in children and youth is associated with a complex set of demographic, environmental, physiological, and psychosocial factors. Expert opinion and available research suggest that physical activity can be best promoted in children and youth by providing physical activity experiences that enhance self-efficacy about exercise. Such experiences should be provided in the home, school, community, and health-care settings. Future research should test the effects of specific intervention strategies in each of these settings and should determine how to best tailor such interventions to the individuals' needs, taking into account the specifics of age, sex, health status, and ethnicity.

References

1. US Department of Health and Human Services. *Healthy People 2000: National Health Promotion and Disease Prevention Objectives.* DHHS publication PHS 91-50212. Washington, DC: US Department of Health and Human Services, 1991.

2. American Academy of Pediatrics Committees on Sports Medicine and School Health. Physical fitness and the schools. *Pediatrics.* 1987;80:449-450.

3. American College of Sports Medicine. Opinion statement on physical fitness in children and youth. *Med Sci Sports Exercise.* 1988;20:422-423.

4. Sallis JF, Patrick K. Physical activity guidelines for adolescents: Consensus statement. *Ped Exerc Sci.* 1994;6:302-314.

5. Pate RR, Long BJ, Heath G. Descriptive epidemiology of physical activity in adolescents. *Ped Exerc Sci* 1994;6:434-447.

6. Ross JG, Gilbert GG. The National Children and Youth Fitness Study: A summary of findings. *J Phys Educ Recreation and Dance.* 1985;56:45-50.

7. Heath GW, Pratt M, Warren CW, Kann L. Physical activity patterns in American high school students. *Arch Pediatr Adolesc Med.* 1994; 148:1131-1136.

8. Sallis JF, Simons-Morton BG, Stone EJ et al. Determinants of physical activity and interventions in youth. *Med Sci Sports Exercise.* 1992;24(suppl): S248-S257.

9. Taylor WC, Baranowski T, Sallis JF. Family determinants of childhood physical activity: A social-cognitive model. In: Dishman RK, ed. *Advances in Exercise Adherence.* Champaign, IL: Human Kinetics, 1994:319-342.

10. US Department of Health and Human Services. *Physical Activity and Health:*

A Report of the Surgeon General. Atlanta, GA: US Department of Health and Human Services, Centers for Disease Control and Prevention, National Center for Chronic Disease Prevention and Health Promotion, 1996.

11. Pate RR, Dowda M, Ross JG. Associations between physical activity and physical fitness in American children. *AJDC.* 1990;144:1123-1129.

12. Pate RR. Physical activity in children and youth: Relationship to obesity. *Contemp Nutr.* 1993;18:Number 2.

13. Higginson DC. The influence of socializing agents in the female sport-participation process. *Adolescence.* 1985;20:73-82.

14. Anderssen N, Wold B. Parental and peer influence on leisure-time physical activity in young adolescents. *Res Q Exerc Sport.* 1992;63:341-348.

15. Sallis JF, Nader PR, Broyles SL et al. Correlates of physical activity at home in Mexican-American and Anglo-American preschool children. *Health Psychol.* 1993;12:390-398.

16. Trost SG, Pate RR, Dowda M et al. Gender differences in physical activity and determinants of physical activity in rural fifth grade children. *J Sch Health.* 1996;66:145-150.

17. Klesges RC, Eck LH, Hanson CL et al. Effects of obesity, social interactions, and physical environment on physical activity in preschoolers. *Health Psychol.* 1990;9:435-449.

18. Simons-Morton BG, Parcel GS, Baranowski T et al. Promoting physical activity and a healthful diet among children: Results of a school-based intervention study. *Am J Public Health.* 1991;81:986-991.

19. McKenzie TL, Sallis JF, Faucette N et al. Effects of a curriculum and in-service program on the quantity and quality of elementary physical education classes. *Res Q Exerc Sport.* 1993;64:178-187.

20. Luepker RV, Perry CL, McKinlay SM et al. Outcomes of a field trial to improve children's dietary patterns and physical activity: The Child and Adolescent Trial for Cardiovascular Health (CATCH). *JAMA.* 1996;275:768-776.

21. Dwyer T, Coonan WE, Leitch DR et al. An investigation of the effects of daily physical activity on the health of primary school students in South Australia. *Int J Epidemiol.* 1983;53:467-471.

22. Killen JD, Robinson TN, Telch MJ et al. The Stanford Adolescent Heart Health Program. *Health Educ Quart.* 1989;16:263-283.

23. Baranowski T, Simons-Morton BG, Hooks P et al. A center-based program for exercise change among Black-American families. *Health Educ Quart.* 1990;17:179-196.

24. Taggart AC, Taggart J, Siedentop D et al. Effects of a home-based activity program: A study with low fitness elementary school children. *Behavior Modification.* 1986;10:487-507.

25. King AC. Clinical and community interventions to promote and support physical activity participation. In: Dishman R, ed. *Advances in Exercise Adherence.* Champaign, IL: Human Kinetics, 1994:183-212.

26. DuRant RH, Hegenroeder AC. Promotion of physical activity among adolescents by primary health care providers. *Ped Exerc Sci.* 1994;6:448-463.

27. Epstein LH, McCurley J, Wing RR et al. Ten-year follow-up of behavioral, family-based treatment for obese children. *JAMA.* 1990;264:2519-2523.

28. Kelder SH, Perry CL, Klepp KI. Community-wide youth exercise promotion: Long-term outcomes of the Minnesota Heart Health Program and the Class of 1989 Study. *J Sch Health.* 1993;63:218-223.

Effectiveness of Physical Activity Intervention in Minority Populations

Andrea M. Kriska

University of Pittsburgh, Pittsburgh, Pennsylvania, USA

I was asked to speak today about the effectiveness of physical activity intervention in minority populations. This was a very difficult talk to pull together since little is known concerning this topic. If the reader gains anything from this presentation, it is the recognition of an urgent need for public-health research to focus in this area.

Unfortunately, one thing that is known is the relatively poor health status of many of the US minority populations. I will use the diabetes literature as an example. In general, diabetes is a major health concern among many of the American Indian communities (Gohdes, 1986) and more recently the Eskimos and Athabascan Indians (Murphy, 1992). As the fastest growing minority population in the United States, Hispanics are at increased risk for many medical conditions, such as diabetes and hypertension (Council on Scientific Affairs, 1991). Likewise, Japanese Americans, African Americans, and more recently, Native Hawaiians have been found to have higher rates of diabetes than do their white counterparts (Burchfiel, 1995; Harris, 1991; Native Hawaiian Health Research Project, 1994).

Since the health status of most of the minority populations is below the national average, one would expect that physical activity levels would mirror this trend. This appears to be the case when examining data from the Strong Heart Study, an epidemiologic study of cardiovascular and diabetes disease in Native American communities from three geographic areas in Arizona, Oklahoma, and the Dakotas (Lee, 1990). The diabetes prevalence in 45- to 74-year- old members of these American Indian communities are several times higher than are national levels (Lee, 1995). Crudely comparing similarly aged individuals who report no leisure physical activity over the past week from the Strong Heart Study participants (Yurgalevitch, submitted manuscript) with those who report no physical activity over the past two weeks from the 1985 National Health Interview Survey (Caspersen, 1986), the American Indian communities from Arizona, Oklahoma, and the Dakotas appear to be at least as inactive, if not more inactive, compared to national levels.

Many other studies in the literature have found minority populations to have relatively lower physical activity levels. Decreased leisure activity levels were found in lower socioeconomic women (90% African American) compared to higher socioeconomic white women (Ford, 1991). An investigation of 15 800 African American and white participants of the Atherosclerosis Risk in Communities Study showed higher sport/leisure activity scores in the latter group (Duncan, 1995). However, this trend was not maintained for work-related activity. Similar African American and white differences have been found in the Minnesota Heart Survey

(Folsom, 1991), the Coronary Artery Risk Development in Young Adults (CAR-DIA) Study (Bild, 1993), and the National Health Interview Survey (Caspersen, 1986). Most recently, examination of national data (NHANES III, 1988-1991) showed that the age-adjusted prevalence of reporting no leisure physical activity over the past month in individuals 20 years or older was higher for non-Hispanic black and Mexican American men and women than their non-Hispanic white counterparts (Crespo, 1996).

Studies done in minority children mirror those of the adults. Based upon data from the Youth Risk Behavior Survey, aerobic activities, such as jogging or swimming, were performed more frequently by white than by Hispanic or black adolescents (Stevens, 1996). Pima children, especially females, were less active and watch more TV than were age-matched Caucasian children (Fontvieille, 1993). Likewise, in a school-based survey of 551 girls, a greater percent of the black, Hispanic, and Asian girls were sedentary (defined as less than one hour of strenuous activity per week) and watched more than five hours of TV compared to white girls (Wolf, 1993). Likewise, in a Pittsburgh school district, non-white 12- to 16-year-old adolescents were less active than were their white counterpart (Aaron, 1993).

Similar results were observed in individuals 70 years and older from the Longitudinal Study of Aging. Older African Americans scored lower on various measures of physical activity compared to white Americans (Clark, 1995). However, this activity difference no longer remained significant after adjusting for the income and education differences between the two groups.

The literature consistently supports the fact that minority populations are among the most sedentary in this country. Perhaps part of this difference in physical activity levels is due to the way in which physical activity has been measured in some of these populations. Part of this difference in activity levels may be due to the fact that occupational activity is often not assessed and can be a major contributor to total energy expenditure in employed lower-economic populations (Mayer, 1991). However, a substantial part of this difference in activity levels appears to be explained by socioeconomic factors, an important point to remember when designing intervention programs.

Since minority populations of this country have relatively poor health and appear to be more inactive than their white counterpart, it is obvious that they would gain the most from physical activity intervention efforts (Kriska, 1994). Described below are some of the physical activity intervention programs that have been implemented in minority populations.

African American Intervention Programs

The Physical Activity for Risk Reduction Project (PARR), was an intervention effort whose goal was to increase physical activity levels in African American residents of low-income rental communities in Alabama (Lewis, 1993a and b). The community played a central role in guiding the project. During the first phase of the project, data was gathered through focus groups, and an interviewer-administered survey in order to assess physical activity levels as well as determinants and barriers to activity. This information was then used to design the intervention program that was administered in eight communities, with two randomly assigned control communities. The intervention efforts included a community-based exercise program, pamphlets on home-based exercises, and behavioral intervention strategies. Effort was made to adequately address the primary barriers to activity, which were access to programs and suitable facilities. Based upon postintervention cross-sectional surveys, the intervention communities did not demonstrate great increases in activity levels. However, increased activity levels were noted in those communities that were organized and maintained commitment to the program, highlighting the importance of community support. Attendance at the exercise sites reflected this finding, with higher group attendance rates in these organized communities. The authors also suggested that insufficient resources to deliver extensive group programs may have limited their success.

The Community Health Assessment and Promotion Program (CHAPP) was designed to reduce the high incidence of cardiovascular risk factors in a black urban community in Atlanta. Specifically, the intervention was comprised of a 10-week exercise and nutrition program targeted to obese women (Lasco, 1989). The exercise component of the intervention consisted of low-impact aerobic dance, walking, and water exercises. Other program strategies included monitoring, contracts, rewards, home visits to help build family support, free transportation and child care, and special-interest sessions. Immediate responses to participants' concerns included increased police protection for the walkers and blinds for privacy in the aerobics class. In the first group of 70 participants to complete the program, 45% significantly lost weight (with 40% remaining the same), and 70% of the participants attended at least half of the 20 sessions. Family involvement and commitment were identified as important factors influencing the participation rates. Since the formal evaluation of that program, the author estimates that over 400 additional community members have participated in this program. The success of the program is attributed to the personal attention received from staff and to ongoing community support.

PATHWAYS is a weight-loss program targeted for obese inner-city diabetic black women that also incorporated activity in its intervention strategy (McNabb, 1993). The design of the study was built upon information obtained from focus groups from the community to identify potential obstacles. The program did not attempt to modify exercise or nutrition at the onset of the study but tried to guide the individuals through active discovery learning. During the 18-week program, women were gradually encouraged to walk for 20 to 30 minutes at least three times weekly. Ten of the original 13 recruited intervention women completed the program and had one-year weight loss significantly greater than that of the control group. The reasons for dropping out included time and family commitments. Unfortunately, no assessment of activity was done in this study.

The Baltimore Church High Blood Pressure Program (CHBPP) offered a be-havioral-oriented weight-control intervention targeted for black women that in-corporated both diet and exercise over the period of eight weeks (Kumanyika, 1992a). The unique feature of this program is the church setting as a natural envi-ronment for support and reinforcement. Each session included both group discus-sion and exercise led by trained exercise leaders. Exercise consisted of low-impact aerobics, with encouragement to exercise twice a week on their own. Behavioral strategies included incentives, self-monitoring, and alumni classes for those who needed support beyond the end of the program. Based upon the first wave of women from 22 churches who participated in this program, it seemed to be relatively suc-cessful. Around 90% lost some weight, and 69% attended at least five of the eight sessions. Unfortunately, no assessment of activity was done in this study either. However, exercise and social support were ranked highest by the participants as the most useful aspects of this program.

A center-based aerobic activity intervention program was developed to promote physical activity among black families with children in 5th to 7th grades (Baranowski, 1990). Based on a listing of 5th- to 7th-grade students in public or private schools in Texas, families were actively recruited to participate and were randomly assigned to either an intervention or control group. Those families ran-domly assigned to the intervention arm were asked to participate in a 14-week program with one education and two fitness sessions per week in a building lo-cated in a convenient community setting. Community advisory council meetings were held to ascertain the optimal location, time of offering, and content of ses-sions. African American staffing, free transportation, and child care were among some of the strategies used in this intervention program as well. Participation to-ward the end of the program dropped to 20%, with reasons for nonattendance including time conflicts. No differences in cardiovascular fitness were detected between the two randomized groups. The authors concluded that possible reasons for the program failure may be the fact that random assignment split families that had desired to attend the exercise sessions together. In addition, randomization within a community precluded the use of media to motivate and inform the partici-pants. Finally the authors suggested that perhaps more emphasis should have been placed on activities that families could participate in together without going to a specific location.

Hispanic Intervention Programs

An exercise/diet program was developed for obese Mexican American women, in which volunteers informed by flyers distributed within the community were ran-domized into an experimental or control group (Avila, 1994). The intervention lasted eight weeks and was composed of both nutrition and exercise classes. Indi-viduals contracted with a fellow participant as well as a family member to com-plete the program. A physician taught all classes and participated in all physical activities. Of the 44 women who began the program, 39 completed the study. Immediate follow-up data indicated increased walking behavior in the intervention group but not the control group at eight weeks based upon questionnaire and the one-mile walk-run. Follow-up reports from the participants mentioned that the strongest motivational factors to exercise were the active exercise component of the program and that they were able to incorporate a new walking routine at home with their spouses, demonstrating the importance of family/friend support when attempting to successfully increase activity levels.

Social support, as an important incentive to exercise, is a recurrent theme in the interventions described above in adults, as well as in several studies examining the correlates to exercise in children. Two such studies in children showed that Mexican American four-year-old children were relatively more sedentary than were their white counterpart and received less prompting from their parents to be active (McKenzie, 1992; Sallis, 1993). Likewise, in high school students (60% Latino), family and friend support were related to exercise participation (Zakarian, 1994). Other important determinants of activity that emerged in these studies were environmental-economic issues, such as time spent outdoors, access to active toys in the four-year-old children, and self-efficacy in the high school students.

Native American Intervention Programs

The Zuni Indian Project of New Mexico is a structured exercise program created in 1983 by a community coalition that provides motivation, guidance, and education to patients with diabetes and, more recently, to the general Zuni community (Heath, 1991; Leonard, 1986). Participants are recruited by recommendation of medical staff and by general community advertisement. This community-based program is owned by the tribe and supports Zuni volunteers trained in exercise and group leadership. A small substudy from this project demonstrated that motivated volunteers with non-insulin-dependent diabetes mellitus (NIDDM) may benefit from the exercise program. A more convincing argument of the success of the program is the fact that there are currently more than 48 aerobic sessions offered at a variety of sites in the community, with attendance varying from 15 to 50 participants. Success of this project is attributed to the fact that it is a community-driven program with technical and organizational support from experts provided as needed.

A pilot feasibility study was recently done among Pima Indians from the Gila River Indian Community in Arizona to test two specific lifestyle interventions over a 12-month period (Narayan, 1996). Ninety-five overweight men and women between the ages of 25 to 64 years were randomly assigned to either a talking group in which culture, lifestyle, and health issues in Pimas were discussed, or to a diet/exercise group. A community task force was organized to guide the development and execution of this pilot study. The exercise goal for the diet/exercise group was 12 hours a month of activity that could be performed either with the group or on their own. Group activities included community litter cleanup, walking, aerobics, and farming a plot of land that was obtained for participant use. At the 12-

month evaluation, both intervention groups reported increased physical activity levels, with no significant physical activity difference found between the two groups. Although quite preliminary, these findings suggest an important role of individual empowerment in activity intervention programs and reiterate the need to design appropriate intervention strategies.

Work Site Intervention Programs

A recent study examined the role of the work site as a potential place to promote health (Brill, 1991). All employees of a Dallas school district were invited to participate in a 10-week intervention that included both activity and health education classes. The exercise classes were held at the schools throughout the week and consisted of stretching, calisthenics, and aerobic activity. Overall, participants showed an improvement due to the program. However, both the initial recruitment and the retention of the African American employees were lower than that of the white or Hispanic participant. This raises the question of whether or not the physical activity intervention was properly marketed for all individuals.

Perceptions and Beliefs About Exercise/Activity

Focus groups comprised of relatively sedentary white, black, and Hispanic individuals with low family income were organized by the Office of Disease Prevention and Health Promotion (White, 1990). An important item that emerged in these discussions was confusion in regard to what counted as exercise. In general, exercise seemed to mean higher levels of activity associated with gyms, exercise equipment, and sweat. Likewise, African American focus groups organized in Pennsylvania identified the fact that many individuals get enough activity in their occupations and daily routine (Airhihenbuwa, 1995). In the case of some of the young males, this seemed to be a valid statement. However, some of the females believed that they get enough activity during a normal day at home, which may or may not be the case at all. Part of the intent of the new ACSM/CDC activity recommendations (Pate, 1995) is to try to clarify the confusion regarding appropriate physical activity levels. Hopefully this message will reach the minority sedentary individuals as well.

In addition, the minority focus groups described above, as well as focus groups led by Carter-Nolan et al. (1996), also identified limited economic resources and safety concerns as barriers to exercise. This serves to remind us of the resounding socioeconomic issues that need to be kept in mind when designing appropriate activity intervention programs for many of the minority groups.

In general, the barriers and incentives to exercise that were identified in this presentation are no different than those identified in general reviews of the exercise compliance literature for any group or population. In a recent quote from the newsletter of the President's Council of Physical Fitness and Exercise (1994), Dr.

James Sallis stated, "Research suggests that the effectiveness of programs will be maximized when participants' confidence about their ability to continue physical activities is nurtured, they enjoy the activities they have chosen, receive encouragement and assistance from other people in their lives, and reside in a supportive environment that provides convenient, attractive, and safe places for physical activity." Yet, although it appears that the lists of barriers and incentives to exercise are generally similar across populations, it is likely that the relative importance of some of the items varies between populations and even within populations.

In conclusion, based on what was presented today, it is painfully obvious that much more work needs to be done in regard to effective physical activity intervention strategies in minority populations. Increasing the physical activity levels of any sedentary group is a tremendous challenge. Reaching our minority populations adds one more dimension to this challenge, that is, designing an appropriate program to fit within the culture of the minority group. In designing an appropriate intervention program, Dr. Kumanyika (1991, 1992b) has pointed out that a culturally appropriate intervention will go beyond simply understanding the characteristics of the minority participant but will also entail an intervention design and delivery that is culturally appropriate.

The Native American culture reminds us that an individual is multidimensional. This is exemplified by the Native American medicine wheel, which includes the physical, mental, emotional, and spiritual self as an integrated whole. In order to stay in balance, all dimensions of the wheel must be addressed. Likewise, in order to be effective in delivering appropriate physical activity interventions to minority groups, it is necessary to consider all dimensions of the individual and his or her culture.

Acknowledgements

To enhance my ability to represent what is currently known on this topic, I sent a request for help to some of my colleagues around the country that work in this field. I would like to thank those individuals who responded to my cry for help: Lucile Adams-Campbell, Barbara Ainsworth, Steve Blair, Pamela Carter-Nolan, Carl Caspersen, Carlos Crespo, Shannon Fitzgerald, Ed Gregg, Jim Hagberg, Tony Henley, Greg Heath, William Knowler, Shiriki Kumanyika, Marjorie Mau, Kelly Mayo, Wylie McNabb, Venkat Narayan, Mark Pereira, Debra Rohm Young, Cynthia Schraer, Kevin Stevens, and the Strong Heart Study Investigators.

References

Aaron DJ, Kriska AM, Dearwater SR, Anderson RL, Olsen TL, Cauley JA, LaPorte RE. The epidemiology of leisure physical activity in an adolescent population. *Med Sci Sports Exercise*, 1993;25:847-853.

Airhihenbuwa CO, Kumanyika S, Agurs TD, Lowe A. Perceptions and beliefs about exercise, rest, and health among African Americans. *Am J Health Promotion*, 1995;9:426-429.

Avila P, Hovell MF. Physical activity training for weight loss in Latinos: A controlled trial. *Intern J Obesity*, 1994;18:476-482.

Baranowski T, Simons-Morton B, Hooks P, Henske J, Tiernan K, Dunn JK, Burkhalter H, Harper J, Palmer J. A center-based program for exercise change among Black-American families. *Health Educ Q*, 1990;17:179-196.

Bild DE, Jacobs DR, Sidney S, Haskell WL, Anderssen N, Oberman A. Physical activity in young black and white women—the CARDIA Study. *AEP*, 1993;3:636-644.

Brill PA, Kohl HW, Rogers T, Collingwood TR, Sterling CL, Blair SN. The relationship between sociodemographic characteristics and recruitment, retention, and health improvements in a worksite health promotion program. *Am J Health Promotion*, 1991;5:215-221.

Burchfiel CM, Curb JD, Rodriguez BL, Yano K, Hwang L, Fong K, Marcus EB. Incidence and predictors of diabetes in Japanese-American men. The Honolulu Heart Program. *AEP*, 1995;5:33-43.

Carter-Nolan PL, Adams-Campbell LL, Williams J. Recruitment strategies for black women at risk for NIDDM into exercise protocols: A qualitative assessment. *J Nat Med Assoc*, 1996.

Caspersen CJ, Christenson GM, Pollard RA. Status of the 1990 physical fitness and exercise objectives—Evidence from the NHIS 1985. *Public Health Rep*, 1986;101:587-592.

Clark, DO. Racial and educational differences in physical activity among older adults. *Gerontologist*, 1995;35:472-480.

Council on Scientific Affairs. Hispanic health in the United States. *JAMA*, 1991;265:248-252.

Crespo CJ, Keteyian SJ, Heath GW, Sempos CT. Leisure time physical activity among US adults: Results from the third National Health and Nutrition Examination Survey. *Arch Intern Med*, 1996;156:93-98.

Duncan BB, Chambless LE, Schmidt MI, Szklo M, Folsom AR, Carpenter MA, Crouse JR. Correlates of body fat distribution. Variation across categories of race, sex, and body mass in the Atherosclerosis Risk in Communities Study. *AEP*, 1995;5:192-200.

Folsom AR, Cook TC, Sprafka JM, Burke GL, Norsted SW, Jacobs DR. Differences in leisure-time physical activity levels between blacks and whites in population-based samples: The Minnesota Heart Study. *Journal of Behavioral Medicine*, 1991;14:1-9.

Fontvieille A, Kriska A, Ravussin E. Decreased physical activity in Pima Indian compared with Caucasian children. *Int J Obesity*, 1993;17:445-452.

Ford E, Merritt R, Heath G, Powell K, Washburn R, Kriska A, Haile G. Physical activity behaviors in lower and higher socioeconomic status populations. *Am J Epidemiol*, 1991;133:1246-1256.

Gohdes DM. Diabetes in American Indians: A growing problem. *Diabetes Care*, 1986;9:609-613.

Harris MI. Epidemiological correlates of NIDDM in Hispanic, whites, and blacks in the US population. *Diabetes Care*, 1991;14:639-648.

Heath GW, Wilson RH, Smith J, Leonard BE. Community-based exercise and weight control: Diabetes risk reduction and glycemic control in Zuni Indians. *Am J Clin Nutr*, 1991;53:1642S-1646S.

Kriska AM, Blair SN, Pereira MA. The potential role of physical activity in the prevention of non-insulin-dependent diabetes mellitus: The epidemiological evidence. *Exercise Sport Sci Rev*, 1994;22:121-143.

Kumanyika SK, Charleston JB. Lose weight and win: A church-based weight loss program for blood pressure control among black women. *Patient Education and Counseling*, 1992a;19:19-32.

Kumanyika SK, Morssink C, Agurs T. Models for dietary and weight change in African-American women: Identifying cultural components. *Ethnicity Dis*, 1992b;2:166-175.

Kumanyika SK, Obarzanek E, Stevens VJ, Hebert PR, Whelton PK. Weight-loss experience of black and white participants in NHLBI-sponsored clinical trials. *Am J Clin Nutr*, 1991;53:1631S-1638S.

Lasco RA, Curry RH, Dickson VJ, Powers J, Menes S, Merritt RK. Participation rates, weight loss, and blood pressure changes among obese women in a nutrition-exercise program. *Public Health Rep*, 1989;104:640-646.

Lee ET, Howard BV, Savage PJ, Cowan LD, Fatsitz RR, Oopik AJ, Yeh J, Go O, Robbins DC, Welty TK. Diabetes and impaired glucose tolerance in three American Indian populations aged 45-74 years. *Diabetes Care*, 1995;18:599-610.

Lee ET, Welty TK, Fabsitz R, Cowan LD, Le N, Oopik AJ, Cucchiara AJ, Savage PJ, Howard BV. The Strong Heart Study. A study of cardiovascular disease in American Indians: Design and methods. *Am J Epidemiol*, 1990;132:1141-1155.

Leonard B, Leonard C, Wilson R. Zuni diabetes project. *Public Health Reports*, 1986;101:282-288.

Lewis CE, Raczynski JM, Heath GW, Levinson R, Cutter GR. Physical activity of public housing residents in Birmingham, Alabama. *Am J Public Health*, 1993a;83:1016-1020.

Lewis CE, Raczynski JM, Heath GW, Levinson R, Hilyer JC, Cutter GR. Promoting physical activity in low-income African-American communities: The PARR Project. *Ethnicity Dis*, 1993b;3:106-118.

Mayer EJ, Alderman BW, Regensteiner JG, Marshall JA, Haskell WL, Baxter J, Hamman RF. Physical-activity-assessment measures compared in a biethnic rural population: The San Luis Valley Diabetes Study. *Am J Clin Nutr*, 1991;53:812-820.

McKenzie TL, Sallis JF, Nader PR, Broyles SL, Nelson JA. Anglo-and Mexican-American preschoolers at home and at recess: Activity patterns and environmental influences. *J Dev Behav Pediatr*, 1992;13:173-180.

McNabb WL, Quinn MT, Rosing L. Weight loss program for inner-city black women with non-insulin-dependent diabetes mellitus: PATHWAYS. *J Am Diet Assoc*, 1993;93:75-77.

Murphy NJ, Schraer CD, Bulkow LR, Boyko EJ, Lanier AP. Diabetes mellitus in Alaskan Yup'ik Eskimos and Athabascan Indians after 25 yr. *Diabetes Care*, 1992;15:1390-1402.

Narayan V, Hoskin M, Kozak D, Kriska A, Hanson R, Pettitt D, Bennett P, Knowler W. Feasibility study of lifestyle interventions in Pima Indians. Accepted abstract, 1996.

Native Hawaiian Health Research Project, RCMI Program. Diabetes mellitus and heart disease risk factors in Hawaiians. *Hawaii Medical Journal*, 1994;53:340-364.

Pate RR, Pratt M, Blair SN, Haskell WL, Macera CA, Bouchard C, Buckner D, Caspersen CJ, Ettinger W, Heath GW, King A, Kriska AM, Leon AS, Marcus BH, Morris J, Paffenbarger R, Patrick K, Pollock M, Rippe JM, Sallis J, Wilmore JH. Physical activity and public health: A recommendation from the Centers for Disease Control and Prevention and the American College of Sports Medicine. *JAMA*, 1995;273:402-407.

Sallis JF, Nader PR, Broyles SL, Berry CC, Elder JP, McKenzie TL, Nelson JA. Correlates of physical activity at home in Mexican-American and Anglo-American preschool children. *Health Psychology*, 1993;12:390-398.

Stevens KC. Nutrition and physical activity status of adolescents by ethnicity: Youth Risk Behavior Survey. Accepted Abstract, 1996.

Yurgalevitch SM, Kriska AM, Welty TK, Go O, Robbins DC, Howard BV. The relation between physical activity and lipids and lipoproteins in American Indians age 45-74 years: The Strong Heart Study. Submitted to *Med Sci Sports Exer*

White SL, Maloney SK. Promoting healthy diets and active lives to hard-to-reach groups: Market research study. *Public Health Rep*, 1990;105:224-231.

Wolf AM, Gortmaker SL, Cheung L, Gray HM, Herzog DB, Colditz GA. Activity, inactivity and obesity: Racial, ethnic, and age differences among schoolgirls. *Am J Public Health*, 1993;83:1625-1627.

Zakarian JM, Hovell MF, Hofstetter CR, Sallis JF, Keating KJ. Correlates of vigorous exercise in a predominantly low SES and minority high school population. *Prevent Med*, 1994;23:314-321.

Physical Activity Interventions in Older Adults

David M. Buchner
University of Washington, Seattle, Washington, USA

Interest in the health effects of physical activity in older adults began with interest in endurance activities in the 1960s to early 1980s. In the past decade, interest broadened to include other activities, including strength training, balance training, and activity programs such as Tai Chi. This paper provides an overview of (1) the evidence of beneficial health effects of physical activity in older adults, and (2) approaches to promoting activity in older adults.

The three major reasons for increasing interest in the health effects of physical activity in older adults are the following:

- The role of physical activity in the prevention and treatment of diseases, including coronary heart disease (CHD)
- The role of physical activity in longevity
- The role physical activity has in preventing age-related disability, including frail health and its sequelae, such as injurious falls

The evidence that physical activity reduces risk of CHD in older adults is discussed elsewhere in this book. The evidence is stronger that physical activity prevents CHD in adults aged 65 to 75, than in adults over age 75. This situation is not surprising because, generally, more is known about the first group (ages 65-75) than the latter (ages 75+).

The evidence from cohort studies strongly supports the conclusion that physical activity increases longevity in older adults.[1-7] These studies are well-designed and several include adults aged 75+. In the population-based Established Populations for Epidemiologic Studies of the Elderly (EPESE) study, physical activity was associated with reduced mortality at six-year follow-up (odds ratios ranged from 0.59 to 0.73 at the three EPESE sites).[7] A recent review of some of these studies notes that measures of activity varied considerably among studies.[8]

Evidence is accumulating that physically active older adults have lower risk of disability.[7,9-14] For example, physically active EPESE adults were less likely to show loss of mobility over time (adjusted odds ratio = 0.6).[11] Because it is difficult to control for the possibility that physical activity levels are simply a marker for other factors affecting rate of decline, experimental trials have been, and are being, done to demonstrate that physical activity prevents disability. Evidence to date is encouraging that physical activity prevents disability.

Health Benefits of Physical Activity

Experimental evidence that exercise has physiologic effects in older adults supports the plausibility that physical activity is healthful. Most evidence comes from small (less than 25 subjects per group), short-term studies. There is conclusive evidence that exercise improves measures of fitness.[15,16] Perhaps 50 or more studies report that endurance exercise increases endurance capacity in older adults, including evidence from a large (N>200) randomized trial of one year of endurance exercise using an intention to treat design.[17] There is some sort of dose-response relationship between observed improvement and the frequency, duration, and intensity of exercise. The typical study reports a 10% to 25% increase in $\dot{V}O_2$max over 3 to 12 months of exercise.

There is also conclusive evidence that strength training increases skeletal muscle strength. A 1993 review found 18 studies reported in enough detail to include in a meta-analysis.[18] The meta-analysis found that high-intensity exercise programs reported much more gain in strength than did low-intensity. High-intensity training is well-tolerated by older adults, even those who are frail.[19] In frail adults, training is reported to improve physical performance on daily tasks.[19]

As in younger adults, there is variability in the response to strength training and endurance training.[18,20,21] The Consensus Statement of the 1988 International Conference on Exercise, Fitness, and Health commented on variability at all ages, noting as much as 75% of individual differences may be caused by the genotype.[22] The statement noted that this situation makes it difficult to predict the exact benefits an individual will derive from regular physical activity. In contrast, the benefits of activity are easier to predict for a population.

Promoting Physical Activity

Programs to increase physical activity in older adults can be successful. The argument that older adults are "too old to change" is disproved by the large number of formal exercise studies that have successfully recruited sedentary older adults for 2- to 12-month exercise trials. The limited data on adherence to regular physical activity beyond one year is encouraging. For example, almost half of veterans who began a two-year exercise study completed the study, with most dropouts due to illness.[23] In a small research study, older participants were more likely than were younger participants to continue exercising after the formal study ended.[24] One year after another exercise study ended, 94% of the older adults available for follow-up were still exercising.[25]

Successful approaches to promoting physical activity in older adults are similar to those for younger adults. The main adaptation needed for older adults deals with addressing barriers to activity. Certainly the broad barriers to activity of poverty, social class, isolation, and educational level act as barriers in both young and old adults. But many barriers are important mainly in older adults, particularly chronic illness. For example, illness was reported as the most common reason for stopping a walking program—the most common form of activity in older adults.[26] Studies by Thompson[27] and by Morey[28] illustrate that illness is usually the most common reason for dropouts in exercise studies that target chronically ill adults. In a survey of inactive Ontario older adults, 39% reported "physical inability" as the reason for inactivity.[29] Hence, interventions designed to help older adults remain active during and after chronic illness episodes are important, and research should continue to address this issue.

Other specific barriers for older adults include ageist views about appropriate activity; the belief that age-related decline is inevitable and irreversible; arthritic pain; depression; time demands from an aging spouse; incontinence; lack of transportation to supervised programs; the typical orientation of fitness clubs to younger adults; lack of funds for supervised exercise classes; lack of supervised, home-based programs; weather; lack of knowledge (e.g., fear of wearing out the body); lack of experience during youth (mainly in women); fear of falling and fall injury; and concern about neighborhood safety.[30]

The public health approach to promoting physical activity in older adults is to have a variety of activity options appropriate for the adults in a particular community. Exercise classes are important, but are not the most important option. Extrapolating from research in middle-aged adults, probably most older adults prefer home-based exercise programs.[31,32] There is a great need for developing and evaluating supervised, home-based options. Walking programs delivered via self-help written materials (e.g., AARP, Canadian National Walking Campaign) are an important option. Walking appears to be the most accessible option in low-income and obese adults.[33]

Nonprofit senior organizations can potentially have a large role in promoting physical activity in older adults. This fact is recognized by a *Healthy People 2000* objective: "Increase to at least 90% the proportion of people age 65 and older who had the opportunity to participate during the preceding year in at least one organized health promotion program through a senior center, life-care facility, or other community-based setting that serves older adults."[34] Promoting physical activity via senior centers merits more study as to feasibility and acceptability.

Risks of Increased Physical Activity

Like younger adults, physically active older adults are at risk for exercise-related injuries. Also like in younger adults, the risk is not excessive, and the benefits of activity far outweigh the risks. Almost all exercise intervention studies in older adults report that no major injuries occurred.[20] Of course, the subjects in these studies were carefully screened and supervised. There is less data on injury risk in community-based programs. One study with denominator data reported that older adults who exercise regularly are not at higher risk of orthopedic problems than are younger adults who exercise.[35] A home-based program in middle-aged adults reported exercise as safe.[36]

There has been particular concern that exercise might exacerbate arthritis and increase fall injuries in older adults. Concern that physical activity causes arthritis to develop is not supported by epidemiologic research.[37,38] Concern that physical activity exacerbates existing arthritis is refuted by recent randomized trials reporting that exercise improves symptoms and function in adults with rheumatoid and osteoarthritis.[39-42] Concern that promoting physical activity will increase fall rates is mitigated by existing theory and data. The present working hypothesis is actually that regular physical activity reduces fall injuries. In a meta-analysis of the Frailty and Injuries: Cooperative Studies of Intervention Techniques (FICSIT) exercise studies, exercise decreased risk of falls.[43] The idea can be illustrated by analogy. For many years cardiologists treated a *surrogate outcome*—incidence of abnormal heart rhythms—because it was assumed abnormal heart rhythms caused sudden death, and medication that reduced abnormal rhythms would decrease risk of death. Mortality then is the *primary outcome*. It turned out medications *decreased* abnormal rhythms (the surrogate outcome), but *increased* risk of death (the primary outcome)! It has never been shown that decreasing falls (the surrogate outcome) actually decreases fall injuries (the primary outcome). The need for continued research is illustrated by a study reporting that members of running clubs have more fractures than do nonrunners.[9] Yet these data are insufficient to raise great concern; their generalizability to older adults is likely limited because the study cases (runners) were a highly selected sample.

Recommendations

The present public-health recommendations for physical activity in older adults are essentially the same as those for younger adults, and are nonspecific as to activity type; that is, the US Preventive Services Task Force simply recommends that clinicians advise their patients to have regular physical activity.[44] Research is needed to clarify (1) which subgroups of older adults need more specific recommendations as to type of activity, and (2) how adherence of these subgroups to regular activity should be promoted. For example, should fall-prone older adults do balance exercises? Do frail adults with *sarcopenia*, age-related loss of muscle mass, mainly need strength training to build muscle mass? Do older adults show the same benefit from cardiac rehabilitation as do middle-aged adults? Inherent in this research agenda are rigorous studies that clarify how to evaluate adults prior to beginning a physical activity program, so as to minimize reliance on expert opinion in recommendations on how to screen older adults prior to exercise. Research is also needed on how to relate the evaluation to each patient's specific activity recommendation.

References

1. Blair SN, Kohl HW III, Paffenbarger RS Jr, Clark DG, Cooper KH, Gibbons LW. Physical fitness and all-cause mortality. A prospective study of healthy men and women. *JAMA*, 1989; 262:2395-401.

2. Blair SN, Kohl HW III, Barlow CD, Paffenbarger RS Jr, Gibbons LW, Macera

CA. Changes in physical fitness and all-cause mortality. A prospective study of healthy and unhealthy men. *JAMA*, 1995; 273:1093-8.

3. Davis MA, Neuhaus JM, Moritz DJ, Lein D, Barclay JD, Murphy SP. Health behaviors and survival among middle-aged and older men and women in the NHANES I Epidemiologic Follow-up Study. *Prevent Med*, 1994; 23:369-76.

4. Kaplan GE, Seeman TE, Cohen RD. Mortality among the elderly in the Alameda County Study: Behavioral and demographic risk factors. *Am J Public Health*, 1987; 77:307-12.

5. Paffenbarger RS Jr, Hyde RT, Wing AL, Hsieh CC. Physical activity, all-cause mortality, and longevity of college alumni. *N Engl J Med*, 1986; 314:605-13.

6. Ruigomez A, Alonso J, Anto JM. Relationship of health behaviours to five-year mortality in an elderly cohort. *Age Ageing*, 1995; 24:113-9.

7. Simonsick EM, Lafferty ME, Phillips CL, Mendes de Leon CF, Kasl SV, Seeman TE et al. Risk due to inactivity in physically capable older adults. *Am J Public Health*, 1993; 83:1443-50.

8. Wagner EH, LaCroix AZ, Buchner DM, Larson EB. Effects of physical activity on health status in older adults I: Observational studies. *Annu Rev Public Health*, 1992; 13:451-68.

9. Fries JF, Singh G, Morfield D, Hubert HB, Lane NE, Brown BW. Running and the development of disability with age. *Ann Intern Med*, 1994; 121:502-9.

10. Hubert HB, Bloch DA, Fries JF. Risk factors for physical disability in an aging cohort: The NHANES I Epidemiologic Follow-up Study. *J Rheumatol*, 1993; 20:480-8.

11. LaCroix AZ, Guralnik JM, Berkman LF, Wallace RB, Satterfield S. Maintaining mobility in late life II. Smoking, alcohol consumption, physical activity, and body mass index. *Am J Epidemiol*, 1993; 137:858-69.

12. Stewart AL, Hays RD, Wells KB, Rogers WH, Spritzer KL, Greenfield S. Long-term functioning and well-being outcomes associated with physical activity and exercise in patients with chronic conditions in the Medical Outcomes Study. *J Clin Epidemiol*, 1994; 47:719-30.

13. Strawbridge WJ, Camacho TC, Cohen RD, Kaplan GA. Gender differences in factors associated with change in physical functioning in old age: A 6-year longitudinal study. *Gerontologist*, 1993; 33:603-9.

14. Wu AW, Damiano AM, Lynn J, Alzola C, Teno J, Landefeld CS et al. Predicting future functional status for seriously ill hospitalized adults. The SUPPORT prognostic model. *Ann Intern Med*, 1995; 122:342-50.

15. Schwartz RS, Buchner DM. Exercise in the elderly: Physiologic and functional effects. In Hazzard WR, Bierman EL, Blass JP, Ettinger WH, Halter JB (eds): *Principles of geriatric medicine and gerontology*. 3d edition. New York: McGraw Hill, 1993; 91-105.

16. Buchner DM, Beresford SAA, Larson EB, LaCroix AZ, Wagner EH. Effects of physical activity on health status in older adults II: Intervention studies. *Annu Rev Public Health*, 1992; 13:469-88.

17. Cunningham DA, Rechnitzer PA, Howard JH, Donner AP. Exercise training of men at retirement: A clinical trial. *J Gerontol*, 1987; 42:17-23.

18. Buchner DM. Understanding variability in studies of strength training in older adults: A meta-analytic perspective. *Top Geriatr Rehabil*, 1993; 8:1-21.

19. Fiatarone MA, O'Neill EF, Ryan ND, Clements KM, Solares GR, Nelson ME et al. Exercise training and nutritional supplementation for physical frailty in very elderly people. *N Engl J Med*, 1994; 330:1769-75.

20. Buchner DM, Coleman EA. Exercise considerations in older adults: Intensity, fall prevention, and safety. *Phys Med Rehabil Clin North Am*, 1994; 5:357-75.

21. Buchner DM, Cress ME, de Lateur BJ, Wagner EH. Variability in the effect of strength training on skeletal muscle strength in older adults. *Facts Res Gerontol*, 1993; 7:143-53.

22. Bouchard C, Shephard RJ, Stephens T, Sutton JR, McPherson BD. *Exercise, fitness, and health. A consensus of current knowledge.* Champaign, IL: Human Kinetics, 1990; 24.

23. Morey MC, Cowper PA, Feussner JR, DiPasquale RC, Crowley GM, Sullivan RJ. Two-year trends in physical performance following supervised exercise among community-dwelling older veterans. *J Am Geriatr Soc*, 1991; 39:549-54.

24. Sheldahl LM, Tristani FE, Hasting JE, Wenzler RB, Levandoski SG. Comparison of adaptations and compliance to exercise training between middle-aged and older men. *J Am Geriatr Soc*, 1993; 41:795-801.

25. Emery CF, Hauck ER, Blumenthal JA. Exercise adherence or maintenance among older adults: 1-year follow-up study. *Psychol Aging*, 1992; 7:466-70.

26. Kriska AM, Bayles C, Cauley JA, Laporte RE, Sandler R, Pambianco G. A randomized exercise trial in older women: Increased activity over two years and the factors associated with compliance. *Med Sci Sports Exercise*, 1986; 18:557-62.

27. Thompson RF, Crist DM, March M, Rosenthal M. Effects of physical exercise for elderly patients with physical impairments. *J Am Geriatr Soc*, 1988; 36:130-5.

28. Morey MC, Cowper PA, Feussner JR, DiPasquale RC, Crowley GM, Kitzman DW et al. Evaluation of a supervised exercise program in a geriatric population. *J Am Geriatr Soc*, 1989; 37:348-54.

29. Myers AM, Gonda G. Research on physical activity in the elderly: Practical implications for program planning. *Can J Aging*, 1986; 5:175-87.

30. O'Brien SJ, Vertinsky PA. Unfit survivors: Exercise as a resource for aging women. *Gerontologist*, 1991; 31:347-57.

31. King AC, Haskell WL, Young DR, Oka RK, Stefanick ML. Long-term effects of varying intensities and formats of physical activity on participation rates, fitness, and lipoproteins in men and women aged 50 to 65 years. *Circulation*, 1995; 91:2596-604.

32. King AC, Taylor CB, Haskell WL, DeBusk RF. Identifying strategies for increasing employee physical activity levels: Findings from the Stanford/Lockheed Exercise Survey. *Health Educ Q*, 1990; 17:269-85.

33. Siegel PZ, Brackbill RM, Health GW. The epidemiology of walking for exercise: Implications for promoting activity among sedentary groups. *Am J Public Health*, 1995; 85:706-10.

34. US Department of Health and Human Services PHS. *Healthy People 2000: National Health Promotion and Disease Prevention Objectives*. DHHS Publication No.(PHS)91-50212. Washington, DC: US Government Printing Office, 1991.

35. Macera CA, Jackson KL, Hagenmaier GW, Kronenfeld JJ, Kohl HW, Blair SN. Age, physical activity, physical fitness, body composition, and incidence of orthopedic problems. *Res Q Exercise Sport*, 1989; 60:225-33.

36. King AC, Haskell WL, Taylor CB, Kraemer HC, DeBusk RF. Group- vs home-based exercise training in healthy older men and women. *JAMA*, 1991; 266:1535-42.

37. Panush RS, Schmidt C, Caldwell JR, Edwards NL, Longley S, Yonker R et al. Is running associated with degenerative joint disease? *JAMA*, 1986; 255:1152-4.

38. Jannan MT, Felson DT, Anderson JJ, Naimark A. Habitual physical activity is not associated with knee osteoarthritis: The Framingham Study. *J Rheumatol*, 1993; 20:704-9.

39. Ekdahl C, Andersson SI, Moritz U, Svensson B. Dynamic versus static training in patients with rheumatoid arthritis. *Scand J Rheumatol*, 1990; 19:17-26.

40. Fisher NM, Pendergast DR. Effects of a muscle exercise program on exercise capacity in subjects with osteoarthritis. *Arch Phys Med Rehabil*, 1994; 75:792-7.

41. Kovar PA, Allegrante JP, KacKenzie CR, Peterson MGE, Gutin B, Charlson ME. Supervised fitness walking in patients with osteoarthritis of the knee. *Ann Intern Med*, 1994; 116:529-34.

42. Minor MA, Hewett JE, Webel RR, Anderson SK, Kay DR. Efficacy of physical conditioning exercise in patients with rheumatoid arthritis and osteoarthritis. *Arthritis Rheumat*, 1989; 32:1396-405.

43. Province MA, Hadley EC, Hornbrook MC, Lipsitz LA, Miller JP, Mulrow CD et al. The effects of exercise on falls in elderly patients. A preplanned meta-analysis of the FICSIT trials. *JAMA*, 1995; 273:1341-7.

44. US Preventive Services Task Force. *Guide to clinical preventive services. An assessment of the effectiveness of 169 interventions.* Baltimore, MD: Williams & Wilkins, 1989.

Supported in part by grants from the Centers for Disease Control and Prevention (R48/CCR002181), and by the Department of Veterans Affairs (Health Services Research and Development Service). The opinions expressed are those of the author, and do not necessarily represent the opinions of the sponsoring institutions or funding agencies.

Physical Activity, Disability, and Cardiovascular Health

James H. Rimmer
Northern Illinois University, Dekalb, Illinois; and University of Illinois at Chicago, Chicago, Illinois, USA

David Braddock
University of Illinois at Chicago, Chicago, Illinois, USA

The increased visibility of persons with disabilities in American society is associated with a strong disability rights movement that led to the passage of three major laws addressing the rights of persons with disabilities: the *Rehabilitation Act of 1973*, the *Individuals With Disabilities Education Act* (formerly called *The Education for All Handicapped Children Act*), and the *Americans With Disabilities Act*. These laws guaranteed that Americans with disabilities would not be discriminated against in entities receiving federal financial assistance, in schools, in the workplace, and in other public settings,[1] and have helped dismantle some of the common myths associated with persons with disabilities.

The rights of persons with disabilities to live, work, and recreate in the same community as their nondisabled peers will continue to be an important component of our national agenda. Despite this, there is a glaring absence of focus on persons with disabilities in the *health promotion and disease prevention movement*, which was established in the late 1980s by the Public Health Service in collaboration with 22 expert health-care groups and all of the state health departments.[2] Persons with disabilities have not been actively involved in physical activity, and there has been little effort on the part of the scientific community to search for ways to improve the cardiovascular health of these persons.[3] The focus of this paper will be to summarize the research literature on physical activity, disability, and cardiovascular health, and to provide recommendations for future research in this area.

Prevalence of Disability

The prevalence of disability in the United States ranges from 38 million to 50 million Americans, depending on which document is cited. The variation in these numbers is largely due to the way *disability* is defined by the different agencies responsible for tracking the number of Americans with physical and cognitive impairments.[4] According to *Disability in America*, published by the Institute of Medicine, a disability is defined as "limitations in physical or mental function, caused by one or more health conditions, in carrying out socially defined tasks and roles that individuals generally are expected to be able to do" (p. 35). The report estimates that there are 35 million Americans (one in seven persons) who have a disability, and that disabilities are disproportionately represented among minorities, the elderly, and persons of low socioeconomic status.[4]

The Bureau of the Census published a report in 1993 entitled *Americans With Disabilities: 1991-92*.[5] The aim of this report was to gather data on the number and types of disabilities in the United States, broken out by age, race, gender, educational level, and socioeconomic and employment status. Disability was defined as "limitations in performing socially defined roles and tasks in such spheres as interpersonal relationships, family life, education, recreation, self-care, and work" (page 1). The report notes that there are 48.9 million Americans with disabilities (one in five persons).

Neither of these reports includes individuals living in nursing homes or other institutional settings, which would increase these estimates by several hundred thousand people. These reports also do not include people with a moderate degree of arthritis, type II diabetes, asthma, obesity, and other health impairments, which would add millions more to this estimate. In any event, it is clear that Americans with disabilities represent one of the largest segments in our society, and this number will continue to increase as medical advances save the lives of the most seriously impaired, and as an unprecedented number of older Americans survive into their 80s and 90s with one or more disabilities.[6]

Health Care, Physical Activity, and Disability

The Institute of Medicine notes that disability ranks as the *largest public health problem* in the nation, which not only affects persons with disabilities but also their immediate family and society as a whole.[4] The day-to-day physical and psychological rigors of living with a disability, or taking care of a loved one with a disability, can be overwhelming to many people.

In a government report published by the National Center for Health Statistics, it was noted that "a large proportion of persons who are in bad health have some disability, and a large proportion of persons who are disabled are in bad health."[7] Almost $200 billion is spent annually treating people with disabilities who have major functional impairments related to restricted mobility, sensory impairments, cognitive deficits, and communication problems.[8] Secondary conditions, such as hypertension, heart disease, pulmonary dysfunction, obesity, diabetes, and depression, appear to take a greater toll on persons with disabilities and are not even factored into this dollar amount.[9,10]

In an effort to build a better health-care system, researchers must begin to study the benefits of physical activity in reducing secondary conditions in persons with disabilities. Despite all the attention that has been given to physical activity and cardiovascular health over the last three decades, information on the activity patterns of persons with disabilities is scarce.[11] This may be related in some way to a general perception on the part of researchers and scientists that people with disabilities are already suffering from a disease or disorder, and so there is no need wasting precious health-care dollars trying to get them "well." Although on the surface this appears to be a cogent argument, there are two underlying problems with this assumption.

First, health care is a right, not a privilege. Everyone should be afforded the opportunity to achieve the highest level of health possible. People with disabilities need to be concerned about their overall health just like any other American, and improving their quality of life should be no less important because of their disability. They should be able to go to public facilities that are *architecturally* and *programmatically* accessible, such as parks, golf courses, swimming pools, health clubs, and recreation centers.

Second, since physical inactivity is a major risk factor for cardiovascular disease, people with disabilities will further compromise their health by leading a sedentary lifestyle. Having spina bifida and becoming obese is clearly a greater threat to a person's health than just having one of these conditions. A person's health could be made much worse or much better—regardless of the disability—by certain alterations in lifestyle.

Research on Physical Activity, Disability, and Cardiovascular Health

Researchers in the fields of physical activity and cardiovascular health have yet to address the needs and concerns of persons with disabilities. There are very few studies on the activity patterns in this population, and there remain many unanswered questions related to their cardiovascular health. What follows is a brief summary of the research that has been published in this area.

Evidence suggests that cardiovascular disease, particularly coronary heart disease, is the leading cause of death in persons with spinal cord injury (SCI).[12,13] In one investigation, Brenes and coworkers[9] reported higher mortality rates from cardiovascular disease in persons with SCI compared to the general population. The investigators concluded that future research must determine the specific amount of physical activity that is necessary to reduce the increased risk for heart attack in this population. In another study, researchers found high levels of body fat (M=28.7%) among men with SCI,[14] and noted that this could have an important influence on the higher levels of heart disease seen in this population.

In the few studies that have focused on the physical activity levels of persons with physical and cognitive disabilities, the data suggest that, as a group, persons with disabilities are an extremely sedentary population.[15-19] Coyle and Santiago[15] reported that there was a high incidence of physical inactivity among persons with physical disabilities. They noted that this may be a contributing factor in the deteriorating *physical* health often seen in adults with physical disabilities. In an earlier study, Santiago, Coyle, and Kinney[18] found that physical inactivity may also be a major contributing factor to the deteriorating *psychological* health seen in persons with physical disabilities, and may be linked to higher levels of depression. In another investigation, researchers found that a sedentary lifestyle made ambulation in a wheelchair a more stressful event when fitness levels were low.[20] This made certain activities of daily living difficult to perform.

In a recent study comparing the physical activity levels of children with cerebral palsy to nondisabled children, investigators reported that children with this disorder were considerably less active than were their age-matched peers.[21] It was concluded that as a result of the low levels of physical activity, the effectiveness of costly rehabilitation programs was compromised because the children regressed once they stopped receiving therapy. It was also noted that activities of daily living became more stressful when activity levels declined.

The cardiovascular health of persons with cognitive disabilities is also very poor. In two studies involving adults with mental retardation, investigators reported a high incidence of obesity and low levels of physical fitness among persons with this condition.[22,23] In this same population, Rimmer, Braddock, and Marks reported that less than 10% of adults with mental retardation participate in physical activity three or more days a week.[24] And in a study comparing the blood lipid levels of adults with mental retardation to the Framingham Offspring data, Rimmer, Braddock, and Fujiura[25] found higher levels of total cholesterol and lower levels of high-density lipoprotein cholesterol (HDL-C) in a sample of adults with mental retardation living in community residences.

Recommended Research Directions

There is a strong need for researchers to begin to study the activity patterns in large cohorts of persons with disabilities. Most of the studies on physical activity and cardiovascular health have had very small sample sizes, thus limiting their generalizability.[26,27] Because there is a great deal of heterogeneity among persons with different disabilities, it is important for researchers to isolate a specific disability and address research questions specifically to that population. One of the problems with the information reported on persons with disabilities in the "Physical Activity and Fitness" section of the *Healthy People 2000* document is that it fails to report data by specific disability. Therefore, it is impossible to know if the goals listed in this document apply to every physical and cognitive disability or just certain types of disabilities.

A similar situation occurred in a recent position paper published in *The Journal of the American Medical Association*. A panel of experts recommended that special populations be included in a consensus statement on physical activity and the nation.[28] However, only two paragraphs addressed the needs of *special populations*, and the term included "older adults, the socioeconomically disadvantaged, the less educated, and persons with disabilities." The problem with lumping all of these groups into one heading is that it is impossible to get a clear picture of what needs to be done for the specific subgroups listed under this broad term. Clearly, in order to make better headway into this new frontier of research, it is important to study specific subgroups of disabilities. What the research literature direly needs are data sets on the activity patterns and cardiovascular health of people with certain physical and cognitive disabilities, so that the research agenda will move in the direction where there is the most need.

Although the barriers to participation in physical activity have not been extensively studied in persons with disabilities, lack of knowledge concerning the importance of exercise to healthy living, limited access to transportation to and from the exercise site, a low interest level, and inaccessible facilities and equipment may be some of the reasons that can be attributed to the inactive lifestyle seen in this population.[3,29] The situation may also be exacerbated by the medical profession's lack of enthusiasm in prescribing exercise to healthy patients,[30] which may be even more pronounced for someone with a disability where safety and medical concerns are an issue, and where there may be little or no understanding of the disability by the physician or the medical staff.

One of the areas that needs a great deal of attention relates to the health promotion/disease prevention goals listed in *Healthy People 2000.*[2] There are 12 objectives listed under the health promotion category labeled "Physical Activity and Fitness." Only two of these objectives include data on persons with disabilities, and they are not broken out by disability. On the other 10 objectives, it is unknown if they are realistic for all individuals with physical and cognitive impairments since there are no baseline data. For example, in Objective 1.1, "Reduce coronary heart disease to no more than 100 per 100 000 people," data are available only on the general population and a separate subgroup of African Americans.

Aside from the *Healthy People 2000* objectives, it is also unknown if persons with disabilities are treated as aggressively as people without disabilities for hyperlipidemia, hypertension, and coronary heart disease. Likewise, there are no data on the number of people with disabilities who have had open-heart surgery or who are involved in cardiac rehabilitation programs.

A major question that must be addressed in future research is, What are the long-term benefits of physical activity for persons with disabilities? The epidemiological studies that have been completed over the last few years demonstrating the enormous health benefits that can be derived from physical activity have not included this population.[31,32] Therefore, it is important for researchers to develop similar studies that track the effects of chronic exercise in persons with disabilities over an extended time frame. It is also important to determine the quantity of exercise that is necessary for improving cardiovascular health, and what the recommended exercise modalities should be to achieve this amount of physical activity.

There is also a strong need to answer the question: Does physical activity have any benefit in terms of reducing levels of obesity, type II diabetes, chronic pain, fatigue, depression, pressure sores, and many other secondary conditions seen in persons with disabilities? Since many individuals with disabilities have one or more of these conditions,[8,10] it would be valuable to know if physical activity has any benefit in terms of reducing the occurrence or severity of any of these conditions.

Disabilities That Need the Most Attention in the Area of Physical Activity and Cardiovascular Health

The disabilities that need the most attention in the area of physical activity and cardiovascular health include the following:

- **Progressive neuromuscular diseases,** including multiple sclerosis, muscular dystrophy, amyotrophic lateral sclerosis, postpolio syndrome, myasthenia gravis, and Guillain-Barre syndrome
- **Physical disabilities**, including spinal cord injury, cerebral palsy, and spina bifida
- **Cognitive disabilities**, including Alzheimer's disease, autism, mental retardation, and Down syndrome
- **Sensory impairments**, including blindness and deafness
- **Traumatic brain injury**

Conclusion

Within the domain of health promotion and disease prevention, the Surgeon General's office has noted that increasing physical activity levels is as important a goal as is getting Americans to quit smoking. Within this paradigm of health, however, persons with disabilities are not adequately represented. We do not know how active or inactive persons with disabilities are, nor do we know the specific amounts of physical activity that persons with disabilities should do to enhance their cardiovascular health.

Since many individuals with physical and cognitive disabilities do not consider physical activity an important component of their overall health, researchers and clinicians must find alternative ways to encourage exercise in this population. The traditional strategies of using employee-wellness programs, exercise support groups, and local health clubs will probably not be effective for persons with physical and cognitive disabilities since they are generally unemployed, socially isolated, at a low socioeconomic level, and lacking transportation.[1,4,5]

As the "health promotion/disease prevention" movement continues, America's largest, poorest, and least educated minority—persons with disabilities—will remain in the background until researchers and epidemiologists begin to study this cohort. Perhaps there is no better time to initiate the study of physical activity, disability, and cardiovascular health than the present era, when the Paralympics are being held in the United States, the Americans With Disabilities Act is in full force, children with disabilities are receiving a public education, people in institutions are moving into the community, and Congress is looking for ways to reduce health-care expenditures. It is time for exercise scientists to open a new frontier of research in the area of physical activity and disability.

References

1. Albrecht GL. *The disability business. Rehabilitation in America.* Newbury, NY: Sage, 1992.

2. Public Health Service. *Healthy People 2000: National health promotion and disease prevention objectives.* Washington, DC: US Dept. of Health and Human Services, 1991.

3. Miller PD. *Fitness programming and physical disability.* Champaign, IL: Human Kinetics, 1995.

4. Institute of Medicine. *Disability in America.* Washington, DC: National Academy Press, 1991.

5. McNeil JM. *Americans with disabilities: 1991-92.* US Bureau of the Census. (Current Populations Reports, P70-33.) Washington, DC: US Government Printing Office, 1993.

6. Ansello EF, Eustis NN (Eds). *Aging and disabilities: Seeking common ground.* Amityville, NY: Baywood, 1992.

7. Ries P. Disability and health: Characteristics of persons by limitation of activity and assessed health status, United States, 1984-88. *Vital Health Stat,* 1991; 197:1-12.

8. National Institutes of Health. *Research plan for the National Center for Medical Rehabilitation Research.* (NIH Pub. No. 93-3509). Washington, DC: US Dept. of Health and Human Services, 1993.

9. Brenes G, Dearwater S, Shapera R, LaPorte RE, Collins E. High density lipoprotein cholesterol concentrations in physically active and sedentary spinal cord injured patients. *Arch Phys Med Rehabil,* 1986; 67:445-50.

10. Lollar DJ (Ed). *Preventing secondary conditions associated with spina bifida and cerebral palsy: Proceedings and recommendations of a symposium.* Washington, DC: Spina Bifida Association of America, 1994.

11. Heath G. Physical activity promotion in persons with disabilities: Clinical applications—Public health implications. *Med Sci Sports Exercise,* 1993; 26(Suppl 5):S1.

12. Geisler WO, Jousse AT, Wynne-Jones M. Survival in traumatic transverse myelitis. *Paraplegia,* 1983; 21:364-73.

13. Le CT, Price M. Survival from spinal cord injury. *J Chronic Dis,* 1981; 35:487-92.

14. Bostom AG, Toner MM, McArdle WD et al. Lipid and lipoprotein profiles relate to peak aerobic power in spinal cord injured men. *Med Sci Sports Exercise,*

1991; 23:409-14.

15. Coyle CP, Santiago MC. Aerobic exercise training and depressive symptomatology in adults with physical disabilities. *Arch Phys Med Rehabil*, 1995; 76:647-52.

16. Painter P, Blackburn G. Exercise for patients with chronic disease. *Postgrad Med*, 1988; 83:185-96.

17. Pitetti, KH. Introduction: Exercise capacities and adaptations of people with chronic disabilities—Current research, future directions, and widespread applicability. *Med Sci Sports Exercise*, 1993; 25:421-22.

18. Santiago MC, Coyle CP, Kinney WB. Aerobic exercise effect on individuals with physical disabilities. *Arch Phys Med Rehabil*, 1993; 74:1192-8.

19. Marcus BH. Exercise behavior and strategies for intervention. *Res Q Exercise Sport*, 1995; 66:319-23.

20. Janssen TWJ, Van Oers CAJM, Van Der Woude LHV, Hollander AP. Physical strain in daily life of wheelchair users with spinal cord injuries. *Med Sci Sports Exercise*, 1994; 26:661-70.

21. Van den Berg-Emons HJG, Saris WHM, de Barbanson DC et al. Daily physical activity of schoolchildren with spastic diplegia and of healthy control subjects. *J Pediatr*, 1995; 127:578-84.

22. Pitetti KH, Tan D. Cardiorespiratory responses of mentally retarded adults to air-brake ergometry and treadmill exercise. *Arch Phys Med Rehabil*, 1990; 71:318-21.

23. Rimmer JH, Braddock D, Fujiura G. Prevalence of obesity in adults with mental retardation: Implications for health promotion and disease prevention. *Ment Retard*, 1993; 31:105-10.

24. Rimmer JH, Braddock D, Marks B. Health characteristics and behaviors of adults with mental retardation residing in three different living arrangements. *Res Dev Dis*, 1995; 16:489-99.

25. Rimmer JH, Braddock D, Fujiura G. Cardiovascular risk factor levels in adults with mental retardation. *Am J Ment Ret*, 1994; 98:510-18.

26. Auchus MP, Wood K, Kaslow N. Exercise patterns of psychiatric patients admitted to a short-term inpatient unit. *Psychsoc Rehab J*, 1995; 18:137-40.

27. Godin G, Shephard RJ, Davis GM, Simard C. Prediction of exercise in lower-limb disabled adults: The influence of cause of disability (traumatic or atraumatic). *J Soc Beh Pers*, 1989; 4:615-23.

28. Pate RR, Pratt M, Blair SN et al. Physical activity and public health. A recommendation from the Centers for Disease Control and Prevention and the American College of Sports Medicine. *JAMA*, 1995; 273:402-7.

29. Rimmer JH. *Fitness and rehabilitation programs for special populations.* Dubuque, IA: Brown & Benchmark, 1994.

30. Patrick K, Calfas K, Long B et al. *The impact of health care providers on physical activity. NIH Consensus Development Conference on physical activity and cardiovascular health.* Bethesda, MD: National Institutes of Health, 1995.

31. Paffenbarger RS Jr, Hyde RT, Wing AL et al. Association of changes in physical-activity level and other lifestyle characteristics with mortality among men. *N Engl J Med*, 1993; 328:538-45.

32. Lee I-M, Hsieh C-C, Paffenbarger RS Jr. Exercise intensity and longevity in men: The Harvard Alumni Health Study. *JAMA*, 1995; 273:1179-84.

The Impact of Health-Care Providers on Physical Activity

Kevin Patrick
University of California, San Diego, La Jolla, California, USA
San Diego State University, San Diego, California, USA

Karen J. Calfas, Wilma J. Wooten
San Diego University, San Diego, California, USA
University of California, San Diego, La Jolla, California, USA

Barbara J. Long
University of Pittsburgh, Pittsburgh, Pennsylvania, USA

James F. Sallis
San Diego State University, San Diego, California, USA

A national health promotion objective identified in *Healthy People 2000* is to in-crease to at least 50% the percentage of primary-care providers who appropriately assess and counsel their patients about physical activity.[1] In 1993, the primary care disciplines of Family Practice, General Practice, Internal Medicine, Pediatrics, and Ob-Gyn accounted for 46% of physicians in active patient care, or approximately 250 000 physicians.[2] Americans average 2.7 office visits per person per year to health-care providers, and 60% of these visits occur in a primary-care setting.[3] The attainment of this objective will result in literally millions of opportunities each year for physicians to address risk behaviors, such as sedentary lifestyle. How-ever, most physicians do not counsel their patients about physical activity.[4-6] Na-tional data from the Missouri Behavior Risk Factor Surveillance Survey showed that of those who had a routine checkup within the preceding 12 months, only 15% reported being told by their physician to exercise more.[7]

Barriers to Promoting Physical Activity

There are many reasons physicians do not routinely counsel their patients about physical activity, including the following:[8-12]

- Lack of resources: Including lack of time, reimbursement, clear-cut recom-mendations and strategies, and insufficient office staff support
- Lack of knowledge: About the value of physical activity, how to counsel and follow up patients, and how to respond to patient concerns
- Lack of motivation: Stemming from a sense of inability to change patient behavior and, perhaps, personal beliefs (and behaviors) related to the health value of physical activity

This array of barriers is compatible with the Lomas and Haynes taxonomy of factors that influence physician behaviors associated with the provision of clinical preventive services: patient, educational, personal, economic, and administrative/ systems factors.[13] However, we[14] and others have found that patients want and expect their physicians to counsel them about physical activity. Patients in an HMO reported greater satisfaction with their medical care if they were offered or received preventive care services, including exercise counseling.[15] Unfortunately, less knowledge exists about effective health-care-provider-based interventions for physical activity than for smoking or other health behaviors.[16-18] Two such interventions are the INSURE project and Project PACE.

Successful Programs

The INSURE (Industry-Wide Network for Social, Urban, and Rural Efforts) project is perhaps the most frequently cited example of a successful health promotion/ disease prevention project that changed physician and patient behaviors.[19] This program and others[20,21] have shown improvement in patient physical activity following physician intervention. They indicate that given the appropriate training, primary-care physicians can provide successful health promotion interventions that can affect large numbers of patients. However, further studies are needed to refine intervention and evaluation methods.

More recently, Project PACE (Physician-Based Assessment and Counseling for Exercise) was undertaken to develop and evaluate a practical counseling approach for primary-care providers. The program was designed to overcome several of the barriers to counseling in primary care by (1) creating structured counseling protocols that can be implemented in a brief time (3-5 minutes), (2) providing basic knowledge about physical activity and health, and (3) training providers in effective behavioral counseling strategies. Counseling was based on the "stages-of-change" model to help tailor interventions to the needs of each patient, whether sedentary or already physically active. Written protocols guide the counseling for each stage of change.[22]

The acceptability of the PACE materials and training program was evaluated in four regions of the United States. Twenty-seven physicians and nurse practitioners were trained, and satisfaction with the program was high. For example, 78% of providers rated the program as good or very good. Thirty-seven percent of providers reported an increase in their own physical activity during the study. Patients also were satisfied with the materials, and over 70% reported that the counseling was helpful.[14]

The PACE materials were then evaluated in a controlled field trial. Control and intervention physicians were matched on medical practice variables. A group of 255 apparently healthy, sedentary, adult patients were recruited from 17 physician offices (mean age=39 years, 84% female, 28% ethnic minority). Intervention physicians delivered three to five minutes of structured physical activity counseling during a well visit or during a follow-up for a chronic condition. A health educator made a 10-minute booster phone call to patients two weeks after receiving physician counseling. Self-reported physical activity and stage of change (i.e., behavioral readiness to adopt or maintain activity) were collected at baseline and at a four- to six-week follow-up. Objective activity monitoring was conducted on a subsample. Fifty-two percent of intervention patients moved from the contemplator (i.e., thinking about it) to action stage of change (i.e., doing activity), compared to 12% of control patients (p<.0001). Intervention patients increased walking for exercise more than did control patients (increase of 37 minutes/week vs an increase of 7 minutes/week, p<.05; see Figure 1). These self-reports were confirmed by an activity monitor, which also showed differential increase in the intervention group (see Figure 2). These results suggest that physician-based counseling for physical activity is efficacious in producing short-term increases in moderate physical activity among previously sedentary patients.[23]

With the exception of the INSURE project, focused research to date on provider-based approaches to physical activity promotion has been limited to small populations of adults. Little is known about unique issues associated with minority populations, children and adolescents, or the elderly (although a group at Brown University is investigating physical activity interventions for this last population and expects to report results soon). As well, little is known about the differences in the efficacy of physical activity intervention by type, or combinations of types, of health-care providers (e.g., physicians, nurse practitioners, health educators).

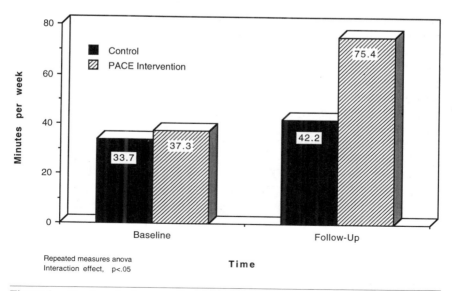

Figure 1. Number of minutes walked for exercise per week at baseline and follow-up (National Health Interview Survey items).

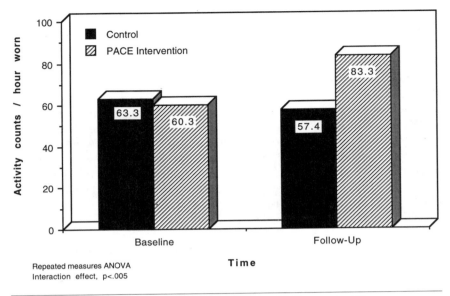

Figure 2.   Caltrac accelerometer scores at baseline and follow-up (n=56).

Evidence to date suggests that characteristics of successful interventions for physical activity based on health-care providers will include the following:

- Brevity: Short length of interaction between provider and patient, primarily for pragmatic reasons but, given adequate patient follow-up, this may be as effective as more lengthy interactions.
- Focus: Through either a stages-of-change or other "patient-centered" approach, messages given to patients should be tailored to their individual needs. Shotgun admonitions to "Just do it" are unlikely to produce meaningful change.
- Follow-up and reinforcement: Follow-up prompting via phone calls after the provider visit has been used by PACE[23] and others[24] to encourage adoption of walking. As with other behavioral interventions, it is likely that repeated attention during subsequent office visits will be necessary.[25]
- A systems approach: Interventions prompted by health-care providers must be embedded in a larger, supportive system of related activities that address predisposing, enabling, and reinforcing factors at the individual, organizational, and community level.[26-28]

Future Considerations

Changes in the structural and financial mechanisms underlying our health-care system may have substantial impact on whether providers will deliver preventive counseling to their patients. As the financing mechanism changes from fee-for-service to prepayment and capitation, the incentive for providers is to shift the focus from illness-care to prevention and health promotion. Managed-care plans provide more preventive services than do traditional indemnity plans, including the types of counseling necessary for physical-activity promotion.[29] Kellie and Griffith[30] predict that managed-care environments will continue to foster the adoption of appropriate preventive services in three ways: (1) increased monitoring of a given organization's population health status, which will influence decisions about services to be provided, (2) increased emphasis on evidence-based practice guidelines and performance indicators, and (3) increased use of tools of quality management and improvement processes to assure that system changes occur. Given the importance of sedentary lifestyle as a risk factor for cardiovascular and other disease, the move to managed care will probably increase the demand for effective interventions aimed at increasing active lifestyles.

Unanswered questions about the role of health-care providers in the promotion of more active lifestyles include the following:

- Effectiveness: What are the essential characteristics of interventions (e.g., length, focus, kind of follow-up) that are capable of producing lasting behavior change and improved health outcomes? What unique issues exist for counseling special populations, and how are these best addressed?
- Efficiencies: Who needs to do what portions of physical activity behavioral intervention and at what cost? What approach is the most cost-effective? How can physical activity interventions be most efficiently combined with interventions aimed at other health risk behaviors?
- Pedagogical: How can health-care providers best learn and maintain the knowledge, skills, and attitudes necessary to support physical activity counseling?
- Systems issues: What impact do different health-care organizational and financing mechanisms have on physical activity counseling? For purposes of supporting the adoption and maintenance of active lifestyles, what relationships need to exist between and among individuals, health-care providers, employers, schools, communities, and others with a stake in public health?

There is considerable potential for primary-care providers to intervene with millions of Americans each year regarding health behaviors such as physical activity. Several studies have documented that counseling by primary-care providers can be effective in promoting physical activity, but many gaps in knowledge remain. While studies to improve outcomes continue, the major current challenge is to improve the quality and quantity of physical activity counseling delivered by the 250 000 primary-care physicians and other providers in the United States.

References

1. US Department of Health and Human Services. *Healthy People 2000: National health promotion and disease prevention objectives.* (US Dept. of Health and Human

Services Publication PHS 91-50212.) Washington, DC: US Dept. of Health and Human Services, 1990.

2. Department of Data Release Services, Division of Survey and Data Resources. *Physician characteristics and distribution in the US*, 1993 edition. Chicago:American Medical Association, 1993.

3. Schappert SM. *National Ambulatory Medical Care Survey: 1991 Summary.* (Advance Data from Vital and Health Statistics No. 230.) Hyattsville, MD: National Center for Health Statistics, 1993.

4. Wells KB, Lewis CE, Leake B, Schleiter MK, Brook RH. The practice of general and subspecialty internists in counseling about smoking and exercise. *Am J Public Health*, 1986;76:1009-1013.

5. Wells KB, Lewis CE, Leake B, Ware JE. Do physicians preach what they practice? A study of physicians' health habits and counseling practices. *JAMA*, 1984;252:2846-2848.

6. Orleans CT, George LK, Houpt JL et al. Health promotion in primary care: A survey of US family practitioners. *Prevent Med*, 1985;14:636-647.

7. Friedman C, Brownson RC, Peterson DE, Wilkerson JC. Physician advice to reduce chronic disease risk factors. *Am J Prevent Med*, 1994;10(6):367-371.

8. Mann KV, Putnam RW. Physicians' perceptions of their role in cardiovascular risk reduction. *Prevent Med*, 1989;18:45-58.

9. Horowitz MM, Byrd JC, Gruchow HW. Attitudes of faculty members, residents, students, and community physicians toward health promotion. *J Med Educ*, 1987;62:931-934.

10. Lewis CE, Clancy C, Leake B, Schwartz JS. The counseling practices of internists. *Ann Intern Med*, 1991;114:54-58.

11. Mullen P, Tabak GR. Patterns of counseling techniques used by family practice physicians for smoking, weight, exercise, and stress. *Med Care*, 1989;27:694-704.

12. Schwartz JS, Lewis CE, Clancy C, Kinosian MS, Radany MH, Koplan JP. Internists' practices in health promotion and disease prevention. *Ann Intern Med*, 1991;114:46-53.

13. Lomas J, Haynes RB. A taxonomy and critical review of tested strategies for the applicaiton of clinical practice recommendations: From "official" to "individual" clinical policy. *Am J Prevent Med*, 1988;4:77-94.

14. Long B, Calfas KJ, Wooten W et al. A multi-site field test of the acceptability of physical activity counseling in primary health care: Project PACE, *Am J Prevent Med*, 1996 (in press).

15. Weingarten SR, Green SE, Pelter M, Nessim S, Huang H, Kristopaitis R. A study of patient satisfaction and adherence to preventive care practice guidelines. *Am J Med*, 1995;99(6):590-596.

16. Okene JK. Physician-delivered interventions for smoking cessation: Strategies for increasing effectiveness. *Prevent Med*, 1987;16:723-737.

17. Kottke TE, Battista RN, DeFriese GH. Attributes of successful cessation interventions in medical practice: A meta-analysis of 39 controlled trials. *JAMA*, 1988;259:2882-2889.

18. Bostick RB, Luepker RV, Kofron PM, Pirie PL. Changes in physician practice for the prevention of cardiovascular disease. *Arch Int Med*, 1991;151:478-484.

19. Logsdon DN, Lazaro MA, Meir RV. The feasibility of behavioral risk reduction in primary medical care. *Am J Prevent Med*, 1989;5:249-256.

20. Lewis BS, Lynch WD. The effect of physician advice on exercise behavior. *Prevent Med*, 1993;22:110-121.

21. Kelly RB. Controlled trial of a time-efficient method of health promotion. *Am J Prevent Med*, 1988;4:200-207.

22. Patrick K, Sallis J, Long BJ, Calfas KJ, Wooten W, Heath G. Project PACE—Physician-based assessment and counseling for exercise. *Phys and Sports Med*, Nov 1994;22(11):45-55.

23. Calfas K, Long BJ, Sallis JF, Wooten WJ, Pratt M, Patrick K. A controlled trial of physician counseling to promote the adoption of physical activity. *Prevent Med* (in press).

24. Lombard DN, Lombard TN, Winett RA. Walking to meet health guidelines: The effect of prompting frequency and prompt structure. *Health Psychol*, 1995;164-170.

25. Ockene JK, Kristeller J, Pbert L et al. The physician-delivered smoking intervention project: Can short-term interventions produce long-term effects for a general outpatient population? *Health Psychol*, 1994;13(3):278-281.

26. Thompson RS, McAfee TA, Stuart ME et al. A review of clinical preventive services at group health cooperative of Puget Sound. *Am J Prevent Med*, 1995;11(6):409-416.

27. Walsh JM, McPhee SH. A systems model of clinical preventive care: An analysis of factors influencing patient and physician. *Health Educ Q*, 1992;19:157-175.

28. Green L, Kreuter M. Applications of PRECEDE/PROCEED in community settings. *Health promotion planning: An educational and environmental approach*. Mt. View, CA: Mayfield, 1991.

29. Miller RH, Luft HS. Managed care plan performance since 1980: A literature analysis. *JAMA*, 1994;271(19):1512-1519.

30. Kellie SE, Griffith H. Emerging trends in assessing performance and managing in health care: Expectations for implementing preventive services. *Am J Prevent Med*, 1995;11(6):388-392.

Community-Based Interventions for Increasing Physical Activity

Deborah Rohm Young

The Johns Hopkins School of Medicine, Baltimore, Maryland, USA

Community-based interventions are conducted in a variety of settings and include a variety of strategies for behavior change. They differ from individual-level interventions in that the intervention goals include changes in social networks, organizational norms, and the physical environment, rather than relying solely on individual behavior change.[1] Interventions that engage the community in the planning phase, encourage community ownership of projects, target multiple settings, and use multiple strategies across the individual, organizational, environmental, and policy levels have the greatest capacity for reaching broad segments of communities and achieving a sustainable change. Few interventions, however, are conducted across all of these levels. This paper will review interventions across community settings and strategies and also will review results from key integrated projects.

Settings

Schools. Schools represent a setting in which lifetime skills can be developed with the goal of maintaining a physically active lifestyle throughout youth and into adulthood. They also represent institutions that have the capacity to reach across personal, environmental, and policy levels and can potentially reach parents and other family members. Several school-based projects have reported positive results for youth, although the ability of school-based programs to influence the physical activity patterns of other family members remains equivocal.

The Class of 1989 Study, part of the Minnesota Heart Health Program (MHHP), conducted yearly screenings of a cohort of children initially in the sixth grade.[2] In addition to the community-wide health education intervention of the MHHP, a school-based intervention was initiated in the 8th and 10th grades that encouraged regular aerobic physical activity. These peer-led programs were conducted in classes other than physical education (PE) classes and incorporated strategies from individual, behavioral, and environmental factors. For example, instruction was given regarding how to monitor heart rate, choose aerobic activities, and exercise safely; weekly group goals were set; exercise skills were taught and positive exercise habits were reinforced; positive role models were encouraged; and cultural norms and expectations were influenced by creating peer, family, and school personnel support. The results showed that, although there was an overall downward trend in exercise participation, the students in the intervention community had higher levels of physical activity that were performed outside of class at all grade levels compared with students in the reference community. Because the MHHP was being conducted in the intervention community, it cannot be determined whether these effects were due to the school-based intervention or to the broader community-based efforts.

The Children and Adolescent Trial for Cardiovascular Health (CATCH) was a three-year, randomized cardiovascular health promotion trial conducted in 96 schools across four states.[3] Over 5,000 children from diverse ethnic and racial backgrounds were enrolled in the project. The physical activity component, or CATCH PE, promoted children's participation in moderate-to-vigorous physical activity in PE classes as well as outside of class. CATCH PE included extensive teacher training, class and curricular materials for grades three to five, and a home/family component. Results indicated that the intervention schools spent a significantly greater percentage of PE class time in moderate-to-vigorous physical activity at all six follow-up semesters relative to the control schools. Further, students from the intervention schools reported spending a significantly greater number of daily minutes in vigorous physical activity compared with those from the control schools. Extended follow-up of this cohort of children or other similar cohorts is needed to determine the effects of aerobic physical activity PE classes on long-term physical activity participation—that is, participation in physical activity throughout adolescence and into adulthood.

Several studies have used schools as a means for identifying children and family members to enroll in community-based physical activity interventions. The San Diego Family Health Project was a one-year experiential and educational intervention that included both Mexican American and non-Hispanic white families.[4] Although there was a significant increase in knowledge of skills required to change exercise habits in the intervention families relative to the control families, no difference in physical activity level or cardiorespiratory fitness level was found. A similar program that recruited African American families resulted in low participation rates, and no difference was found in cardiorespiratory fitness between intervention and control groups.[5]

The CATCH Feasibility Study was a home-based program that consisted of two programs lasting five and twelve weeks, respectively, and included activities that families could participate in together.[6] Of the 424 families who provided pre- and postintervention information, 75% reported participating in the home activities. Moreover, frequency of reported exercise behavior increased in both children and parents from the preintervention levels. Interventions that occur in more natural family settings, such as the home or neighborhood, may have greater appeal to families and should continue to be investigated.

Work sites. Work sites represent an important setting for developing effective physical activity interventions. One-third of work sites with 50 to 99 employees and 83% of work sites with greater than 750 employees offer programs, exceeding the *Healthy People 2000* target for physical activity and fitness activities at work sites.[7] Systematic evaluation of these programs is not common, however, and many interventions that have been conducted in this setting are limited by the lack of appropriate control groups, inadequate representation of the work-site population, or single strategy interventions. The most common interventions are conducted on the individual level, although environmental interventions, such as providing conveniently located stairways, and policy-level interventions, such as providing compensatory time for physical activity participation, can be readily implemented in this setting.

Of work sites that offer physical activity programs, 41% provide information or physical activity promotion activities, while only 12% provide on-site exercise facilities.[7] Lack of facilities may not be a barrier to employee physical activity participation, however. This was demonstrated by Heirich et al.,[8] who reported on the effectiveness of three different approaches to increase employee participation in physical activity and reduce cardiovascular risk. They found that, after three years, the work site with a staffed physical fitness facility had physical activity participation rates that were comparable to the control site (29% reported exercising three or more times per week compared with 35% at the control site) and had participation rates substantially below the sites that offered either one-to-one counseling (43%) or one-to-one counseling combined with work-site organized fitness activities and environmental approaches (41%). These results, taken in combination with the many studies that report low employee participation at work-site facilities,[9] indicate that multilevel strategies conducted across individual, environmental, and organizational levels may be more effective in sustaining physical activity participation than do the presence of fitness facilities.

The postulated benefits of work-site fitness programs include reduced employee turnover, increased productivity, decreased absenteeism, and decreased health-care costs. However, these benefits have not been systematically evaluated. Formal evaluation of the effectiveness of the programs is conducted in only 12% of work sites.[7] Of work sites that conduct evaluations, about one-half compile data on health-care costs and employee disability, with information collected less often on employee health status, absenteeism, and productivity. Furthermore, true evaluation of effectiveness is hampered by the following issues:[10]

- Individuals are rarely randomly assigned to groups; thus, self-selection bias is of concern.
- Increased productivity is hard to quantify and is usually based on subjective ratings.
- Definitions of absenteeism are inconsistent across studies.
- Analysis of medical costs is complicated by positive skewing, in which a large percentage of costs are incurred by a small number of workers.

Nonetheless, studies evaluating absenteeism have found work-site program participants to have 0.5 to 2 days less yearly absenteeism than nonparticipants, which can translate into up to 1.4% of payroll costs. Some studies suggest that medical costs savings can be up to $450 per employee per year.[10]

As stated by Shephard,[10] the benefits of work-site fitness programs should be evaluated by performing economic analyses in which the programs are viewed as a method of maximizing benefits to employees and of increasing the effectiveness of available resources. Issues that are addressed with this type of analysis include attributing costs to the appropriate sector of the economy, determining the opportunity costs of program participants and the marginal costs of adding or altering existing services, calculating discount rates, performing sensitivity analyses, and choosing between cost-benefit or cost-effectiveness analyses. For example, reduced employee turnover should be evaluated relative to alternative strategies to retain employees.

To adequately evaluate the benefits of work-site fitness programs and make valid comparisons across work sites, standard methods of determining cost-effectiveness and standard record-keeping in a greater number of work sites are necessary. In addition, investigations are needed to determine effective strategies for work sites with less than 50 employees and to determine innovative methods to maximize work-site health promotion reach. The potential use of information networks to reach a greater number of employees should be investigated. Finally, the impact of including retirees and family members in programs should be evaluated.

Places of worship. Places of worship are effective settings for attracting minority and low-income, urban populations. Several projects, including The Fitness Through Churches Project in North Carolina,[11] the Health and Religion Project in Rhode Island,[12] and the Living in God's Healthy Temple, or LIGHT, Way Project in Baltimore,[13] promoted aerobic exercise in conjunction with other healthy behaviors to African American and other urban residents. These projects demonstrated that programs in this setting are feasible and attractive to church pastors and to their congregations, and that lay leaders can be successfully trained as volunteers to conduct physical activity classes.

Residential housing facilities. Senior residential facilities and public housing developments are communities in which comprehensive physical activity programs can be conducted. One such intervention in low-income housing developments in Birmingham, Alabama (which primarily consisted of African American women) resulted in wide variability in the effectiveness of the intervention.[14] The intervention was multifocused and included hiring and training community residents to conduct classes, disseminating exercise pamphlets that met literacy levels of the residents, and conducting intra- and intercommunity competitions. Specific support from community and church leaders was solicited, and attempts were made to reduce barriers to attendance, such as providing for child care. Change in physical activity participation was site-specific and, in the communities with high levels of organization, physical activity increased from pre- to postintervention. Increased community organization and commitment may be necessary to influence physical activity patterns of low-income, urban populations.

Other community facilities. Settings such as YMCAs and YWCAs, senior centers, community centers, parks and recreational centers, health clubs, and community colleges all typically provide either formal exercise programs or exercise facilities. Passive approaches in community settings, such as restricting downtown centers to foot or bicycle traffic, placing parking lots at a distance from buildings, providing extensive bicycle paths, and making public stairways convenient and safe, may be more successful in achieving population-wide changes than would those approaches that require individuals to sign up and attend classes.[15] Systematic evaluation of these settings are rarely attempted, precluding determination of their effectiveness.

Strategies

Contests, competitions, and incentives. These can be conducted across individual, group, population, and environmental levels. Contests, competitions, and providing incentives and lotteries have been implemented in work-site as well as other community settings. Contests and competitions have been successful in increasing physical activity participation in the short-term, although their long-term effects have not been investigated.

Classes and self-help programs. Direct education through classes or self-help materials that teach the benefits of regular physical activity, as well as provide individuals with the skills to make necessary behavioral changes, can be implemented successfully in some groups of people. The San Diego Medicare Preventive Health Project[16] provided participants with a health-promotion program that included feedback on individual risk, face-to-face counseling supplemented with telephone calls, and eight-week informational sessions. Results showed a 21% increase in energy expenditure and significant increases in stretching and strengthening exercises in the intervention group over a one-year period, although no change was found in the control group. Marcus et al.[17] found that a community-wide campaign that delivered self-help written materials matched to an individual's stage of readiness for change in exercise behavior was associated with an increase in stage of exercise adoption over a six-week period.

Mass media. In 1990 and 1991, the National Heart Foundation in Australia conducted two nationwide mass media campaigns to promote physical activity.[18] The campaigns were broad-based, including television advertisements, radio public service announcements, distributions of posters, T-shirts, magazine articles, and even messages in a television drama series. Results from 1990 indicated that physical activity message recall increased from 46% precampaign to 77% postcampaign. Prevalence of walking for exercise increased postcampaign for those who were older than 40 years of age. No additional changes in physical activity were found in the second year, although the behavioral change made in the first year was maintained. These data suggest that mass media efforts are effective in some target groups, such as older adults, but may need to be combined with other more extensive strategies to reach a broader segment of the population.

Environmental change. Providing bicycle and walking paths in the community, closing roads down to motor vehicles during certain times of the day to facilitate pedestrian and bicycle use, and changing the environmental milieu of work sites by encouraging the use of stairs instead of elevators are examples of environmental approaches to changing a community's physical activity levels. Posting signs promoting stair use in public places more than doubled stair use over a two-week period, although use returned to baseline after three months.[19]

A more extensive environmental approach was tested in active-duty personnel at a US Navy airfield, the majority of whom were enlisted personnel, and compared with a similar control group at another site.[20] The environmental intervention included strategies such as building bicycle paths along roadways, extending hours at fitness facilities, and organizing exercise clubs and athletic events. In addition, social changes were incorporated into the airfield structure, in which personal responsibility for fitness was stressed by higher-level commanders and high performance on fitness tests was rewarded. After one year, active-duty personnel significantly improved their times on the mandatory 1.5 mile run and the physical-readiness test relative to personnel from the control site. There was no change in leisure time energy expenditure over time, however.

Screening. Creating awareness regarding the need to be more active, without providing the requisite skills associated with behavior change, generally is not thought to influence physical activity patterns. However, one study found that participants who attended subsequent direct screening/education programs had a 500 kcal per week increase in energy expenditure at one-year follow-up.[21]

Certain strategies appear to be effective in some groups of people but not others. Class-based educational programs may appeal to older, highly educated persons,[16] but not to families with different time constraints.[4,5] Combining a variety of strategies that may appeal to different groups of people may result in a broader reach than might single-strategy interventions. Strategies that intervene on the environmental and policy levels rarely have been systematically investigated and warrant further study.

Comprehensive, Multilevel, and Multistrategy Interventions

Several comprehensive cardiovascular risk-reduction interventions, along with the Stanford Five-City Project,[22] the Minnesota Heart Health Program,[23] and the Pawtucket Heart Health Program,[24] included community-wide efforts to increase physical activity. As shown in Table 1, these interventions covered multiple intervention targets, multiple channels, and settings. Individuals, schools, work sites, and neighborhoods were targeted. Volunteers and community coordinators were trained to plan and implement programs. Information was delivered through a variety of sources, including distributing booklets and self-help kits, printing newspaper articles and newsletters, and airing television and radio announcements. Direct education was provided through classes, demonstrations, and lectures. Community contests and challenges were organized, and community organizational activities were established to influence local policies.

Results from the Stanford Five-City Project indicated that not all physical activity measures were significantly improved relative to the control communities. However, positive treatment effects were found for men for estimated daily energy

Table 1.   Examples of Targets and Strategies of Comprehensive, Multilevel, Multistrategy Interventions

Levels and strategies	Example
Levels	
Individuals	Community audience segments, health-care professionals, community leaders
Organizations	Schools, work sites, places of worship, volunteer groups
Communities	Neighborhoods
Strategies	
Face-to-face	Classes, demonstrations, lectures
Mass media	Print materials, newspaper columns, television and radio public service announcements
Community Activation	Consensus building coalitions, advisory committees, community planning for program institutionalization
Environmental/policy	Organizational regulations

expenditure and percent participation in vigorous activities. For women, there was a significant increase in the number who engaged in moderate activities, and a nonsignificant trend was found for men.[22] Results from the Minnesota Heart Health Program indicated that regular physical activity increased significantly in experimental relative to control communities.[23] Follow-up analyses indicated that this increase was primarily due to an increase in the proportion of the population who engaged in light, as opposed to moderate or vigorous, activities. Results from the two projects suggest that community-wide strategies aimed at increasing moderate-intensity activities may have greater appeal to adults than would messages encouraging more vigorous forms of activity. The Pawtucket Heart Health Program has not yet published results specific to physical activity.

Specific portions of the physical activity campaigns were highly effective. The Stanford Five-City Project's organized walking events attracted nearly 1,000 participants, and some groups that were formed continued for at least five years.[22] The work-site exercise program involved 87 work sites and included approximately 3,000 participants. Process evaluation from the Minnesota Heart Health Program indicated that the community-wide campaigns were highly visible: 93% of the population were aware of at least one of the six campaigns, and awareness did not differ by education or habitual physical activity level.[21] An exhibition and demonstration fair conducted by community institutions that offered physical activity programs was attended by 500 people.

Detecting significant effects in large-scale, diffuse interventions is difficult due to low-power, diffuse interventions, changing secular trends, and changes in the economic climate, such as migration patterns and availability of community resources. Program participation and other process evaluation may be more realistic outcomes for community-based projects and can provide information on effective strategies for reaching populations considered to be hard to reach.[25] While some targeted interventions have shown promise in the short term, little is known about the effectiveness of long-term, community-based strategies to increase and maintain physical activity over a lifetime.

In summary, effective interventions that reach across individual, organizational, environmental, and policy levels; engage the community in the planning phase; and encourage community ownership of projects have the greatest capacity for reaching broad segments of communities and for achieving a sustainable change. Multiple strategies are necessary to appeal to a variety of target groups. Future research is needed to determine effective strategies for low-income and minority groups. Understanding minority cultures and the role culture plays in the practice of healthy lifestyle behaviors is critical for developing effective interventions. The cost-effectiveness of community-based strategies in the work site and in other community settings has not been determined. Finally, strategies that are effective in increasing physical activity levels over the long term should be planned and evaluated.

References

1. King AC. Community and public health approaches to the promotion of physical activity. *Med Sci Sports Exercise*, 1994; 26:1405-12.

2. Kelder SH, Perry CL, Klepp K-I. Community-wide youth exercise promotion: Long-term outcomes of the Minnesota Heart Health Program and the Class of 1989 Study. *J School Health*, 1993; 63:218-23.

3. Luepker RV, Perry CL, McKinlay SM et al. Outcomes of a field trial to improve children's dietary patterns and physical activity: The Child and Adolescent Trial for Adolescent Health (CATCH). *JAMA*,1996; 275: 768-76.

4. Nader PR, Sallis JF, Patterson TL et al. A family approach to cardiovascular risk reduction: Results from The San Diego Family Health Project. *Health Educ Q*, 1989; 16:229-44.

5. Baranowski T, Simons-Morton B, Hooks P et al. A center-based program for exercise change among Black-American families. *Health Educ Q*, 1990; 17:179-96.

6. Hearn MD, Bigelow C, Nader PR et al. Involving families in cardiovascular health promotion. The CATCH Feasibility Study. *J Health Educ*, 1992; 23:22-31.

7. US Department of Health and Human Services: Public Health Service. 1992 National survey of worksite health promotion activities: Summary. *Am J Health Promotion*, 1993; 7:452-64.

8. Heirich MA, Foote A, Erfurt JC, Konopka B. Work-site physical fitness programs. Comparing the impact of different program designs on cardiovascular risks. *J Occup Med*, 1993; 35:510-17.

9. Lovato CY, Green LW. Maintaining employee participation in workplace health promotion programs. *Health Educ Q*, 1990; 17:73-88.

10. Shephard RJ. A critical analysis of work-site fitness programs and their postulated economic benefits. *Med Sci Sports Exercise*, 1992; 24:354-70.

11. Hatch JW, Cunningham AC, Woods WW, Snipes FC. The Fitness Through Churches Project: Description of a community-based cardiovascular health promotion intervention. *Hygie*, 1986; 5:9-12.

12. DePue JD, Wells BL, Lasater TM et al. Vounteers as providers of heart health programs in churches: A report on implementation. *Am J Health Promotion*, 1990; 4:361-6.

13. Miller KW, Alford A, Mason J et al. The LIGHT Way Project: Nutrition education and exercise promotion in an urban African-American church-based partnership. Unpublished paper presented at the 122d Annual Meeting and Exhibition of the American Public Health Association, Washington, DC, October 30-November 3, 1994.

14. Lewis CE, Raczynski JM, Heath GW et al. Promoting physical activity in low-income African-American communities. The PARR Project. *Ethnicity Dis*, 1993; 3:106-18.

15. King AC, Jeffrey RW, Fridinger F et al. Environmental and policy approaches to cardiovascular disease prevention through physical activity: Issues and opportunities. *Health Educ Q*, 1995; 22:499-511.

16. Mayer JA, Jermanovich A, Wright BL et al. Changes in health behaviors of older adults: The San Diego Medicare Preventive Health Project. *Prevent Med*, 1994; 23:127-33.

17. Marcus BH, Banspach SW, Lefebvre RC et al. Using the stages of change model to increase the adoption of physical activity among community participants. *Am J Health Promotion*, 1992; 6:424-9.

18. Owen N, Bauman A, Booth M et al. Serial mass-media campaigns to promote physical activity: Reinforcing or redundant? *Am J Public Health*, 1995; 85:244-8.

19. Brownell KD, Stunkard AJ, Albaum JM. Evaluation of modification of exercise patterns in the natural environment. *Am J Psychiatry*, 1980; 137:1540-5.

20. Linenger JM, Chesson CV, Nice DS. Physical fitness gains following simple environmental change. *Am J Prevent Med*, 1991; 7:298-310.

21. Crow R, Blackburn H, Jacobs D et al. Population strategies to enhance physical

activity: The Minnesota Heart Health Program. *Acta Med Scand*, (Suppl) 1986; 711:93-112.

22.   Young DR, Haskell WL, Taylor CB et al. Effect of community health education on physical activity knowledge, attitudes, and behavior: The Stanford Five-City Project. *Am J Epidemiol*, 1996; 144: 264-74.

23.   Luepker RV, Murray DM, Jacobs DR Jr et al. Community education for cardiovascular disease prevention: Risk factor changes in the Minnesota Heart Health Program. *Am J Public Health*, 1994; 84:1383-93.

24.   Carleton RA, Lasater TM, Assaf AR et al. The Pawtucket Heart Health Program: Community changes in cardiovascular risk factors and projected disease risk. *Am J Public Health*, 1995; 85:777-85.

25.   Mittelmark MB, Hunt MK, Heath GW et al. Realistic outcomes: Lessons from community-based research and demonstration programs for the prevention of cardiovascular diseases. *J Public Health Policy*, 1993; 14:437-62.

Appendix A Consensus Development Panel

Lester Breslow, MD, MPH
Professor and Dean Emeritus
School of Public Health
University of California, Los Angeles

Aram V. Chobanian, MD
Dean and Professor of Medicine
Boston University School of Medicine
Boston, Massachusetts

Clarence Edward Davis, PhD
Professor of Biostatistics
Director, Collaborative Studies
Coordinating Center
Department of Biostatistics
School of Public Health
University of North Carolina at
Chapel Hill

Brian R. Duling, PhD
Professor of Molecular Physiology
and Biological Physics
University of Virginia Medical School,
Charlottesville

Suzanne Bennett Johnson, PhD
Professor and Program Director
Center for Pediatric Psychology
Research
University of Florida, Gainesville

Shiriki Kumanyika, PhD, MPH
Professor and Associate Director for
Epidemiology
Center for Biostatistics and
Epidemiology
Pennsylvania State University College
of Medicine
Hershey, Pennsylvania

Ronald M. Lauer, MD
Professor of Pediatrics, Preventive
Medicine, and Occupational Health
Director, Division of Pediatric

Cardiology
University of Iowa Hospitals and
Clinics, Iowa City

Punkie Lawson, MBA
Senior Vice President
Nations Bank
Charlotte, North Carolina

Russell V. Luepker, MD
Panel and Conference Chairperson
Professor and Head
Division of Public Health
University of Minnesota, Minneapolis

Patrick E. McBride, MD, MPH
Associate Professor
Division of Preventive Cardiology
Departments of Family Medicine and
Medicine
University of Wisconsin, Madison

Suzanne Oparil, MD
Director, Vascular Biology and
Hypertension Program
Division of Cardiovascular
Disease Department of Medicine
University of Alabama,
Birmingham

Ronald J. Prineas, MD, PhD
Professor and Chair
Department of Epidemiology
University of Miami School of
Medicine
Miami, Florida

Reginald L. Washington, MD
Vice President
Rocky Mountain Pediatric
Cardiology
Denver, Colorado

Appendix B Planning Committee

Anne Bavier, MN
Deputy Director for Research on
Women's Health
Office of Research on Women's
Health
National Institutes of Health
Bethesda, Maryland

Steven N. Blair, PED
Director of Research
Director, Epidemiology and Clinical
Applications
Cooper Institute for Aerobics
Research
Dallas, Texas

Karen A. Donato, MS, RD
Coordinator, NHLBI Obesity
Education Initiative
Office of Prevention, Education, and
Control
National Heart, Lung, and Blood
Institute
National Institutes of Health
Bethesda, Maryland

Thomas J. Doubt, PhD
Scientific Group Leader
Division of Heart and Vascular
Diseases
National Heart, Lung, and Blood
Institute
National Institutes of Health
Bethesda, Maryland

Chhanda Dutta, PhD
Director of Musculoskeletal Research
Geriatrics Program
National Institute on Aging
National Institutes of Health
Bethesda, Maryland

Jerry M. Elliott
Program Analyst
Office of Medical Applications

Research
National Institutes of Health
Bethesda, Maryland

John H. Ferguson, MD
Director
Office of Medical Applications
Research
National Institutes of Health
Bethesda, Maryland

Gilman D. Grave, MD
Chief, Endocrinology, Nutrition, and
Growth Branch
Center for Research for Mothers and
Children
National Institute of Child Health and
Human Development
National Institutes of Health
Bethesda, Maryland

William H. Hall
Director of Communications
Office of Medical Applications of
Research
National Institutes of Health
Bethesda, Maryland

Stephen P. Heyse, MD, MPH
Director, Office of Prevention,
Epidemiology, and Clinical Applica-
tions
National Institute of Arthritis and
Musculoskeletal and Skin Diseases
National Institutes of Health
Bethesda, Maryland

Van S. Hubbard, MD, PhD
Chief, Nutritional Sciences Branch
Director, Division of Nutrition
Research Coordination
National Institute of Diabetes and
Digestive and Kidney Diseases
National Institutes of Health
Bethesda, Maryland

John Kalberer, PhD
NIH Coordinator for Disease
Prevention
Office of the Director
National Institutes of Health
Bethesda, Maryland

James Kiley, PhD
Director, Airway Biology and Disease
Program
Division of Lung Diseases
National Heart, Lung, and Blood
Institute
National Institutes of Health
Bethesda, Maryland

Russel V. Luepker, MD
Conference and Panel Chairperson
Professor and Head
Division of Epidemiology
School of Public Health
University of Minnesota,
Minneapolis

Gregory J. Morosco, PhD, MPH
Associate Director for Prevention,
Education, and Control
National Heart, Lung, and Blood
Institute
National Institutes of Health
Bethesda, Maryland

Eva Obarzanek, PhD, RD
Nutritionist, Prevention Scientific
Research Group
Division of Epidemiology and Clinical
Applications
National Heart, Lung, and Blood
Institute
National Institutes of Health
Bethesda, Maryland

Ralph S. Paffenbarger, Jr, MD,
FACSM
Professor of Epidemiology, Emeritus

Division of Epidemiology
Department of Health Research and
Policy
Stanford University School of
Medicine
Stanford, California

Russell R. Pate, PhD
Professor and Chairman,
Department of Exercise Science
School of Public Health
University of South Carolina,
Columbia

Debra Rothstein, PhD
Senior Prevention Policy Advisor
Office of Disease Prevention and
Health Promotion
Washington, District of Columbia

Hilary D. Sigmon, PhD
Physiologist and Nurse Scientist
Acute and Chronic Illness Branch
Division of Extramural Programs
National Institute of Nursing Research
National Institutes of Health
Bethesda, Maryland

Denise Simons-Morton, MD, PhD
Leader, Prevention Scientific Research
Group
Division of Epidemiology and Clinical
Applications
National Heart, Lung, and Blood
Institute
National Institutes of Health
Bethesda, Maryland

Christine G. Spain, MA
Director, Research, Planning, and
Special Projects
President's Council on Physical
Fitness and Sports
Washington, District of Columbia

Index

About the Editor

Arthur S. Leon, MD, is the Henry L. Taylor professor and director of the Laboratory of Physiological Hygiene and Exercise Science in the Division of Kinesiology as well as adjunct professor and Chief Cardiologist in the Department of Medicine's Heart Disease Prevention Clinic at the University of Minnesota in Minneapolis.

Dr. Leon, who earned his MD in 1957 from the University of Wisconsin at Madison, has studied the effects of physical activity on cardiovascular health for more than 32 years. His research has contributed significantly to recent recommendations by the Centers for Disease Control and Prevention and the Surgeon General's Report on the health benefits of regular physical activity.

A Fellow of the American College of Sports Medicine, the American Association of Cardiovascular and Pulmonary Rehabilitation, and the Epidemiology and Prevention Cardiology Council, Dr. Leon also is a member of the editorial board for the Surgeon General's Report. He won the AAHPERD's William G. Anderson ward in 1981 and ACSM Citation Award in 1995.

Dr. Leon lives in Minnetonka, Minnesota, with his wife, Gloria. He enjoys jogging and exercise, gardening, and watching University of Minnesota basketball s.

About the Editor

Arthur S. Leon, MD, is the Henry L. Taylor professor and director of the Laboratory of Physiological Hygiene and Exercise Science in the Division of Kinesiology as well as adjunct professor and Chief Cardiologist in the Department of Medicine's Heart Disease Prevention Clinic at the University of Minnesota in Minneapolis.

Dr. Leon, who earned his MD in 1957 from the University of Wisconsin at Madison, has studied the effects of physical activity on cardiovascular health for more than 32 years. His research has contributed significantly to recent recommendations by the Centers for Disease Control and Prevention and the Surgeon General's Report on the health benefits of regular physical activity.

A Fellow of the American College of Sports Medicine, the American Association of Cardiovascular and Pulmonary Rehabilitation, and the Epidemiology and Prevention Cardiology Council, Dr. Leon also is a member of the editorial board for the Surgeon General's Report. He won the AAHPERD's William G. Anderson Award in 1981 and ACSM Citation Award in 1995.

Dr. Leon lives in Minnetonka, Minnesota, with his wife, Gloria. He enjoys jogging and exercise, gardening, and watching University of Minnesota basketball games.